Zuspan and Quilligan's

MANUAL OF OBSTETRICS AND GYNECOLOGY

Zuspan & Quilligan's

MANUAL OF OBSTETRICS AND GYNECOLOGY

ob/gyn

Obstetrics Editor

JAY D. IAMS, M.D.

Associate Professor
Division of Maternal Fetal Medicine
Department of Obstetrics and Gynecology
Ohio State University College of Medicine
Columbus, Ohio

Gynecology Editor

FREDERICK P. ZUSPAN, M.D.

Professor
The Richard Lewis Meiling Chair in Obstetrics and Gynecology
Ohio State University College of Medicine
Columbus, Ohio

Consulting Editor

EDWARD J. QUILLIGAN, M.D.

Vice Chancellor Health Science
Dean of California College of Medicine;
Professor
Division of Maternal Fetal Medicine
Department of Obstetrics and Gynecology
University of California, Irvine
Irvine, California

Second Edition

*With **90** illustrations*

The C. V. Mosby Company

St. Louis • Philadelphia • Baltimore • Toronto   1990

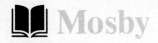

Editor: Stephanie Bircher Manning
Assistant Editor: Anne Gunter
Project Manager: Mark Spann
Production Editor: Janet R. Livingston
Designer: Rey Umali

Second Edition

The C. V. Mosby Company
11830 Westline Industrial Drive, St. Louis, Missouri 63146

Library of Congress Cataloging-in-Publication Data

Manual of obstetrics and gynecology.
    Zuspan and Quilligan's manual of obstetrics and gynecology/
obstetrics editor, Jay D. Iams; gynecology editor, Frederick P.
Zuspan; consulting editor, Edward J. Quilligan.— 2nd ed.
      p. cm.
    Rev. ed. of: Practice manual of obstetric care. 1982.
    Includes bibliographical references.
    ISBN 0-8016-5476-9
    1. Obstetrics—Handbooks, manuals, etc. I. Zuspan, Frederick P.,
1982-   . II. Quilligan, Edward J., 1925-   . III. Iams, Jay D.
IV. Practical manual of obstetric care. V. Title. Vi. Title:
Manual of obstetrics and gynecology.
    [DNLM: 1. Gynecology—handbooks. 2. Obstetrics—handbooks.   WQ
39 M2943]
RG531.M293 1990
618—dc20
DNLM/DLC
for Library of Congress   89-12934
                                                     CIP

C/C/D 10 9 8 7 6 5 4 3 2

Contributors

Susan W. Aucott, M.D.
Fellow in Neonatology
Case Western Reserve University School
of Medicine
Cleveland Metropolitan General Hospital
Cleveland, Ohio

David Bell, M.D.
Clinical Instructor
Department of Obstetrics and Gynecology
Ohio State University College of Medicine
Columbus, Ohio

Michael Blumenfeld, M.D.
Assistant Professor
Department of Obstetrics and Gynecology
Ohio State University College of Medicine
Columbus, Ohio

John G. Boutselis, M.D.
Professor
Division of Gynecologic Oncology
Department of Obstetrics and Gynecology
Ohio State University College of Medicine
Columbus, Ohio

Christopher Copeland, M.D.
Clinical Assistant Professor
Department of Obstetrics and Gynecology
Ohio State University College of Medicine
Columbus, Ohio

Larry J. Copeland, M.D.
Professor
Division of Gynecologic Oncology
Department of Obstetrics and Gynecology
Ohio State University College of Medicine
Columbus, Ohio

William G. Dodds, M.D.
Assistant Professor
Division of Endocrinology and Infertility
Department of Obstetrics and Gynecology
Ohio State University College of Medicine
Columbus, Ohio

Garth Essig, M.D.
Associate Professor
Department of Obstetrics and Gynecology
Ohio State University College of Medicine
Columbus, Ohio

Michael Foley, M.D.
Fellow
Division of Maternal Fetal Medicine
Department of Obstetrics and Gynecology
Ohio State University College of Medicine
Columbus, Ohio

Chad Friedman, M.D.
Associate Professor
Division of Endocrinology and Infertility
Department of Obstetrics and Gynecology
Ohio State University College of Medicine
Columbus, Ohio

Steven G. Gabbe, M.D.
Professor and Chairman
Division of Maternal Fetal Medicine
Department of Obstetrics and Gynecology
Ohio State University College of Medicine
Columbus, Ohio

Jeffrey M. Goldberg, M.D.
Assistant Professor
Division of Endocrinology and Infertility
Department of Obstetrics and Gynecology
Ohio State University School of Medicine
Columbus, Ohio

Lindsey Grossman, M.D.
Assistant Professor
Department of Pediatrics
Ohio State University College of Medicine
Columbus, Ohio

Jay D. Iams, M.D.
Associate Professor
Division of Maternal Fetal Medicine
Department of Obstetrics and Gynecology
Ohio State University College of Medicine
Columbus, Ohio

Moon Kim, M.D.
Professor
Division of Endocrinology and Infertility
Department of Obstetrics and Gynecology
Ohio State University College of Medicine
Columbus, Ohio

Mark B. Landon, M.D.
Assistant Professor
Division of Maternal Fetal Medicine
Department of Obstetrics and Gynecology
Ohio State University College of Medicine
Columbus, Ohio

John J. Moore, M.D.
Assistant Professor
Department of Pediatrics
Case Western Reserve University School
of Medicine
Cleveland Metropolitan General Hospital
Cleveland, Ohio

Richard O'Shaughnessy, M.D.
Associate Professor
Division of Maternal Fetal Medicine
Department of Obstetrics and Gynecology
Ohio State University College of Medicine
Columbus, Ohio

Stephen F. Pariser, M.D.
Associate Professor
Department of Obstetrics and Gynecology
Ohio State University College of Medicine
Columbus, Ohio

Edward J. Quilligan, M.D.
Vice Chancellor Health Science
Dean of California College of Medicine;
Professor
Division of Maternal Fetal Medicine
Department of Obstetrics and Gynecology
University of California, Irvine
Irvine, California

Rosemary E. Reiss, M.D.
Assistant Professor
Division of Maternal Fetal Medicine
Department of Obstetrics and Gynecology
Ohio State University College of Medicine
Columbus, Ohio

Philip Samuels, M.D.
Assistant Professor
Department of Obstetrics and Gynecology
Jerrold R. Golding Division of Maternal
Fetal Medicine
Hospital of the University of Pennsylvania
Philadelphia, Pennsylvania

Jiri Sonek, M.D.
Fellow, Division of Maternal Fetal Medicine
Department of Obstetrics and Gynecology
Ohio State University College of Medicine
Columbus, Ohio

Nicholas J. Teteris, M.D.
Professor
Department of Obstetrics and Gynecology
Ohio State University College of Medicine
Columbus, Ohio

Frederick P. Zuspan, M.D.
Professor
The Richard Lewis Meiling Chair
in Obstetrics and Gynecology
Ohio State University College of Medicine
Columbus, Ohio

Kathryn J. Zuspan, M.D.
Clinical Assistant Professor
Department of Anesthesia
University of Minnesota
Hennepin Faculty Associate
Minneapolis, Minnesota

Preface

The first edition of the *Practical Manual of Obstetric Care* was published in 1982. There were 12 contributors and 136 illustrations in this 414-page handbook.

This second edition contains information that is needed to treat both the obstetric and gynecologic patient. Information regarding gynecology has been added. The book is not intended to replace other texts whose reference lists and contents are extensive. It is intended to supply information that will assist the clinician in arriving at a diagnosis by the application of deductive reasoning and by the application of tests and procedures. The dosages of commonly used drugs are provided, but the drug list is not meant to be inclusive nor overly extensive.

The make-up of this book is different since Dr. Jay Iams and I serve as editors of the book and we called upon many collaborators to assist us. Most of the collaborators are from either The Ohio State University College of Medicine or the University of California at Irvine, where Dr. Quilligan resides.

Each chapter identifies the author of the text, and an extensive index and cross references are provided to assist the reader to quickly find the information.

This edition differs from the last edition in that we have limited the number of references to those we think are most useful; thus the reference lists are not intended to be all inclusive. Additionally, we have included National Board or CREOG-type questions at the end of each chapter, with appropriate indexing of answers. The illustrations and tables have been expanded, and this edition is written in a more abbreviated outline form instead of a totally narrative form, as was the first text.

The editors and authors hope that this manual will be useful in direct patient care. Every effort has been made to make the text error-free. Comments regarding format, usefulness, and other information are welcomed by the editors and the authors.

Frederick P. Zuspan, M.D.

Contents

Anatomy and Physiology

Michael Foley
William Dodds

An understanding of reproductive medicine begins with a base of knowledge about the anatomy and physiology of the female reproductive system. The anatomy will be extensively reviewed here, along with an introduction to physiology, which is discussed further in Chapters 3 (maternal physiology in pregnancy), 20 (lactation), 21 (contraception), 27 (abnormal uterine bleeding), 28 (amenorrhea), and 32 (menopause).

ANATOMY
External Genital Organs
Mons pubis (mons veneris)

The *mons pubis* is situated in the lower abdomen just above the symphysis pubis. It is covered with a thick tuft of hair, the distribution of which differs in males and females (Fig. 1-1). The female pattern is more sharply demarcated on the upper border than the male pattern.

Labia majora

The *labia majora* form the lateral boundaries of the pudendal cleft, the area into which the urethra and vagina open. The labia themselves consist of an outer pigmented layer of skin covered with hair and an inner smooth layer that contains large sebaceous follicles. Areolar and adipose tissues are sandwiched between these layers, as are blood vessels and nerves.

Labia minora

The *labia minora* form a bilateral cutaneous fold that unites anteriorly to split and ensheathe the clitoris. The anterior fold forms the prepuce and the posterior fold forms the frenulum of the clitoris. Posteriorly, the labia minora unite to form the posterior commissure, or fourchette. It is devoid of hair follicles and rich in sebaceous glands. The labia minora correspond morphologically with the proximal part of the corpus cavernosum urethrae of the male.

Clitoris

The *clitoris* is situated between the anterior ends of the labia minora and consists of two corpora cavernosa that are structured primarily of erectile tissue enclosed in a fibrous membrane. These unite along their medial surfaces in an incomplete fibrous septum, forming the body of the clitoris. The posterior extensions of the corpora cavernosa form two crura, which compose the root of the clitoris and anchor it to the inferior rami of the pubic ischium. The free end of the clitoris (the glans) is richly supplied

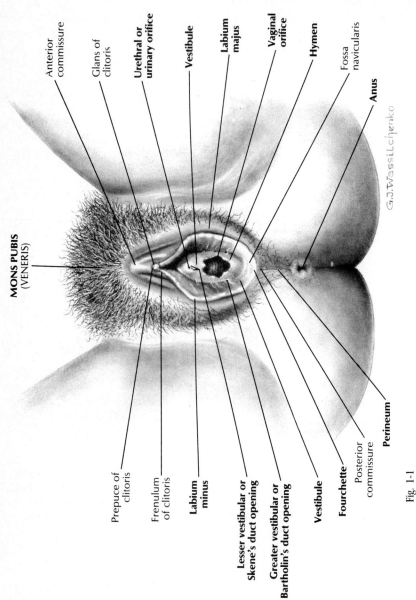

Fig. 1-1
External female genitals.
(From Bobak IM: Maternity and gynecologic care, ed. 4, St. Louis, 1989, The CV Mosby Co.)

with nerve endings and is extremely sensitive. It is composed of erectile tissue and covered by squamous epithelium. The clitoris corresponds morphologically with the male glans penis.

Vestibule of the vagina

The *vestibule of the vagina* is a shallow depression bounded on either side by the labia minora and posteriorly by the vaginal orifice. The opening of the ducts of the greater vestibular (Bartholin's) glands drain into the vestibule.

External urethral orifice

The *external urethral orifice* is located in the anterior vestibule, and the vagina is located below and behind the opening of the urethra. The orifice opens in the midst of the vestibule of the vagina about 2.5 cm posterior to the base of the clitoris and is bordered bilaterally by two small paraurethral (Skene's) ducts, which are rudimentary homologs of the prostate gland in the male.

Bulb of vestibule

The *bulb of the vestibule* consists of two erectile bodies lying on either side of the vaginal orifice in contact with the inferior surface of the urogenital diaphragm and covered by the bulbocavernosus (sphincter vaginae) muscles. Each structure is 3 to 4 cm long and 1 to 2 cm wide. The bulb of vestibule is the homolog of the bulb and the adjoining part of the corpus cavernosum urethrae of the male.

Greater vestibular glands (Bartholin's glands)

Bartholin's glands are a pair of compound glands located on either side of the vaginal orifice, each under cover of the corresponding bulb. They are small round bodies ranging in size from 0.5 to 1 cm. Each gland opens by means of a duct (Bartholin's gland duct), is approximately 2 cm long, and drains between the labia minora in the vaginal orifice. The gland is a homolog of the bulbourethral (Cowper's) gland in the male.

Vaginal orifice

The *vaginal orifice* is located below and posterior to the urethral orifice. The contour and degree of the opening depends on virginity, age, and parity of the woman. In nulliparous women, the vaginal orifice is usually partially occluded by the hymen.

Hymen

The *hymen* is a thin fold of mucous membrane attached around the circumference of the vaginal orifice. There are various types of openings in the hymen: annular, crescentic, cribriform, septate, and imperforate. It is invariably ruptured during coitus or after first parturition, and the shrunken nodular hymenal tags remaining at the margins of the vaginal orifice are called the *carunculae hymenales* (Fig. 1-2).

The Perineum and Pelvic Diaphragm

The perineum

The *perineum* is bounded by the mons pubis in front, the buttocks behind, and the thighs laterally.

The perineal floor

The *floor of the perineum* is composed of skin and two layers of superficial fascia: a superficial fatty layer (fascia of camper) and a deeper membranous layer limited to the anterior half of the perineum (Colles' fascia).

Annular   Septate   Cribriform   Parous introitus

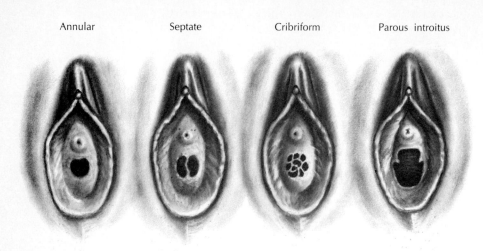

G. J. Wassilchenko

Fig. 1-2
Hymen and parous introitus.
(From Bobak IM: Maternity and gynecologic care, ed. 4, St. Louis, 1989, The CV Mosby Co.)

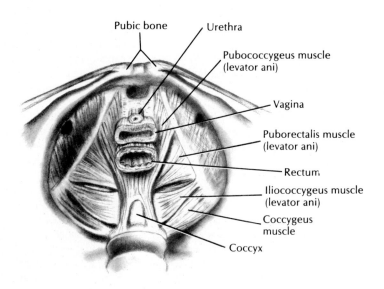

G. J. Wassilchenko

Fig. 1-3
Upper pelvic diaphragm viewed from above.
(From Bobak IM: Maternity and gynecologic care, ed. 4, St. Louis, 1989, The CV Mosby Co.)

The urogenital diaphragm

The *urogenital diaphragm* is a strong musculomembranous partition stretched across the anterior half of the pelvic outlet between the ischiopubic rami. There is a superior and inferior fascial layer, between which are the deep perineal muscles, sphincter of the membranous urethra, and the pudendal vessels and nerves.

The muscles of the perineum include the bulbocavernous, the ischiocavernous, and the superficial and deep transverse perineal muscles, the sphincter muscle of membranous urethra, and the external sphincter muscle of the anus. The central point of the perineum lies at the base of the urogenital diaphragm between the vaginal and anal orifice. It is a common place of attachment for the bulbocavernous, the superficial and deep transverse perineal, and the levator ani muscles and the external sphincter muscle of the anus.

The pelvic diaphragm

The *pelvic diaphragm* is a musculotendinous funnel-shaped partition between the pelvic cavity and the perineum and serves as one of the principal supports of the pelvic viscera. It is composed of the levator ani (anterior pubococcygeal and posterior iliococcygal) and coccygeal muscles sheathed in a superior and inferior layer of fascia. The muscles of the pelvic diaphragm extend from the lateral walls downward and medially to fuse with each other and are inserted into the terminal portions of the urethra and anus (Fig. 1-3).

Internal Genital Organs
Vagina

The *vagina* is a musculomembranous canal that extends from the vestibule to the uterus. The anterior wall of the vagina is usually about 6 to 7.5 cm long, with the posterior wall extending 1.5 to 3 cm longer. The cervix projects into the upper portion of the vagina, forming a circular cul de sac, the *fornix,* which is arbitrarily divided into four regions: anterior fornix, posterior fornix, and two lateral fornices. The vagina is bordered anteriorly by the bladder and trigone and posteriorly by the rectum. The vaginal wall behind the posterior fornix is covered by the peritoneum of the rectovaginal pouch of Douglas and may be in contact with coils of intestine entering this pouch. Laterally, the lateral fornix lies just under the root of the broad ligament and is 1 to 1.5 cm from the point where the uterine artery crosses the ureter. The middle half of the vagina lies in close apposition to the ampulla of the rectum. In this area the contents of the rectum can be easily palpated through the vaginal wall. The wall of the vagina consists of a lining of stratified squamous epithelium, a muscular coat, and an outer layer of connective tissue. The muscular coat consists of two layers: an outer layer composed of longitudinal fibers and an inner circular layer.

There are no true glands in the vagina. The mucus lubricating the vagina originates from vaginal wall transudate and cervical secretions. The acidic nature of the mucus results from fermentative action of bacteria on glycogen from vaginal epithelium. The normal pH of the vagina is 3.5 to 4.5, with a tendency in pregnancy to move in an alkaline direction. The vagina functions as the female copulatory organ, a passageway for drainage from the uterus (i.e., menses), and the birth canal.

Uterus

The *uterus* is a thick, hollow, muscular organ situated between the bladder anteriorly and the rectum posteriorly. The uterine cavity extends from the vagina below to the fallopian tubes above, which open into its upper portion on either side at its lateral superior angle. The main function of the uterus is to serve as a receptacle for the fetus. The fertilized ovum becomes embedded in the uterine wall where it is retained until prenatal development is completed. The uterus, meanwhile, undergoes changes in size and structure to accommodate itself to the needs of the embryo. The uterus is about 7.5 cm in length, is 4 to 5 cm at its widest point, and weighs about 60 g on average.

The uterus has three physiologic demarcations: the cervix at its most distal end, the body or fundus proximally, and an area of constriction situated between the cervix and body, the *isthmus*. The uterus is usually inclined forward so that the body is in intimate relation with the upper surface of the bladder—a pouch of peritoneum intervenes between them. This is the normal anteversion and anteflexion position. Numerous variations in position and flexion exist. Thus, the uterus may be displaced backward (retroversion) or to one side (lateral version). There also may be forward flexure in the region of the isthmus (anteflexion). Correspondingly, there may be retroflexion or lateral flexion.

The *cervix,* as noted, extends from the inferior end of the body of the uterus at the constricted isthmus to the upper part of the vagina, into which it protrudes and forms an angle that varies from 45 to 90 degrees. Important relationships to the cervix include the paracervical nerve plexus on either side of the cervix; the uterine arteries, which run along the margins of the cervix in the parametrium; and the ureters, which course downward and forward approximately 2 cm from the cervix. The internal os is the opening of the cervix into the uterine cavity at the area of the uterine isthmus. The external os opens into the vagina at the most distal portion of the cervix. The cavity between these openings is called the cervical canal and is approximately 2 cm in length. The mucous membrane of the cervix is composed of cylindrical and ciliated epithelium in its upper two thirds, or supravaginal portion, but below this it looses its cilia and changes abruptly to stratified squamous epithelium close to the external orifice.

In the mucosa of the cervix, numerous large glands are present. These glands are extensively branched and lined with mucus-secreting tall columnar epithelium. Frequently, some of the cervical glands become obstructed and are transformed into cysts, the *nabothian follicles.*

The muscle layer of the cervix consists chiefly of circular bundles. An outer longitudinal layer is continuous with the smooth muscle of the vagina. The serous coat derived from the peritoneum covers the anterior surface of the uterus only as far as the junction of the uterine body and cervix (isthmus). The anterior surface of the cervix is not covered and is therefore functionally retroperitoneal. The structure of the uterus is composed of three coats: the external serosa derived from the peritoneum, the muscular layer, and the endometrium.

The muscular coat forms the chief bulk of the uterine structure. It has three layers—external, middle, and internal:

1. The external layer, beneath the peritoneum, consists of fibers that pass transversely across the fundus and converge at each lateral angle of the uterus, forming extensions into the tubes and the ovarian and round ligaments and to each side of the broad ligament.
2. The middle layer consists of fibers that are circularly arranged and include the most vascular layer of the muscular coat.
3. The internal layer consists mainly of longitudinal fibers, occasionally with circular and oblique bundles.

These three muscle layers of the myometrium often are not sharply demarcated because fibers frequently pass from one layer into another (Fig. 1-4).

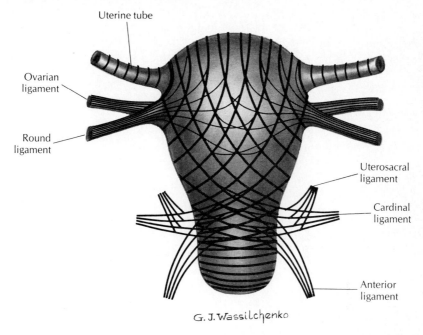

Fig. 1-4
Schematic arrangement of directions of muscle fibers. Note that uterine muscle fibers are continuous with supportive ligaments of uterus.
(From Bobak IM: Maternity and gynecologic care, ed. 4, St. Louis, 1989, The CV Mosby Co.)

The endometrium

The *endometrium*, the interior lining of the uterus, consists of a soft spongy layer that contains many tubular glands lined by ciliated columnar epithelium. After menstruation, the layer is only 1 to 2 mm thick, but before menstruation it increases to as much as 4 to 7 mm. In the early phase of the cycle, the glands are straight, the epithelium is low cuboidal, and the stroma is dense. Before menses, the glands are convoluted, the cells are columnar with marked secretory activity, and the stroma is abundant and loose in the superficial layers (Fig. 1-5).

Uterine Ligaments and Supports

There are eight ligaments of the uterus: one anterior (uterovesical fold of peritoneum), one posterior (retrovaginal fold of peritoneum), two lateral (broad), two uterosacral, and two round. In addition, there are also the transverse ligaments of the cervix, *Mackenrodt's cardinal ligaments*. Together with the surrounding retroperitoneal connective tissue, they function to support the uterus and pelvic viscera.

Uterosacral ligaments of the uterus

These *uterosacral ligaments* are suspensory ligaments of the uterus; they are a pair of ligamentous bands, extending in a curve from the posterior lateral surface of the sacrum, suspending the cervix from the sacrum, and forming a modified hammock.

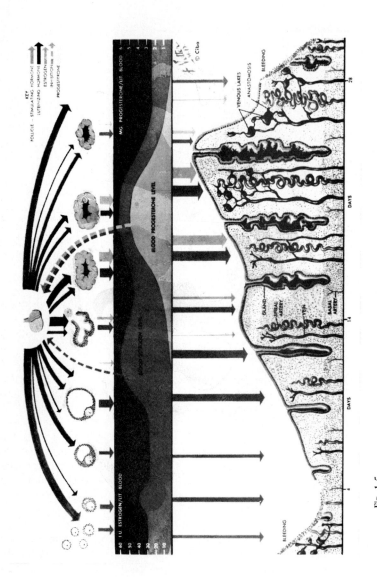

Fig. 1-5

Changes in the endometrium throughout the menstrual cycle, correlated with ovarian activity and blood estrogen and progesterone levels.

Broad ligaments

The *broad ligaments* compose the peritoneal fold, which covers and supports the uterus and its adnexa, and comprise the mesometrium, the mesovarium, and the mesosalpinx, which arise from the uterus, the ovary, and the tube, respectively.

Round ligaments of the uterus

The *round ligaments* consist of two flattened bands approximately 10 to 12 cm in length situated between the layers of the broad ligament in front and below the uterine tubes. They are primarily composed of muscular tissue that extends from the uterus, in addition to fibrous and areolar tissue, blood vessels, and lymphatics.

Cardinal ligaments of the uterus (Mackenrodt's)

The *cardinal ligaments* extend from the cervix to the parietal pelvic fascia as a bulky, ill-defined mass of fibrous tissue located on either side of the cervix at the base of the broad ligament. Along with the pelvic diaphragm and its endopelvic fascial extensions, the cardinal ligaments provide the majority of uterine support. They contain the uterine artery, vein, and nerve plexus.

Parametrium

The cervix and upper vagina are embedded in a mass of fibrous tissue that contains scattered bundles of smooth muscle; this area is termed the *parametrium*. Both the uterosacral and cardinal ligaments are continuous with the parametrium, forming the principal means of fixation and support of the uterus (Fig. 1-6).

Fallopian tube

There are two fallopian tubes, which are convoluted muscular canals that extend from the superior angles of the uterus to the side of the pelvis. Each tube is about 10 to 12 cm long, and their cavities connect the uterus with the peritoneal cavity. The tube is divisible into five segments beginning at the uterus: the interstitium, the isthmus, the ampulla, the infundibulum, and the fimbria (see Fig. 1-6, *A*).

The tube consists of three coats or layers: serous, muscular, and mucous. The external, or serous, coat is peritoneal. The middle, or muscular, coat consists of an external longitudinal and an internal circular layer of muscular fibers continuous with those of the uterus. The inner, or mucosal, layer of the tube is lined with a single layer of high columnar epithelium, which extends outward over the fimbria. A portion of these cells are ciliated. The motile cilia produce a current directed toward the uterus that aids in the passive transport of the ova to the uterus. Fertilization of the ovum is believed to occur in the ampulla of the tube. The ampulla is the most common site for the implantation of an ectopic pregnancy.

The ovaries

The *ovaries* are paired, almond-shaped bodies situated on either side of the uterus in close apposition to the lateral wall of the pelvis. They are set in the posterior layer of the broad ligament located behind and below the uterine tubes. The ovaries are approximately 2.5 to 5 cm in length and 1.5 to 3 cm in width.

The ovary lies in a shallow depression, the *ovarian fossa,* on the lateral wall of the pelvis. This fossa is bounded above by the external iliac vessels, in front by the obliterated umbilical artery, and behind by the ureter. The medial surface is partly overhung by the fimbriated end of the tube and partly related to coils of the intestine. The anterior border is straight, directed toward the obliterated umbilical artery, and at-

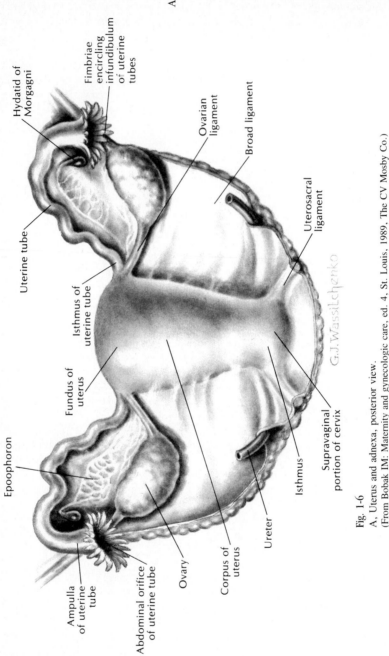

Fig. 1-6

A, Uterus and adnexa, posterior view.
(From Bobak IM: Maternity and gynecologic care, ed. 4, St. Louis, 1989, The CV Mosby Co.)

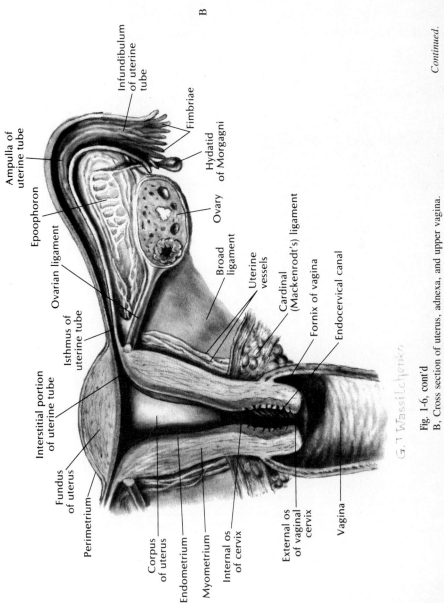

Ampulla of
uterine tube

Epoophoron

Ovarian ligament

Isthmus of
uterine tube

Interstitial portion
of uterine tube

Fundus
of uterus

Perimetrium

Corpus
of uterus

Endometrium

Myometrium

Internal os
of cervix

External os
of vaginal
cervix

Vagina

Infundibulum
of uterine
tube

Fimbriae

Hydatid
of Morgagni

Ovary

Broad
ligament

Uterine
vessels

Cardinal
(Mackenrodt's) ligament

Fornix of vagina

Endocervical canal

B

G. J. Wassilchenko

Fig. 1-6, cont'd
B, Cross section of uterus, adnexa, and upper vagina.

Continued.

Fig. 1-6, cont'd
C, Levator ani muscles of upper pelvic diaphragm and urogenital (lower pelvic) diaphragm, anterior view.

tached to the posterior layer of the broad ligament by a short fold, the *mesovarium*. Between the two layers of this fold, the blood vessels and nerves pass to reach the hilum of the ovary. The posterior border projects into the pelvic cavity, coming into direct contact with loops of intestine.

The epithelium covering the ovary is cuboidal or low columnar and is a persisting portion of the germinal epithelium of the genital ridge of the embryo. Beneath this germinal epithelium is a layer of dense connective tissue, the *tunica albuginea*.

Immediately beneath the superficial covering of the ovary is a layer (cortex) of stroma, in which early follicles are found. Beneath the superficial stratum, other large and more mature follicles are embedded. These follicles increase in size as they recede from the surface toward a highly vascular stroma in the center of the organ, the *medulla*.

The suspensory ligament of the ovary, also called the *infundibulopelvic ligament*, is a triangular fold of peritoneum that is actually the upper lateral corner of the broad ligament as it becomes confluent with the peritoneum at the pelvic brim. It contains the ovarian artery, veins, and nerves after they pass over the pelvic brim and before they enter the mesovarium.

The *ovarian ligament* proper is a musculofibrous cord connecting the lower pole of the ovary with the lateral wall of the uterus. It runs in the substance of the mesovarium

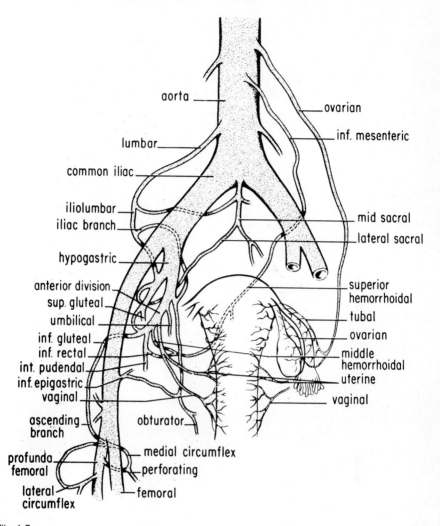

Fig. 1-7
Blood supply to the uterus, fallopian tube, and ovary.
(From Mattingly R, and Thompson JD, editors: TeLinde's operative gynecology, ed. 6, Philadelphia, 1985, JB Lippincott Co.)

and broad ligament. Within the wall of the uterus, the ovarian ligament is continuous with the round ligament of the uterus. Together, they represent the gubernaculum of the fetal ovary.

Blood Supply to the Pelvis
Internal iliac arteries

The major portion of the blood supply to the pelvis is derived from the internal iliac (hypogastric) arteries (Fig. 1-7 and box on p. 14).

Branches of the Internal Iliac Artery

Visceral branches	**Anterior Division** *Parietal branches*	**Posterior Division** *Parietal branches*
Uterine	Obturator	Iliolumbar
Superior vesical	Inferior gluteal	Lateral sacral
Middle vesical	Internal pudendal	Superior gluteal
Inferior vesical		
Middle hemorrhoidal		
Inferior hemorrhoidal		
Vaginal		

Collateral arterial circulation

Branches from the aorta include the ovarian arteries, which anastomose freely with the uterine arteries. The inferior mesenteric artery continues as the superior hemorrhoidal artery to anastomose with the middle and inferior hemorrhoidal arteries from the internal iliac and internal pudendal. The lumbar and vertebral arteries anastomose with the iliolumbar artery of the internal iliac. The middle sacral artery anastomoses with the lateral sacral artery of the internal iliac.

Branches from the external iliac artery include the deep iliac circumflex arteries, which anastomose with the iliolumbar and superior gluteal of the internal iliac. The inferior epigastric artery gives origin to the obturator artery in approximately 25% of cases and provides additional anastomoses with the external iliac by way of the medial femoral circumflex and communicating pelvic branches.

Branches from the femoral artery include the medial circumflex artery, which anastomoses with the inferior gluteal artery from the internal iliac, and the lateral femoral circumflex arteries, which anastomose with the superior gluteal and the iliolumbar arteries from the internal iliac.

Lymphatic system of the pelvis

The lymphatic vessels of the major pelvic organs drain primarily to the hypogastric and other iliac nodes. The efferent vessels of the urethra, bladder, and intrapelvic portion of the ureter pass chiefly to the hypogastric group. Those from the bladder pass to the external iliac and common iliac groups. The lymphatics of the cervix, uterus, and major portions (superior) of the vagina primarily drain to the internal iliac group. The lymphatics from the fundus of the uterus and the broad ligament usually anastomose with those of the fallopian tubes and ovaries and ascend with the ovarian vessels to the aortic nodes. There are a few, however, that may pass to the iliac groups. The lymphatics from the rectum pass upward toward the iliac nodes. The lymphatics of the anus end with those of the lower vagina, vulva, and perineum in the inguinal group (Fig. 1-8).

Innervation of the Pelvis

The innervation of the pelvic organs is from both sympathetic and parasympathetic nerves. Both the sympathetic and parasympathetic systems are accompanied by afferent sensory fibers. The sympathetic innervation is primarily by the hypogastric plexus. The parasympathetic system is composed of the pelvic visceral nerves (S2, S3, S4)

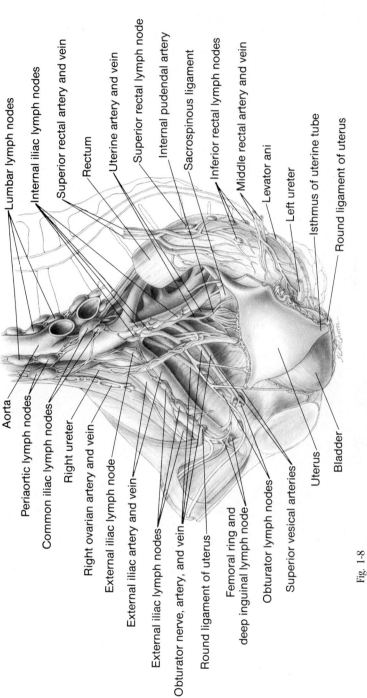

Lumbar lymph nodes

Internal iliac lymph nodes

Superior rectal artery and vein

Rectum

Uterine artery and vein

Superior rectal lymph node

Internal pudendal artery

Sacrospinous ligament

Inferior rectal lymph nodes

Middle rectal artery and vein

Levator ani

Left ureter

Isthmus of uterine tube

Round ligament of uterus

Aorta

Periaortic lymph nodes

Common iliac lymph nodes

Right ureter

Right ovarian artery and vein

External iliac lymph node

External iliac artery and vein

External iliac lymph nodes

Obturator nerve, artery, and vein

Round ligament of uterus

Femoral ring and
deep inguinal lymph node

Obturator lymph nodes

Superior vesical arteries

Uterus

Bladder

Fig. 1-8
A lateral view of the female pelvis demonstrating the extensive lymphatic network. Note that most of the lymphatic channels follow the courses of the major vessels. (Redrawn from Clemente CD: Anatomy: A regional atlas of the human body. Philadelphia, 1975. Lea & Febiger.)

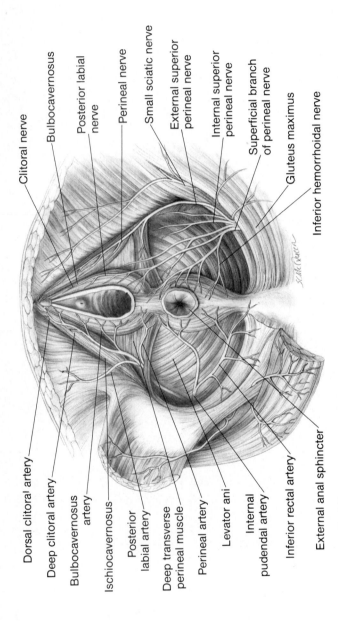

Clitoral nerve

Bulbocavernosus

Posterior labial nerve

Perineal nerve

Small sciatic nerve

External superior perineal nerve

Internal superior perineal nerve

Superficial branch of perineal nerve

Gluteus maximus

Inferior hemorrhoidal nerve

Dorsal clitoral artery

Deep clitoral artery

Bulbocavernosus artery

Ischiocavernosus

Posterior labial artery

Deep transverse perineal muscle

Perineal artery

Levator ani

Internal pudendal artery

Inferior rectal artery

External anal sphincter

Fig. 1-9
A posterior view of the female perineum, demonstrating the pudendal nerve emerging externally. The nerve divides into three segments as it passes out of the pelvis: the inferior hemorrhoidal nerve and the deep and superficial perineal nerves. The clitoral nerve is the terminal branch of the deep perineal nerve.
(Redrawn from Mattingly RF, Thompson JD: Te Linde's operative gynecology, ed 6, Philadelphia, 1985, JB Lippincott Co., p. 49.)

and their synaptic connection with the ganglia in or near the walls of the viscera. The innervation of the external genitalia and peritoneum is primarily by the pudendal nerve and its branches. However, the anterior labial branch of the ilioinguinal nerve (L1), the perineal branch of the posterior femoral cutaneous nerve (S1, S2, S3), and the external spermatic branch of the genitofemoral nerve (L1, L2) all contribute to the innervation of the perineal skin (Fig. 1-9).

The Course of the Ureter

The abdominal ureter is approximately 13 cm in length and courses along the anterior-medial aspect of the psoas muscle throughout its abdominal route to the pelvis. The ureter crosses over the common iliac artery just beyond its bifurcation. The pelvic ureter, which is also approximately 13 to 15 cm in length, passes posteriorly and inferiorly to the anterior division of the hypogastric artery. At that point it courses along the

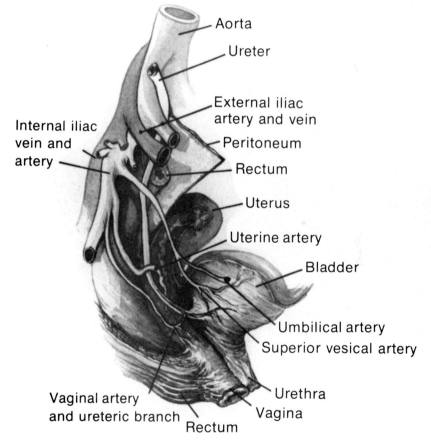

Fig. 1-10
Anatomic relationship of ureter to arterial vessels supplying major pelvic viscera. Note the course of ureter lateral to the uterine body and posterior to the uterine artery. The relative fixation of the pelvic ureter by vascular structures is evident.
(From Buchsbaum, HF and Schmidt, JD: Gynecologic and obstetric urology, Philadelphia, 1978, WB Saunders Co.)

anterior surface of the levator muscles and passes beneath the uterine artery ("water under the bridge") approximately 1 to 1.5 cm laterally to the internal cervical os.

The ureter continues inferiorly for approximately 1 to 2 cm and comes in close approximation with the anterior vaginal fornix where it passes medially to enter the base of the bladder at the trigone (Fig. 1-10).

PHYSIOLOGY
The Menstrual Cycle

At birth, females are endowed with a surplus number of oocytes arrested in diplotene meiotic prophase. With puberty, the hypothalamic-pituitary-ovarian axis is established, and normal cyclic follicle development and ovulation occurs. The pattern of estrogen and progesterone production that accompanies folliculogenesis, ovulation, and corpus luteum development stimulates the endometrium, resulting in the menstrual cycle.

Menstrual cycle overview

The menstrual cycle is best understood, as shown in Fig. 1-11, by dividing it into three phases: the follicular phase, ovulation, and the luteal phase.

The mean menstrual-cycle length is 28 days. Variation from this mean is usually secondary to a change in the length of the follicular phase. Luteal-phase length is generally constant at between 12 to 14 days. The cyclic changes in follicle-stimulating hormone (FSH), luteinizing hormone (LH), estradiol (E_2), progesterone, and 17-hydroxyprogesterone are depicted in Fig. 1-12.

Follicular phase. At the time of menstruation, a cohort of primordial follicles is recruited. The mechanism that determines which follicles are recruited and the number recruited is unknown. Elevated FSH levels in the early follicular phase, as depicted in Fig. 1-12, stimulate follicle development. FSH stimulates both mitotic division of the

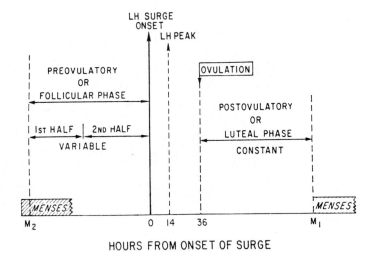

Fig. 1-11

Phases of the menstrual cycle.

(From Yen, SC and Jaffe, R: Reproductive endocrinology: physiology, pathophysiology and clinical management, ed. 2, Philadelphia, 1986, WB Saunders Co.)

granulosa cells surrounding the oocyte and granulosa-cell aromatization of androgen to E_2. E_2 is the key hormone in follicle development. Fig. 1-13 depicts the "two-cell theory" of E_2 production.

As depicted in Fig. 1-13, LH stimulates thecal cell production of androstenedione. Androstenedione is taken up by the granulosa cell, and under FSH stimulation, it is aromatized to E_2. E_2 and FSH both stimulate an increase in the number of FSH receptors on the granulosa cells. The follicle most efficient in E_2 production will be selected to become the dominant follicle, with the other follicles undergoing atresia. The follicle that is best at producing estrogen increases the number of FSH receptors on its granulosa cells, thereby further increasing its ability to respond to FSH through further E_2 production and follicle development. As depicted in Fig. 1-12, as E_2 begins to increase, it feeds back to the hypothalamus and pituitary in a negative fashion to decrease FSH output. The follicle that has produced estrogen efficiently and developed the most granulosa FSH receptors will be able to best sequester and use the decreasing FSH resource. That follicle will dominate while the others undergo atresia.

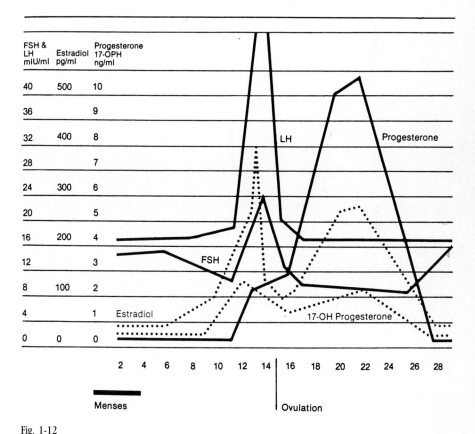

Fig. 1-12
Changes in estradiol progesterone, follicle stimulating hormone (FSH), and luteinizing hormone (LH) during the menstrual cycle.
(From Speroff, L, et al: Clinical gynecologic endocrinology and infertility, ed. 3, Baltimore, 1983, Williams & Wilkins Co.)

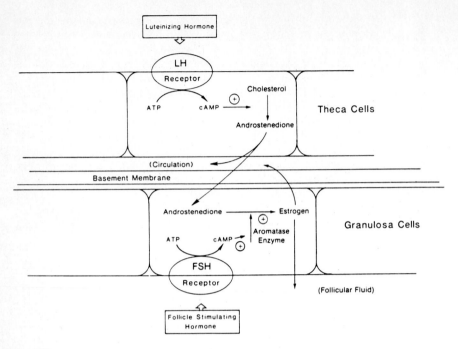

Fig. 1-13
Diagrammatic representation of the two-cell theory of follicle estrogen production.

Ovulation. Ovulation is triggered by the LH surge. The LH surge initiates meiotic resumption, follicle prostaglandin synthesis, and progesterone production. Prostaglandin production is essential for follicle rupture and oocyte release. As shown in Fig. 1-11, ovulation occurs approximately 24 to 36 hours after the LH surge.

Luteal phase. The ruptured follicle under LH stimulation reorganizes as the corpus luteum. Progesterone and E_2 are produced by the corpus luteum, with progesterone being the predominant hormone of the luteal phase. As shown in Fig. 1-12, serum progesterone levels peak by day 8 or 9 after ovulation. The corpus luteum will begin degeneration at that point unless rescued by a pregnancy's hCG production.

REVIEW QUESTIONS

True or False

1. The skene's glands are homologs of the bulbourethral (Cowper's) gland in the male and open by way of a 2 cm long duct between the labia minora and the vaginal orifice.
2. The muscles of the perineum include the bulbocavernosus, the ischiocavernosus, the superficial and deep transverse perineal muscles, the sphincter of the membranous urethra, and the external anal sphincter.
3. The mucus lubricating the vagina originates from vaginal wall transudate and cervical secretions.
4. The major support of the uterus is provided by which of the following ligaments?
   a. Uterosacral ligaments
   b. Broad ligaments
   c. Round ligaments
   d. Cardinal ligaments
5. Which of the following branches of the internal iliac artery arise from the posterior division?
   a. Uterine
   b. Vaginal
   c. Inferior hemorrhoidal
   d. Superior gluteal
6. Which of the following statements is false concerning the course of the ureter?
   a. The ureter runs along the antero-medial aspect of the psoas muscle.
   b. The ureter crosses over the common iliac just beyond the bifurcation.
   c. The ureter passes over the uterine artery approximately 1.0-1.5 cm. lateral to the internal cervical os.
   d. The ureter turns medially at the anterior vaginal fornix to enter the base of the bladder at the trigone.
7. According to the two cell hypothesis of ovarian estrogen production:
   a. FSH stimulates thecal cell androstendione production.
   b. Estradiol inhibits FSH receptor development.
   c. Thecal cells aromatize androstenedione to estradiol.
   d. FSH stimulates Granulosa cell aromatase activity.
   e. FSH inhibits LH receptor development on Granulosa cells.
8. Which of the following statements is false concerning periovulatory hormonal events?
   a. Estradiol positive feedback stimulates the LH surge.
   b. The LH surge initiates resumption of meiosis in the oocyte.
   c. A preovulatory rise in progesterone facilitates the positive feedback action of estradiol.
   d. LH surge inhibits follicle prostaglandin production.
   e. A small FSH surge occurs with the LH surge and may be important in inducing LH receptors on Granulosa cells.

ANSWERS:

1. False (Bartholin's gland)
2. True
3. True
4. d

5. d
6. c
7. d
8. d

BIBLIOGRAPHY

Gould SF: Anatomy. In Gabbe SG, Niebyl JR, and Simpson JL, editors: Obstetrics: normal and problem pregnancies, New York, 1986, Churchill Livingstone, Inc.

Mattingly R, editor: TeLinde's operative gynecology, ed 6, Philadelphia, 1985, JB Lippincott Co, p. 25.

Netter F: The reproductive system. In The Ciba collection of medical illustrations, vol 2.

Speroff L, Glass R, and Kase N: Clinical gynecologic endocrinology and infertility, ed 3, Baltimore, 1983, Williams & Wilkins Co, Inc, p. 75.

Zuspan FP, and Quilligan EJ, editors: Douglas-Stromme operative obstetrics, ed 5, (pp. 1-35) 1988 Appleton Lange, East Norwalk CT.

Diagnosis of Pregnancy

2

William Dodds

The diagnosis of pregnancy requires careful attention to menstrual history, patient symptoms, physical examination, and pregnancy tests. Often the diagnosis of pregnancy is not made because it was not considered. The first step in the evaluation of all females of reproductive age who present with oligomenorrhea and amenorrhea is to rule out pregnancy. Symptoms and physical findings that occur with pregnancy are listed in the box below.

Physical Examination

Cervical mucus will be thick, have poor spinnbarkheit, and be nonferning in both the normal luteal phase and pregnancy. Cervical mucus that is thin and clear and that ferns is consistent with either a normal proliferative phase or an anovulatory state. Physical examination should reveal an enlarged uterus after 6 weeks from the last menstrual period (LMP). Before 12 to 14 weeks gestation, uterine size can give a fairly accurate estimate of the gestational age. Softening of the cervix and uterine isthmus may be appreciated. Auscultation of heart tones is generally first appreciated between 17 to 20 weeks.

Pregnancy Signs and Symptoms

Amenorrhea
Breast enlargement and tenderness
Nausea
Increased urinary frequency
Fatigue and irritability
Increased skin pigmentation
Blue discoloration of vaginal mucosa

Table 2-1 Detection methods for hCG

Test	Sensitivity
Direct hemagglutination	200 mIU/ml
Indirect hemagglutination and latex agglutination inhibition	200 mIU/ml
Radioimmunoassay	5-10 mIU/ml
Enzyme-linked immunoassay	40-50 mIU/ml

Pregnancy Tests

The discovery of human chorionic gonadotropin (hCG) and development of monoclonal antibodies to its B subunit have led to very sensitive and specific pregnancy tests. The major techniques currently used to measure hCG are summarized in Table 2-1.

Today, many of the home pregnancy tests use monoclonal antibody immunoassay techniques, and therefore their sensitivity can be as low as 40 to 50 mIU/ml. These tests detect pregnancy as early as 8 to 10 days after ovulation. False-positive results can occur from one of three main causes: (1) cross-reaction with pituitary gonadotropin (luteinizing hormone [LH], follicle-stimulating hormone [FSH]); (2) local and systemic diseases (e.g., urinary tract infection [UTI], proteinuria, hematuria, systemic lupus erythematosus [SLE], or hCG-producing neoplasms); or (3) drugs (e.g., phenothiazines, barbiturates, methadone, or penicillin).

Ultrasonography

Ultrasonography has revolutionized the obstetrician-gynecologist's ability to diagnose and evaluate early gestations. In particular, it is important in differentiating a normal intrauterine pregnancy from a blighted ovum or an ectopic pregnancy. A transabdominal-sector scan ultrasonogram can usually identify an intrauterine gestational sac at 6 to 7 weeks. A fetal pole and, later, cardiac activity are detected at 7 to 8 weeks. Transvaginal ultrasonographic (TVU) techniques have allowed even earlier detection of pregnancy. With TVU, a gestational sac is seen at 5 weeks menstrual age and a fetal pole at 5½ to 6 weeks gestation. Cardiac activity is seen with TVU at 6½ to 7 weeks gestation.

In a normal intrauterine pregnancy, early ultrasonography gives good confirmation of menstrual dates. Between 7 to 12 weeks, a crown-rump measurement has an accuracy of ±3 days in dating the gestation. Ultrasonography has also become important in evaluating patients with suspected ectopic pregnancy and threatened abortion.

DIAGNOSIS AND MANAGEMENT OF ECTOPIC AND ABORTING GESTATIONS
Ectopic Pregnancy
    Epidemiology

Ectopic pregnancy is one of the most important clinical problems that obstetrician-gynecologists manage. According to figures from the Centers for Disease Control (excluding trauma), ectopic pregnancy is the fourth leading cause of maternal mortality, after pulmonary embolism, hypertensive disease, and obstetric hemorrhage. The maternal mortality of ectopic pregnancy is approximately 1 per 1000 ectopic pregnancies. Ectopic pregnancy has increased in frequency over the past 25 years from approximately 1:200 live births to 1:90 live births. Reasons for the increase are not clear but may include (1) an increase in sexually transmitted disease; (2) better pelvic inflammatory disease treatment that prevents total tubal obstruction and sterility but leaves compromised fallopian tubes; (3) an increase in tuboplasty and tubal reanastomosis procedures; and (4) an increase in maternal age at first pregnancy attempt.

In addition to the above, the increase in the abortion rate has decreased the live-birth rate. This in effect has increased the ratio of ectopic pregnancies to live births.

    Location

Approximately 96% of all ectopic gestations are tubal (see Fig. 2-1). Two thirds of ectopic pregnancies occur in the ampulla.

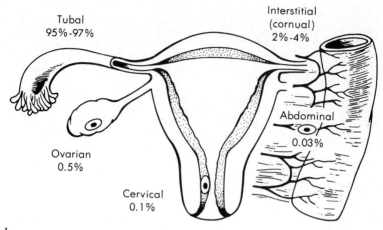

Tubal
95%-97%

Interstitial
(cornual)
2%-4%

Abdominal
0.03%

Ovarian
0.5%

Cervical
0.1%

Fig. 2-1
Location of ectopic pregnancies.
From Mattingly R, and Thompson JD, editors: Te Linde's operative gynecology, ed 6, Philadelphia, 1985, JB Lippincott Co.

Diagnosis

The diagnosis of ectopic pregnancy from clinical criteria alone is not accurate before rupture. Before laparoscopy was developed, approximately 80% of ectopic pregnancies were not diagnosed until after rupture. Today, only 20% of ectopic pregnancies are found ruptured at the time of surgery.

Clinical symptoms. Clinical symptoms and their frequency of presentation with ectopic pregnancy are given in Table 2-2. The classic triad of pelvic pain, amenorrhea, and vaginal bleeding is present in only 50% of all patients with ectopic pregnancy.

Physical findings. Physical findings and their relative frequency are given in Table 2-3.

Culdocentesis. Culdocentesis is a useful diagnostic test to identify the presence of intraperitoneal bleeding. If copious nonclotting blood is aspirated in a patient who is suspected to have an ectopic pregnancy, that patient should be taken directly to surgery. The problem with culdocentesis is that before rupture, many patients' results may be negative.

Laboratory diagnosis of ectopic pregnancy. The use of serial quantitative hCG levels and ultrasonography has provided a vast improvement in accurate diagnosis of ectopic pregnancy before rupture. Serum radioimmunoassay for hCG has a sensitivity to 5 mIU/ml. This means a negative quantitative hCG is essentially 100% accurate in ruling out any gestation, including an ectopic pregnancy. The normal increase in hCG levels

Table 2-2   Ectopic pregnancy symptoms

Symptom	Percent
Abdominal pain	98
Amenorrhea	75
Vaginal bleeding	56
Nausea and vomiting	36
Faintness and syncope	24

From Alsuleiman SA, and Grimes EM: J Reprod Med 27:101, 1982.

Table 2-3   Physical signs with ectopic pregnancy

Physical Sign	Percent
Adnexal tenderness	98
Abdominal tenderness	97
Fullness in the cul-de-sac	70
Rebound tenderness	53
Adnexal mass	32
Enlarged uterus	23

From Alsuleiman SA, and Grimes EM: J Reprod Med 27:101, 1982.

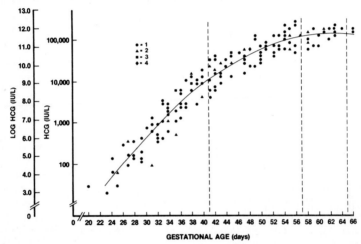

Fig. 2-2
Serum levels of human chorionic gonadotropin by gestational age in four normal pregnancies.
Notice the 2-day "doubling time" before day 42. Quadratic regression line equation is as follows:
log hCG = −8.8695 + 0.6530 (gestational age) − 0.0052 (gestational age)^2. Symbols correspond to indicated number of data points.
From Daya S: Am J Obstet Gynecol 156:286, 1987.

through week 10 of pregnancy has allowed definition of hCG *doubling times* (see Fig. 2-2). This information is used to identify abnormal gestations, including ectopic pregnancies. The doubling time of hCG increases with gestational age. From onset of hCG production through day 42 (i.e., the beginning of gestation week 7), the doubling time is approximately 2 days. The doubling time increases to 4.75 days between days 42 and 57 (i.e., weeks 7 and 8). Approximately two thirds of ectopic pregnancies will demonstrate an inadequate hCG increase. An intrauterine sac should be visualized on ultrasonography when the hCG level reaches the 6500 mIU/ml *discriminatory zone.* The absence of an intrauterine sac on the ultrasonogram when the hCG level has reached the discriminatory zone is suggestive of an ectopic pregnancy. Fig. 2-3 outlines a diagnostic approach for ectopic pregnancy, using both serial quantitative hCG levels and ultrasonography. This approach provides close to 100% accuracy in diagnosing ectopic pregnancy and leads to early diagnosis before rupture so that a conservative procedure to preserve fertility can be performed.

SURGICAL MANAGEMENT OF ECTOPIC PREGNANCY

Surgical management is dictated by the patient's desire to preserve fertility, history of previous tubal pregnancy, past history of tubal surgery, status of the contralateral fallopian tube, specific tubal site of the present ectopic pregnancy, and, of course, whether the ectopic pregnancy is ruptured or unruptured at surgery. For patients who have an unruptured ectopic pregnancy and who desire fertility preservation, a conservative surgical approach is best.

Ampullary Ectopic Gestations

Unruptured ampullary ectopic gestations can be managed by linear salpingostomy. This conservative approach is possible because ampullary ectopic gestations are generally extraluminal in position. Ampullary ectopic gestations erode through the luminal

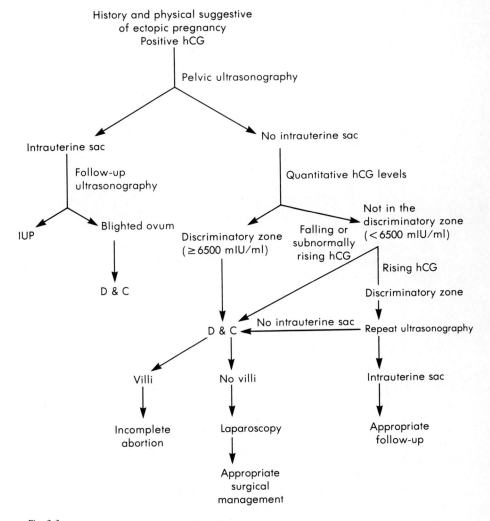

Fig. 2-3
Ectopic pregnancy diagnosis.

epithelium and their muscularis in the ampulla early on, propagating in a subserosal position. This means there is limited luminal epithelium damage, thus reducing the chance of luminal scarring and possible obstruction. A linear incision on the anti-mesenteric surface of the tube can be made with a scalpel, needle cautery, or carbon dioxide or argon laser. The extraluminal products of conception will generally extrude spontaneously and can be gently pulled free. Do not debride the base of the tube because this may cause tubal damage. Hemostasis can be accomplished with needle cautery or a running circumferential 6-0 polyglycolic acid (Vicryl or Dexon) suture. The tube will heal by secondary intent or may be closed with interrupted 6-0 Vicryl or Dexon suture, closing the muscularis and serosa in separate layers. Linear salpingostomy can be performed through the laparoscope with results equal to laparotomy, provided the following criteria are met:
1. Less than 3 cm unruptured ampullary ectopic gestation
2. Stable vital signs
3. Ectopic gestation in easily accessible site
4. Adequate operative laparoscopic skill and experience

Isthmic Ectopic Gestations

Isthmic ectopic gestations are best treated conservatively by segmental resection. One can perform reanastomosis at the time of resection or await healing and do reanastomosis at a later date. Linear salpingostomy is not as successful with isthmic ectopic gestations as it is with ampullary ectopic pregnancies. This is because isthmic ectopic gestations propagate intraluminally until overt tubal rupture. This causes damage of the luminal epithelium, which leads to scarring and tubal obstruction. For this reason, it is best to segmentally resect the damaged tubal portion and reanastomose the healthy portions of tube back together.

Fimbrial Ectopic Gestations

Fimbrial, or infundibular, ectopic gestations are uncommon. They should be managed by gentle removal of the ectopic gestation. "Milking" the ectopic gestation from the distal tubal end is not the recommended approach because it can lead to increased tubal injury and the chance of scarring and recurrent ectopic gestation.

Interstitial Ectopic Gestations

Interstitial, or cornual, ectopic pregnancy is a rare condition that accounts for only 2% to 4% of all tubal ectopic pregnancies. Interstitial ectopic pregnancies generally rupture later in gestation than ampullary ectopic pregnancies. Because they are near the most vascular region of the female pelvis, they usually cause rapid and profound shock with rupture. Mortality with interstitial ectopic pregnancy is approximately 2%. In patients with unruptured cornual ectopic pregnancies with minimal cornual damage, a cornual resection can be performed. Hysterectomy is performed when cornual damage is extensive and bleeding is uncontrollable.

THREATENED AND MISSED ABORTION
Diagnosis and Management of Threatened Abortion

Threatened abortion is diagnosed when the patient has an intrauterine pregnancy and presents with uterine bleeding and a closed cervical os. Ultrasonography is used to confirm the pregnancy as being intrauterine and still viable if it is of sufficient gestational age to evaluate fetal cardiac activity. If the gestation is less than 6 weeks, serial quantitative hCG levels can help to diagnose an abnormal pregnancy. Falling hCG levels would be indicative of either an early pregnancy demise or ectopic gestation; when hCG levels are falling, a dilation and curettage (D & C) is performed to differentiate between these two possibilities. A threatened abortion should be expectantly managed, with the patient advised to avoid vigorous physical activity and intercourse. Approximately 50% will carry the gestation and deliver at or near term.

Inevitable abortion is when the patient has prolonged uterine bleeding, uterine cramping, and dilation of the cervical os. These patients are managed by a D & C. *Missed abortion* is defined as a nonviable pregnancy retained in utero. If such a pregnancy is retained beyond 3 to 4 weeks, maternal hypofibrinogenemia may ensue. Patients with missed abortions require D & C, and coagulation studies should be obtained if the missed abortion has progressed longer than 3 weeks.

REVIEW
QUESTIONS

1. Which of the following is *not* a risk factor for ectopic pregnancy?
   a. Previous ectopic pregnancy
   b. Previous oral contraceptive use
   c. Pelvic inflammatory disease history
   d. Previous tubal reanastomosis
   e. Previous tuboplasty procedure
2. Which of the following statements is true?
   a. Patients with threatened abortion should have a coagulation profile.
   b. Threatened abortions with viable pregnancies on ultrasound should be managed expectantly.
   c. A negative culdocentesis rules out ectopic pregnancy.
   d. Vaginal bleeding with pelvic cramps constitutes a diagnosis of an inevitable abortion.
   e. Less than 25% of patients with threatened abortion will deliver at or near term.
3. Which of the following are criteria to determine when linear salpingostomy can be performed laparoscopically?
   a. Less than 3 cm in diameter
   b. Ampullary in position
   c. Ectopic pregnancy must not be ruptured
   d. Adequate operator experience with laparoscopic surgery
   e. All of the above

True or False

4. Radioimmunoassay hCG measurement can detect pregnancy as early as 8 to 10 days after ovulation.
5. A negative quantitative hCG virtually rules out the possibility of ectopic pregnancy.
6. A fetal pole with heart beat on abdominal ultrasound should be appreciated when the quantitative hCG level is approximately 6500 mIU/ml.
7. The most common site for ectopic pregnancy is the isthmic tubal area.
8. Before the seventh week from LMP, the hCG doubling time is approximately 2 days.

ANSWERS

1. b		5. T	
2. b		6. F	
3. e		7. F	
4. T		8. T	

BIBLIOGRAPHY

Alsuleiman SA, and Grimes EM: Ectopic pregnancy: a review of 147 cases, J Reprod Med 27:101, 1982.

Gabbe SG, Niebyl JR, and Simpson JL, editors: Obstetrics: normal and problem pregnancies, New York, 1986, Churchill Livingstone Inc.

Mattingly R, and Thompson JD, editors: Te Linde's operative gynecology, ed 6, Philadelphia, 1985, JB Lippincott Co.

Pittaway DE, Reish RL, and Wentz AC: Doubling times of human chorionic gonadotropin increase in early viable intrauterine pregnancies, Am J Obstet Gynecol 152:299, 1985.

Romero R et al: The effect of different human chorionic gonadotropin assay sensitivity on screening for ectopic pregnancy, Am J Obstet Gynecol 153:72, 1985.

Smith JC et al: An assessment of the incidence of maternal mortality in the United States, Am J Public Health 74:780, 1984.

Physiologic Changes in Pregnancy

Jay D. Iams

Maternal physiologic adaptation to pregnancy presents many challenges to the obstetric care provider. Physiologic changes perceived by the pregnant woman or detected through routine prenatal surveillance may be either normal for pregnancy or the first manifestation of a medical or obstetric disorder. Distinguishing normal changes from abnormal changes constitutes a large part of obstetric care. This chapter reviews the common normal physiologic alterations of pregnancy.

GASTROINTESTINAL TRACT

1. Appetite. The caloric requirement increases by 200 to 300 kcal/day, leading to increased appetite. The nausea and vomiting of early pregnancy affects 70% of pregnant women and usually begins within 2 weeks of conception and continues through 14 to 18 weeks gestation. It is distinguished from hyperemesis gravidarum by severity and degree of weight loss and is often triggered by food odors or strong smells. Nausea and vomiting can be minimized by frequent meals and carbonated, nonsweetened beverages. The fetus drains calories from the mother, leading to hypoglycemia in the absence of frequent meals.
2. Effects of high maternal progesterone on gastrointestinal tract. Relaxed smooth-muscle tone, a relaxed lower esophageal sphincter, and delayed gastric emptying lead to increased gastroesophageal reflux and esophagitis. The patient can treat this herself by elevating the head of the bed and taking liquid antacids. Delayed small and large bowel transit time leads to increased water resorption and a firm, constipated stool. Gallbladder distention and a propensity for stones are found in susceptible individuals.
3. Hepatic function changes. Alkaline phosphatase increases twofold to fourfold and fibrinogen increases 1½ times, mostly because of placental production. Steroid-binding globulins and cholesterol and lipids also increase. Albumin shows a decrease. The hepatocellular enzymes remain unchanged. Increased estrogen produces physical findings normally seen in liver disease, such as spider angiomata and palmar erythema.

SKIN

1. Increased pigmentation. Increased pigmentation is seen especially in the nipples, areolae, umbilicus, axillae, perineum, and linea nigra and is caused by increased levels of melanocyte-stimulating hormone, estrogen, and progesterone. Pigmented nevi may become darker and should be evaluated as for a nonpregnant woman.

2. Vascular changes. Palmar erythema and skin warmth become apparent and are caused by increased peripheral blood flow resulting from increased estrogen. Spider angiomata appear usually on the anterior upper chest.
3. Hair. Postpartum, an increase in the telogen phase leads to increased hair loss— sometimes alarmingly so.
4. Striae gravidarum. These silvery-pink violaceous "stretch marks" may occur on the abdomen, breasts, and thighs.

RESPIRATORY SYSTEM

1. Upper airway changes (Fig. 3-1). Changes noted in the upper airway include hyperemia and congestion and an increased frequency of epistaxis and sinusitis.
2. Lung volume and pulmonary function changes. These changes are apparently secondary to elevated progesterone levels. There is also a 30% to 40% increase in both tidal volume and minute ventilation and a slight increase in the respiratory rate. Both the functional residual capacity and the inspiratory reserve volume can decrease by 20%. Alteration in blood gases occurs as follows: pO_2 increases above 100 mm/Hg, pCO_2 decreases to 27 to 32 mm Hg, and the pH remains normal with increased renal bicarbonate excretion.
3. Symptoms. Dyspnea is common in 60% to 70% of women.

RENAL FUNCTION

1. Anatomic changes. Dilation of the ureters and renal pelves begins in the first trimester, becoming marked by 20 to 22 weeks gestation. It is a result of progesterone-mediated smooth-muscle relaxation. The right-sided collecting system is usually more dilated than is the left side because of anatomic compression of ovarian vessels and dextrorotation of the gravid uterus. Urinary stasis may lead to increased frequency and/or severity of pyelonephritis in bacteriuric women during pregnancy.

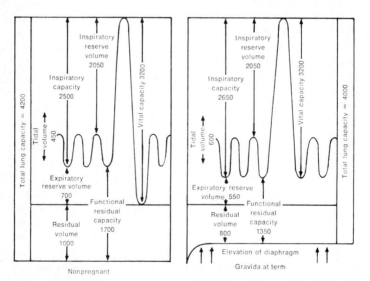

Fig. 3-1
Respiratory changes during pregnancy.
From Bonica J: Principles and practice of obstetric Analgesia and Anesthesia, Philadelphia, 1972, FA Davis Co.

2. Physiologic changes. Effective renal plasma flow increases 75% by the early second trimester, secondary to increased cardiac output and decreased renovascular resistance. Glomerular filtration increases by 50% by the end of the first trimester. The increased filtered load of glucose presented to the kidney may exceed tubular maximum for reabsorption, leading to a "physiologic" glycosuria despite normal blood-sugar levels. Therefore blood sugar levels must be used to detect and follow maternal diabetes; *urine sugar levels cannot be used.* Laboratory correlates of increased glomerular filtration show decreased serum creatinine (<.9 mg) and blood urea nitrogen (<15) and increased creatinine clearance (125 to 200 ml/min). Renin, renin substrate, and aldosterone all increase because of increased estrogen. Decreased sensitivity to the pressor effect of angiotensin is normal during pregnancy.
3. Salt and water metabolism. Factors promoting sodium loss include increased glomerular filtration and increased filtered load of sodium, and high progesterone levels are antagonistic to aldosterone. Factors promoting sodium retention include twofold to fivefold increases in aldosterone, increased estrogen, and increased deoxycorticosterone. The net effect is 1000 mEq sodium retention.

CARDIOVASCULAR SYSTEM

1. Cardiac output (CO). This increases 30% to 50%, from 4.5 to 6.0 L/minute. Increased CO is seen by the end of the first trimester and remains elevated through delivery. It is the result of increases in both stroke volume and heart rate. Increased CO is not accompanied by an increase in blood pressure, therefore resistance must fall. The fall in peripheral resistance is caused by progesterone and induces vascular smooth-muscle relaxation.

   Aortocaval compression by the gravid uterus in the late second and early third trimester when the mother is supine leads to supine hypotension in a fourth to a third of women who lack adequate collateral venous return. Compression can be quickly relieved by the left lateral recumbent position.
2. Blood pressure (Figs. 3-2 to 3-4). A modest fall in mean arterial pressure in the early second trimester is followed by a gradual return to normal by term. Increased venous pressure in the lower extremities caused by prolonged standing or sitting can lead to varicose veins, hemorrhoids, and dependent edema as pregnancy progresses.
3. Cardiac function in labor and delivery. Labor produces a 30% to 40% increase in CO over late third trimester prelabor values. An increase in CO during labor can be minimized to approximately 5% with the lateral recumbent position and epidural anesthesia (Fig. 3-5). Each contraction produces an autotransfusion of 300 ml of blood into maternal circulation from the uteroplacental vasculature. Both the systolic and diastolic pressure rise about 10 mm Hg with each contraction. This is blocked by epidural anesthesia.

   During delivery, the Valsalva maneuver leads to increased central venous pressure. Blood is brought from the legs into central circulation when the mother is in the dorsolithotomy position. Delivery ends the low-resistance uteroplacental circulation. This, along with the normal 300 to 400 ml blood loss, leads to a 10% to 20% increase in cardiac output during and immediately following delivery. Again, this increase can be minimized, if necessary, by epidural anesthesia.
4. Findings of normal pregnancy that mimic heart disease (Fig. 3-6). Some symptoms that appear during normal pregnancy and mimic heart disease include dyspnea, which is seen in 30% to 40% of pregnant women, a reduced tolerance to exercise, and cardiac awareness. Signs to watch for include peripheral edema, lateral dis-

placement of the cardiac apex, increased S_1 and splitting of S_1 and S_2, S_3 gallop, and a systolic flow murmur in 90% of normal pregnant women. Chest radiographs may show changes, including a straightened left-heart border, an elevated diaphragm, and increased heart size and pulmonary vascularity. Electrocardiographic changes include a left axis deviation, ST-T wave changes, and increased frequency of atrial extrasystole; these normal changes are often erroneously read as left ventricular hypertrophy.

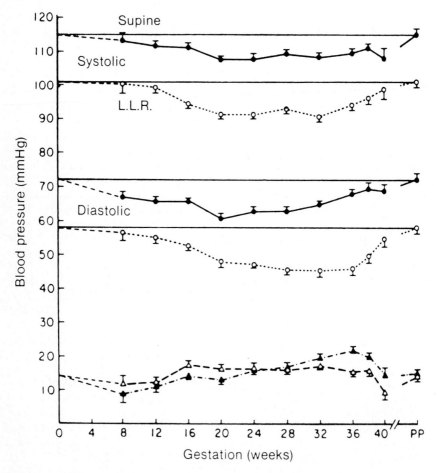

Fig. 3-2
Sequential changes in blood pressures throughout pregnancy with subjects in supine and left lateral recumbent positions (n, 69 patients with standard errors of the mean). The change in systolic (open triangles) and diastolic (closed triangles) blood pressures produced by movement from the left lateral recumbent position is illustrated.
From Wilson M et al: Am J Med 68:99, 1980.

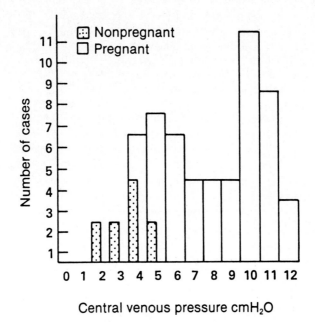

Fig. 3-3
Central venous pressure recorded in 10 nongravid women and 53 gravid women.
From Clark, S.L., Phelan, JP & Cotton DB, (eds) Critical Care Obstetrics, Medical Economics Books, Oradell, NJ, 1987; modified from O'Driscoll KO, and McCarthy JR: J Obstet Gynaecol Br Cwlth 73:923, 1966.

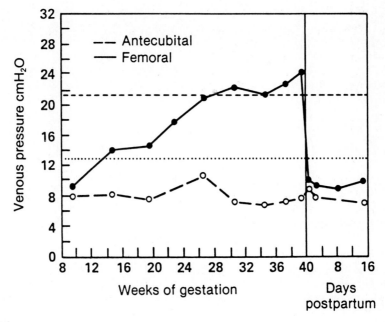

Fig. 3-4
Femoral and antecubital venous pressure during pregnancy.
From McClennan CE: Am J Obstet Gynecol 45:578, 1943.

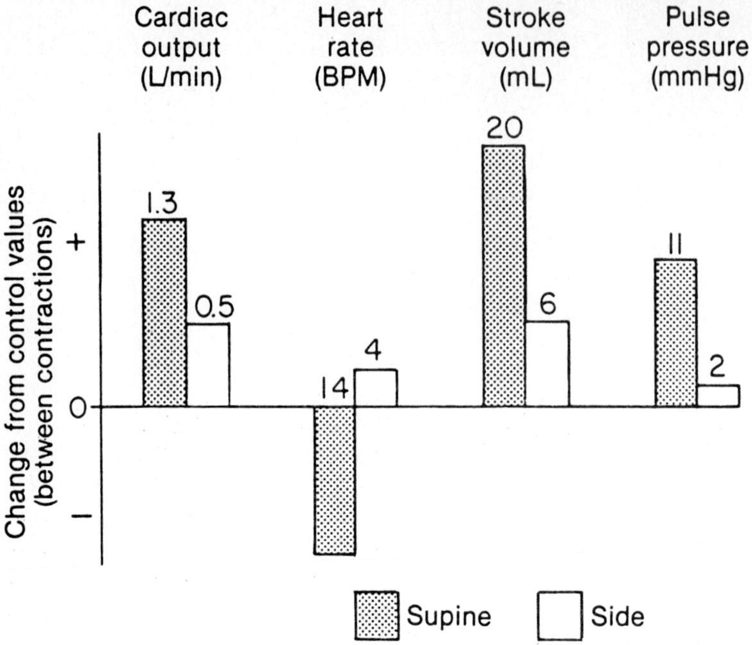

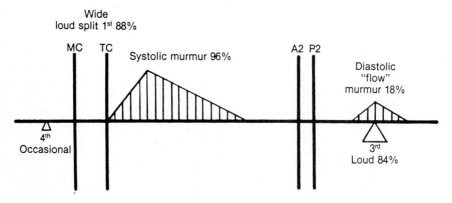

Fig. 3-5
Effect of posture on the maternal hemodynamic response to uterine contractions in early labor.
From Ueland K, and Metcalfe J: Clin Obstet Gynecol 18:41, 1975.

Fig. 3-6
Summarization of cardiac auscultatory findings in 50 pregnant women. *MC*, Mitral closure; *TC*, tricuspid closure; A_2 and P_2, aortic and pulmonary closure element of the second sound.
From Cutforth R, and MacDonald CB: Am Heart J 71:747, 1966.

HEMATOLOGIC SYSTEM

1. Plasma. Plasma volume increases by 50%. This happens slowly from the first tri-mester through 34 weeks gestation (Fig. 3-7).
2. Red cells. Red blood cell (RBC) mass increases by 40% to 50% but more slowly than does plasma, so there is a transient fall in hematocrit in the late second trimes-ter that returns to normal in the third trimester if adequate iron stores are present. Iron supplementation augments the rise in RBC mass. Iron absorption doubles in pregnancy, which results in a requirement for 1000 mg of iron, or about 3.5 mg each day. Supplementation is recommended to prevent depletion of stored iron, es-pecially in women with heavy menses or short (<2 years) interpregnancy intervals.
3. White cells. Increased white blood cell (WBC) counts are normal from 9000 to 12,000, with further increases normally seen in labor from 12,000 to 15,000 and occasionally higher postpartum.
4. Coagulation. Changes in coagulation are evidenced by shorter platelet survival times, although no appreciable effect is seen in the platelet count (a slight decrease to no change). Factors I, VII, VIII, IX, and X show an increase, whereas factors II, V, and XII remain unchanged. Bleeding and clotting times remain normal. The hypercoagulability of pregnancy is caused by venous stasis in the pelvis and legs, vascular injury associated with delivery—especially if by cesarean section—and increased fibrinogen.

ENDOCRINE PHYSIOLOGY

1. Thyroid. An increase in the thyroid gland size is easily palpable during pregnancy. There is also an increase in thyroid-binding globulin (TBG) resulting from high es-trogen levels and increased iodine excretion. The total T_4 rises because of increased TBG, but the *free* T_4 and T_3 levels remain normal, with maintenance of the euthy-roid state. Also, warm skin, increased pulse, and hair loss are normal findings of pregnancy that mimic altered thyroid function.

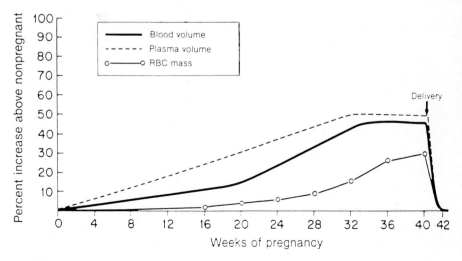

Fig. 3-7
Blood volume changes during pregnancy.
From Scott DE: Obstet Gynecol Annu 1:219, 1972.

2. Adrenal. Corticosteroid-binding globulin (CBG) increases, as do total and free cortisol.
3. Pancreas and fuel metabolism. Fetal and maternal demand for fuel creates a state of "accelerated starvation." Exaggerated-fasting hypoglycemia and starvation ketosis are common. To avoid symptomatic hypoglycemia, several small meals (six per day) with complex carbohydrates are recommended during pregnancy. Insulin resistance increases with advancing gestation primarily because of insulin antagonism by human placental lactogen, and peptide hormone is produced by the placenta in proportion to its mass.

BREASTS

1. Hormonal influences. In the breasts, estrogen produces ductal proliferation, and progesterone leads to alveolar growth.
2. Physical changes. Symptomatic tenderness is common in early pregnancy. In late pregnancy, enlargement of the nipple, the areola, and Montgomery's tubercle are normal. Also in late pregnancy, colostrum is produced (see Chapter 21, Breastfeeding).

REVIEW QUESTIONS

Key: A = Increased
     B = Decreased
     C = Unchanged

1. Maternal cardiac output in pregnancy is _____ by 30% compared with non pregnant levels. This is due to _____ stroke volume and _____ heart rate.
2. Plasma insulin is _____ in pregnancy, while fasting blood sugar is typically _____ .
3. Serum creatinine is _____ in pregnancy, because of _____ glomerular filtration, which is due in large part to _____ renal plasma flow. The net effect is that the serum sodium is_____.
4. The thyroid gland is _____ in size, associated with _____ levels of free T3 and T4, and _____ levels of thyroid binding globulin.
5. _____ smooth muscle tone in pregnancy is thought to be the result of _____ levels of _____ .
   a. Estrogen
   b. Progesterone
   c. Both

ANSWERS

1. A, A, A
2. A, B
3. B, A, A, C
4. A, C, A
5. A, A, B

BIBLIOGRAPHY

Brinkman CR: Biologic adaptation to pregnancy. In Creasy RK, and Resnik R, editors: Maternal fetal medicine, ed 2, Philadelphia 1989, WB Saunders Co.
Cruikshank DP, and Hays PM: Maternal physiology in pregnancy. In Gabbe SG, Niebyl JR, and Simpson JL, editors: Obstetrics: normal and problem pregnancies, New York, 1986, Churchill and Livingstone.

Antenatal Care

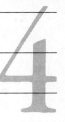

Jiri Sonek
Jay D. Iams

Routine antenatal care is an example of preventive health care at its best. Perinatal morbidity and mortality correlate closely with the availability and quality of antenatal care. Unfortunately, even when quality care is available, it is not always used appropriately because of social or educational problems. Good antenatal care, therefore, includes the ability to involve the pregnant woman in her care through education on good health practices. The ultimate goals of antenatal care are the reduction of maternal and perinatal morbidity in an environment that provides a positive beginning to the parent-child relationship.

Regular antenatal visits are advisable because complications in pregnancy are often present for some time before becoming overtly manifest. Especially, in the third trimester, complications may develop suddenly in previously healthy women, necessitating regular, frequent visits. Approximately a third of high-risk problems are present before pregnancy, another third develop during pregnancy, and the remainder arise during labor, at delivery, or immediately postpartum. Many disorders involve alterations in fetal growth and either premature or delayed onset of labor.

Early and regular care is necessary to establish the duration of pregnancy with confidence. The estimated gestational age (EGA) becomes the benchmark by which the various changes seen in both normal and complicated pregnancies are judged. Therefore, careful assessment of the duration of pregnancy is the single most important task of the first antenatal visit.

ASSESSMENT OF GESTATIONAL AGE

1. Last menstrual period (LMP). The first day of the last normal menses is the traditional starting point for assessing the duration of pregnancy. The estimated date of confinement (EDC) (hospitalization), is derived through Nägele's rule: subtract 3 from the month and add 7 to the day of the LMP to produce the EDC (e.g., an LMP of October 14 produces an EDC of July 21). This method of gestational age assessment will yield reasonably accurate dates in women with regular 28-day cycles who have not recently used oral contraceptives. More than 25% of the time, however, this method will be in error because of a history of irregular menses, a cycle length of more or less than 28 days, the recent use of hormonal contraceptives, or, most commonly, the simple inability to recall the LMP with confidence.
2. Milestones of pregnancy. These milestones are a group of physical and historical findings that can be used to support the dates derived by other methods. They generally are not sufficient to establish the EDC with certainty.

a. Uterine size
  (1) At the pubic symphysis at 12 weeks.
  (2) At the umbilicus at 20 weeks.
  (3) At 28 cm fundal height with a tape at 28 weeks.
b. Maternal perception of fetal activity (quickening). This generally occurs at about 20 weeks in primigravidas and at 16 to 20 weeks in multiparas.
c. Auscultated fetal heart tones. The ability to hear the fetal heartbeat with a "fetoscope," a stethoscope using both bone and air conduction, generally occurs by 20 weeks. The Doppler ultrasound stethoscopes can detect fetal heart sounds as early as 8 to 10 weeks gestation.
3. Neonatal assessment of gestational age is performed through physical examination of the newborn, emphasizing various physical and neurologic findings. These are typically scored to produce an estimate of the duration of pregnancy. Until relatively recently, these examinations were the gold standard, with an accuracy of ±14 days for infants born at or near term. (The scoring systems are less accurate for preterm infants.) Although still invaluable for determining the gestational age of babies born to women who made their first prenatal visit late in the third trimester, neonatal assessment examinations are less precise than either early pregnancy hormone assays or ultrasound estimation of fetal age during the first half of pregnancy (see Chapter 6).
4. Ultrasound examination of multiple fetal physical parameters before 20 weeks gestation has an accuracy of ±10 days, and ultrasound done in the first trimester has an accuracy of ±4 to 5 days. Obviously, neonatal assessment examinations are useful only after delivery, so the ultrasound exam has become the principal dating tool.

INITIAL ANTENATAL EVALUATION

A complete history and physical examination should be performed, with special focus on those factors which might complicate pregnancy.
1. Medical history. Major and/or chronic illness in any organ system may adversely affect pregnancy, either directly through effects on mother or fetus, or indirectly through necessary medications, associated nutritional problems, surgical procedures, or laboratory evaluations. These are comprehensively reviewed in Chapter 7. Hypertension, diabetes, various renal diseases and infections, anemia, and autoimmune disorders are among the most common illnesses. Sexually transmitted diseases are particularly important and merit special attention.
2. Teratogenic exposures. Recreational, occupational, or pharmacologic exposures to any potential teratogens must be carefully documented. This includes both licit drugs, whether prescribed or over the counter, and illicit drugs. Recreational exposure to alcohol and tobacco, both known to harm the developing fetus, should be specifically documented. Occupational exposures are dealt with less easily: the patient wishes to avoid any potential harm to the fetus, no matter how unlikely, whereas the employer wishes to simultaneously retain the employee's services while avoiding any responsibility for adverse fetal outcome. Both parties look to the physician for assistance, but the available literature is largely unhelpful. A cautious policy is best.
3. Demographic data. Various demographic data about the patient may serve to identify those at increased risk of adverse outcome (e.g., preterm delivery or poor fetal growth). A list of demographic risk factors is given in the accompanying box on p. 41.

Demographic Risk Factors for Adverse Pregnancy Outcome

Maternal age of <17 or >35 years.
Low socioeconomic status/limited education.
Nonwhite race—blacks have an increased rate of preterm delivery as compared with whites, regardless of socioeconomic status; the reasons are not clear.
Interpregnancy interval of <1 year.
Low prepregnancy weight <100 pounds.
Cigarette smoking.
Previous premature birth, low birth-weight infant <2500 g, stillbirth or neonatal death.

PREVIOUS OBSTETRIC HISTORY

The patient's previous pregnancy(ies) should be reviewed in detail; spontaneous and therapeutic abortions should always be included. The duration of each pregnancy, the length and character of labor, and the delivery process should be recorded, as each may be repeated in the current pregnancy. Problems during pregnancy, labor, delivery, or occurring postpartum should be sought. *Patients with a history of previous gestational diabetes, gestational hypertension, preterm delivery, prolonged labor and/or difficult delivery, and postpartum hemorrhage are particularly likely to suffer similar complications in the current pregnancy.*

If a previous delivery was performed by cesarean section, the operative report needs to be reviewed. Those whose cesarean delivery was performed via a low cervical transverse incision are candidates for vaginal delivery in subsequent pregnancies, whereas those with a vertical incision entering the myometrium should undergo a repeat cesarean section.

The previous infant's birth weight and immediate newborn course are also important. For instance, an infant with a birth weight of 1500 g who displayed no evidence of respiratory distress but had hypoglycemia and hypothermia suggests intrauterine growth retardation, whereas an infant of the same birth weight with severe hyaline membrane disease is more typical of prematurity.

CURRENT PREGNANCY PROBLEMS

Common problems elicited at the first visit include nutritional deficits, vaginal and urinary tract infections, anemia, teratogenic exposures, and uncertain dates. All should be addressed promptly. Bleeding of any sort occurring since the last normal menses should be evaluated, usually with ultrasound. As the pregnancy progresses, routine surveillance includes regular maternal weight measurement gain as a guide to nutrition; blood pressure measurement; urine dipstick tests for protein, sugar, and nitrite; and fundal height measurement to assess fetal growth. Patients should be educated about the early warning symptoms of common complications of pregnancy such as preeclampsia and preterm labor, which are given in the box on p 42.

The frequency of visits for normal women is customarily monthly until 28 weeks gestation, every 2 to 3 weeks until 36 weeks gestation, and then weekly until delivery. The goal of these visits is not only the early identification, treatment, and prevention of complications, but also to allow the pregnant woman to develop trust in the health care team that will act as her agent when she is in labor. Therefore, it is important for

---

Common Complications of Pregnancy

Early Symptoms of Preeclampsia

Headache
Swelling of the hands or face
Blurred vision or photosensitivity
Epigastric pain
Nausea

Early Symptoms of Preterm Labor

Menstrual-like cramps
Frequent (>4 or 5/hour) uterine contractions, with or without pain
Change or increase in vaginal discharge
Pelvic pressure
Backache

---

the caregivers to know and understand the birth experience each woman desires. For some this means a minimum of medication or an avoidance of episiotomy if possible. For others this means an avoidance of as much of the pain of labor as safety will allow. The role of the health provider is to help each woman have the birth experience she and her family prefer within the guidelines of safety for mother and baby.

ROUTINE LABORATORY EVALUATION IN PREGNANCY

1. At the initial visit
   a. Complete blood count
   b. Blood type and Rh, indirect Coombs' test
   c. Rubella, syphilis, and hepatitis serology
   d. Pap smear
   e. Urinalysis and culture or nitrite stix
   f. Gonorrhea and chlamydia cultures, for those at increased risk of preterm birth group B streptococci culture
2. At 15 to 18 weeks
   a. Maternal serum α-fetoprotein, offered to all as an elective screen for various birth defects
3. At 24 to 28 weeks
   a. 50 g glucose load as screen for diabetes for all patients
   b. Hemoglobin/hematocrit
   c. Urine culture or nitrite stix
4. At 36 weeks
   a. Hemoglobin/hematocrit

DIET AND WEIGHT GAIN IN PREGNANCY

Adequate nutrition during pregnancy in the woman who is neither obese nor nutritionally deficient before pregnancy can be achieved with common sense. All four basic food groups (i.e., fruits and vegetables, grains and cereals, milk and dairy products, meats and fish) should be amply represented. The only dietary supplement currently recommended is iron, in the form of ferrous sulfate, 325 mg 2 to 3 times daily. In the

---

Content of Routine Antenatal Education

Normal physiologic changes of pregnancy, including common physical complaints in
   pregnancy
Fetal development
Labor process, including hospital routines and delivery
Postpartum changes and infant nutrition
Family and infant development and choice of medical care for the infant

---

teenage mother, dietary requirements should be adjusted upward to allow for the increased needs of adolescence.

The optimal weight gain is 20 to 35 lbs., depending on prepregnancy weight and body habitus. Most physicians receive a minimum of education in nutrition; liberal consultation with a registered dietician is recommended whenever special considerations occur.

Prenatal vitamins are not a substitute for a well-balanced diet and may be unnecessary in women who maintain good nutrition before and during pregnancy. There is some recent evidence that routine *prepregnancy* use of prenatal vitamin supplements may decrease the rate of open spina bifida in some populations. On the other hand, large doses of some vitamins, especially vitamin A, are known to be teratogenic.

The box above lists the variety of new information that the mother-to-be will need as she prepares for childbirth and the months to follow. Certified childbirth educators are often the best source of independent and up-to-date information in most areas. These educators are usually anxious to work with physicians and hospitals in achieving a safe and positive childbirth experience.

REVIEW QUESTIONS

1. Maternal mortality is defined as number of maternal deaths per:
   a. 1,000 terminated pregnancies
   b. 10,000 terminated pregnancies
   c. 100,000 terminated pregnancies
2. Maternal death is defined as death of a woman
   a. During a pregnancy
   b. During delivery
   c. While pregnant or within 42 days of termination of pregnancy irrespective of site or duration of the pregnancy
3. Perinatal mortality is defined as
   a. Number of stillborn infants per 1,000 infants born
   b. Number of neonatal deaths (first 28 days of life) per 1,000 live births
   c. Number of fetal deaths plus the number of neonatal deaths per 1,000 births

Match the following common antenatal tests with the most usual time in pregnancy when they would be performed (each may be used more than once)—applies to questions 4-10.
   a. CBC
   b. Platelets
   c. Blood type, rhesus state, indirect Coombs
   d. Rubella, VDRL or RPR

    e. Urine culture
    f. GC culture (cervical and rectal)
    g. Pap smear
    h. Maternal serum AFP
    i. Glucola test
    j. Chorionic villus biopsy
    k. Genetic amniocentesis
    l. Level II ultrasound
    m. Hemoglobin and hematocrit

4. Initial visit
5. 9-12 Weeks
6. 14-18 Weeks
7. 20-22 Weeks
8. 24-28 Weeks
9. 28 Weeks
10. 36 Weeks
11. The earliest gestational age at which fetal heart movement can be detected by dop-tone is:
    a. 6-8 Weeks
    b. 10-12 Weeks
    c. 14-16 Weeks
12. The earliest gestational age at which fetal heart sounds can be detected by feto-scope is:
    a. 14-16 Weeks
    b. 18-20 Weeks
    c. 22-24 Weeks

ANSWERS

1. c
2. c
3. c
4. a, b, c, d, e, f, g
5. j
6. h, k
7. l
8. i
9. m
10. f, m
11. b
12. b

BIBLIOGRAPHY

1. Guidelines for perinatal care, ed 2, Chicago, 1988, American Academy of Pediatrics and American College of Obstetricians and Gynecologists.
2. Johnson TRB, Walker MA, and Niebyl JR: Prenatal care. In Gabbe SG, Niebyl JR, and Simpson JL, editors: Obstetrics: normal and problem pregnancies, New York, 1986, Churchill Livingstone, Inc.

Birth Defects, Genetics, and Teratology

5

Jay D. Iams

Most infants are born healthy. Maldevelopment affects only 2% to 5% of infants born at term. The percentage increases in preterm infants and spontaneously aborted, second-trimester fetuses. Despite their relatively infrequent occurrence, the consequences of birth defects are great: 10% of perinatal mortality and 20% of infant mortality are attributable to congenital anomalies. This chapter reviews the multiple causes of birth defects and highlights their typical presentation in obstetric practice.

ETIOLOGY OF BIRTH DEFECTS

The various causes of birth defects, along with their relative frequency, are outlined in Table 5-1. It is important to note that a given defect (e.g., a facial cleft) may be caused by any of the factors on the list, with widely varying risks of recurrence.

CHROMOSOMAL ANOMALIES

Abnormalities in chromosomes may be *numerical,* in which entire chromosomes are missing or present in more than the normal pairs. They may also be *structural,* in which fragments of chromosomes are excessive or missing (see Table 5-2).

Numerical

1. May involve autosomes (chromosomes 1 to 22) or sex chromosomes (X and Y).
2. A chromosomal complement that is not a multiple of the haploid number of 23 is called *aneuploidy.*
   a. Trisomy—47,XX,+21 or Down syndrome; 47,XXX—Triple X.
   b. Monosomy—45,X or Turner's syndrome; autosomal monosomies are lethal.
3. A chromosomal complement that involves an entire haploid set of 23 (e.g., tetraploidy—92 chromosomes; triploidy—69 chromosomes) is called *polyploidy.*

Structural

1. Rearrangement of chromosomes that may or may not produce phenotypic abnormality, depending upon whether genetic information is missing or excessive.
2. Balanced rearrangements yield phenotypically normal individuals who have an increased risk of producing unbalanced gametes, leading to reproductive loss or abnormal children.

SINGLE GENE DISORDERS

There are more than 1000 known mendelian disorders, which may be either dominant or recessive and may involve either autosomal or sex chromosomes. A general knowledge of inheritance patterns is necessary for accurate historical screening.

45

Table 5-1   Frequency of various causes of birth defects

Causes	Frequency		Examples
	Incidence 1000 Total Births	Percentage of Malformations	
Chromosomal	6	5	Trisomy 21, 18
Single gene defects	6-10	20	Meckel-Gruber syndrome, thrombocytopenia-absent radius (TAR) syndrome
Disruption/deformation	1	1	Amniotic band syndrome
Multifactorial/ polygenic/unknown	10-20	65	Most neural tube and cardiac anomalies, cleft lip/palate, renal anomalies, müllerian fusion defects
Teratogenic	1-3	10	Irradiation, rubella syndrome, thalidomide, Accutane

Autosomal Disorders

1. Both sexes are equally affected.
2. Dominant
   a. Expression may be variable from one individual to another. This is called *penetrance* and *expressivity*.
   b. Affected individuals will produce offspring who are either normal or affected, in a 1:1 ratio.
   c. Affected individual either has an affected parent or represents a new mutation.
   d. Obstetric presentation—these disorders confront the obstetrician in several ways:
      (1) Affected parent—50% risk.
      (2) Previously affected child born to unaffected parents means that the child represents a new mutation—no increase in recurrence risk.
      (3) Older fathers (older than 50 years of age) have an increased risk of new mutations involving autosomal dominant disorders.
      (4) Birth of child with anomalies.
   e. Examples include achondroplasia, tuberous sclerosis, and osteogenesis imperfecta (some types).
3. Recessive
   a. Both parents of affected infant must be carriers.
   b. Offspring of carrier parents will be normal, carriers, or affected in 1:2:1 ratio.
   c. Siblings may be affected, but other affected relatives are uncommon unless there is consanguinity in the pedigree.
   d. Obstetric presentation:
      (1) A couple with a previous affected child has a 1 in 4 chance of recurrence in each pregnancy.
      (2) For women with other affected relatives, the risk depends on frequency of gene in population. The Hardy-Weinberg equation may be used to estimate gene frequency from incidence of disease:

$$p^2 + 2\,pq + q^2 = 1$$

where p^2 is the frequency of noncarriers (nearly always slightly less than 1), q^2 is the frequency of affected individuals, and $2\,pq$ is the frequency of carriers.

(3) Birth of child with rare or unusual anomalies should always prompt consideration of an autosomal recessive disorder.

  e. Examples of autosomal recessive disorders include the following:
  (1) Cystic fibrosis is the most common autosomal recessive disorder in whites, with a gene frequency of 1:25 whites.
  (2) Sickle cell anemia is the most common autosomal recessive disorder in blacks, with a gene frequency of 1:12 blacks.
  (3) Tay-Sachs disease is the most common genetic disorder in the Jewish community, with 1:30 Jews of Ashkenazi origin being carriers.
  (4) Many inborn metabolic errors.
  (5) Many rare malformations such as thrombocytopenia-absent radius (TAR) syndrome and Meckel-Gruber syndrome.

X-Linked Disorders

1. No father-to-son transmission.
2. Dominant
  a. Males and females may both be affected.
  b. An affected male will have all normal sons and all daughters will be affected.
  c. Offspring of an affected female will be normal or carrier, in a 1:1 ratio.
  d. Examples include vitamin D–resistant rickets.
3. Recessive
  a. Only males are affected (there is the possibility of a rare homozygous female).
  b. An affected male will have all normal sons, and all his daughters will be carriers.
  c. Examples include hemophilia and Duchenne's muscular dystrophy.

TERATOGENS

Teratogens are important because they are potentially avoidable causes of birth defects, both as the primary cause of malformation and as cofactors in defects and syndromes of multifactorial origin. They may exert their effect at *any* time in pregnancy. Effects between conception and the eighteenth postconceptional day, during the period of fertilization and implantation, typically produce spontaneous abortion. Organogenesis may be affected during the embryonic period (18 to 55 days after conception), and growth and maturation may be altered thereafter.

Definition

A teratogen is an agent extrinsic to the embryo or fetus that causes an increased risk of the following:

1. Malformation—physical malformation
2. Carcinogenesis—increased risk of cancer
3. Mutagenesis—increased risk of genetic disease
4. Altered function (e.g., mental retardation)
5. Growth deficiency (intrauterine growth retardation [IUGR])
6. Pregnancy wastage (i.e., miscarriage or stillbirth)

Teratogens may produce no effect at all in exposed pregnancies; only the most potent human teratogens typically affect 20% to 70% of exposed fetuses.

Table 5-2 Frequency and presentation of chromosomal anomalies

	Incidence/1000		Obstetric Presentation	Prenatal Diagnosis	Recurrence after One Affected Infant (%)
	Spontaneous Abortions	Live Births			
Aneuploidy					
Trisomy 21: 47,+21, Down syndrome	21	1.25	MS-AFP, abnormal US, thick nuchal skin, short limbs, high BPD/FL ratio, brachycephaly, hydramnios, "double bubble," duodenal atresia, cardiac anomalies, AMA	CVS, amniocentesis, cordocentesis	1
Trisomy 18: 47,+18, Edwards' syndrome	12	0.125	Symmetric IUGR, abnormal US, hydramnios, omphalocele, club foot, multiple anomalies, MS-AFP, AMA	CVS, amniocentesis, cordocentesis	1
Trisomy 16: 47,+16	73	0	Spontaneous first- or second-trimester abortion, AMA	CVS	—
Trisomy 13: 47,+13, Patau's syndrome	11	0.05	MS-AFP, symmetric IUGR, abnormal US, cardiac anomalies, facial clefts, NTD, holoprosencephaly, AMA	CVS, amniocentesis, cordocentesis	1

Sex chromosome anomalies

Monosomy X: 45,X, Turner's syndrome	86	0.1(females)	MS-AFP?, abnormal US, IUGR, cystic hygroma, cardiac anomaly	CVS, amniocentesis, cordocentesis	1
47,XXY: Klinefelter's syndrome	1.5	1(males)	—	CVS, amniocentesis, cordocentesis	1
Polyploidy					
Triploidy: 69,XXX, XYY, and XXY	77	rare	MS-AFP?, abnormal US, IUGR, hydropic placenta, NTDs, facial clefts, omphalocele, polyhydramnios or oligohydramnios, spontaneous first- or second-trimester abortion	CVS, amniocentesis, cordocentesis	1
Tetraploidy: 92,XXXX, XXYY	26	0	Early spontaneous abortions	—	—

MS-AFP, Maternal serum α-fetoprotein; *US*, ultrasonogram; *BPD/FL*, biparietal diameter/femur length; *CVS*, chorionic villus sampling; *AMA*, advanced maternal age; *IUGR*, intrauterine growth retardation; *NTD*, neural tube defect.

Classes of Teratogenic Agents

1. Drugs and chemicals
2. Paternal exposures
3. Infectious agents
4. Radiation
5. Mechanical compression, deformation, or disruption of fetal development

General Principles of Teratogenesis

1. Teratogenic effect depends on:
   a. Dose administered
   b. Gestational age at exposure
   c. Duration of exposure
   d. Maternal and fetal genotype
   e. Simultaneous exposure to other agents:
      (1) Agent A—defect 1
      (2) Agents A+B—defect 2
      (3) Agents A+B+C—no defect
      (4) Agents A+B at different gestational age—no defect
2. Consequences of above:
   a. A given *agent* may have no effect or cause abortion, malformation, altered growth, mutagenesis, or carcinogenesis in a given individual
   b. A given *defect* may result from several different agents
   c. Proof of teratogenicity or safety is very difficult

Mechanisms of Teratogenesis

1. Cell death or reduced proliferative rate (e.g., viral infection)
2. Altered biosynthetic pathways (e.g., chromosomal or genetic disorders)
3. Abnormal cellular and tissue interactions during critical time periods (a possible example is diabetes)
4. Extrinsic factors (e.g., hypoxia or tissue compression)
5. Threshold interaction of multiple genes with known and/or unknown environmental factors (e.g., drugs or radiation)

Drugs as Teratogens (Tables 5-3 and 5-4)

1. *Any* drug given to *any* pregnant woman at *any* time in pregnancy may be teratogenic.
2. Always consider risk versus benefits before advising the use or avoidance of use of a drug by the pregnant patient. Use reference texts, such as Briggs et al, before counseling a patient or colleague about drug use.
3. When drug therapy is chosen, use the lowest effective dose for the shortest effective duration.

Paternal Teratogens

1. Effect is principally on fertility, not on incidence of anomaly.
2. Agent Orange is a common concern among Vietnam War veterans. There are multiple studies showing no effect on the anomaly rate in the offspring of exposed males.
3. Chemotherapy for malignancy is another common concern. Recent research has shown an effect on fertility but not on anomaly rate.

Table 5-3   Common teratogenic drugs and chemicals

Agent	Indication	Fetal Effects	Suggested Alternate Medication
Alcohol	None	Fetal alcohol syndrome	Alcoholics Anonymous, abstinence
Androgens, diethylstilbestrol	Morning after abortifacient	Adenosis, clear cell adenocarcinoma of vagina	—
Cigarettes, nicotine	None	IUGR	—
Coumadin	Anticoagulation	Facial and bone anomalies, CNS hemorrhage	SQ heparin
Folic acid antagonist	Cancer	Spontaneous abortion	—
Lithium	Bipolar mood disorder	Ebstein's anomaly (10%)	Tricyclics
Phenytoin	Anticonvulsant (grand mal)	IUGR, cardiac, facial dysmorphism, (10%-25%)	Carbamazepine, phenobarbital
Isotretinoin	Recalcitrant cystic acne	Major anomaly (25%-50%)	Topicals, erythromycin, or none
Tetracycline	Various infections	Tooth staining	Pencillins, erythromycin
Thalidomide	Sedative/hypnotic	Phocomelia (25%-35%)	Tryptophan
Trimethadione	Anticonvulsant (petit mal)	Facial dysmorphism, mental retardation	Ethosuximide, carbamazepine
Valproic acid	Anticonvulsant	NTD	Phenobarbital, carbamazepine

CNS, Central nervous system.

Infectious Agents as Teratogens (Table 5-5)

1. An approach to counseling for infectious exposures in pregnancy:
   a. This problem rarely presents as a confirmed diagnosis—school, neighborhood, or family exposures are not often documented. Confirming the diagnosis in the supposedly infected individual is necessary before the risk to the exposed pregnant woman can be estimated.
   b. IgG antibody to toxoplasmosis and rubella indicate past infection. Though presence of antibody does not necessarily mean complete immunity, the presence of antibody indicates there is essentially no risk for future pregnancies.
   c. IgG antibody to cytomegalovirus (CMV) indicates past maternal infection. Recurrent maternal infection is possible, which may produce sensorineural damage in the fetus. Major brain, liver, and adrenal infection, producing an infant with IUGR, petechiae, microcephaly, or adrenal/hepatic hemorrhage, is seen only with primary maternal CMV infection.

Table 5-4   Drugs to avoid in late pregnancy

Agent	Indication	Effect	Alternate
Acetylsalicylic acid	Many	Delayed onset of labor, platelet dysfunction	Acetaminophen
Coumadin	Anticoagulation	Fetal anticoagulation	SQ heparin
Diazepam	Tranquilizer	Delayed neurobehavioral adaption	Hydroxyzine
Phenytoin, phenobarbital	Anticonvulsants	Neonatal coagulopathy, neonatal folate deficiency	Carbamazepine
Sulfa	Antibiotic	Bilirubin binding, jaundice	Erythromycin, penicillin
Tetracycline	Antibiotic	Tooth staining	Erythromycin, penicillin

Table 5-5   Teratogenic effects of infectious agents

Infectious Agent	Congenital Abnormality
Toxoplasma gondii	Prematurity, cerebral calcification, microcephalus, mental retardation, hydrocephalus, cerebral palsy, chorioretinitis, hepatosplenomegaly
Syphilis	Cutaneous lesions, saddle nose, hydrocephalus, deafness, osseous lesions, mental retardation, dental anomalies, meningitis
Rubella	IUGR, deafness, cataracts, cardiovascular, chorioretinitis, autism, microcephalus, mental retardation, hepatosplenomegaly, osseous defects
Cytomegalovirus	IUGR, hydrocephalus, microphthalmia, cerebral calcification, blindness, deafness, chorioretinitis, hepatosplenomegaly
Varicella zoster	"Scalded skin," limb deformities

    d. Primary maternal herpes only rarely causes congenital transplacental infection, with a picture similar to primary maternal CMV infection.

    e. Recent TORCH infections can be detected by documenting seroconversion or by using tests for detection of IgM antibody. For a critical review and discussion of the use of TORCH tests, see Sever (see bibliography). It is a good strategy to

Table 5-6 Range of fetal radiation doses from common diagnostic procedures (mrad per examination, not including fluoroscopy)*

Procedure	Estimated Mean Uterine Dose (mrad)	Reported Range (mrad)
Dental	0.06	0.03-0.1
Head, cervical spine	0.5	0.5-3
Extremities	0.5	0.5-18
Shoulder	0.5	0.5-3
Thoracic spine	11.0	10-55
Chest	1	0.2-43
Upper GI series	171	5-1230
Cholecystogram	78	14-1600
Lumbosacral spine	721	20-2900
Pelvis	210	40-1600
Hip and femur	124	53-1000
IVP or retrograde urogram	588	50-4000
Barium enema	900	20-9200
Abdomen	221	18-1400
Pelvimetry	600	160-4000
Hysterosalpingogram	1200	200-6700

Modified from National Council on Radiation Protection and Measurements: NCRP Rep No 54, Washington, DC, 1977, US Government Printing Office.
GI, Gastrointestinal; *IVP,* intravenous pyelogram.
*This table cannot be used in place of individual calculation of radiation exposure because of the wide range of fetal irradiation.

draw blood first and ask questions later. Baseline blood samples may be obtained before the exact nature of the infective exposure is known and then analyzed once the infection is identified.

Radiation as a Teratogen (Table 5-6)

1. The time of exposure after conception is important.
   a. In the first week after conception, there is an "all or none" period (sensitive to lethal effect but low probability of sustaining teratogenic or growth-retarding effects).
   b. Between 2 to 7 weeks after conception is the most sensitive period, during which there is potential for teratogenic, growth-retarding, lethal, or postnatal effects of radiation.
   c. Between 8 and 40 weeks, there is decreased radiosensitivity for multiple organ teratogenesis, but growth retardation, functional abnormalities (e.g., CNS dysfunction), and postnatal neoplastic effects may occur.
2. Assessing the risk from radiation exposure.
   a. Consider gestational age at time of exposure.
   b. Type of radiodiagnostic examination (x-ray or radionuclide). Does the isotope concentrate on the fetal side of the placenta?
   c. Radiation dosage estimate by radiologist or radiation physicist is mandatory.
3. Counseling about risks of radiation exposure.
   a. Less than 5 rad (5000 mrad)—no increased risk of malformation, but other teratogenic effects may occur (e.g., carcinogenesis, mutagenesis)
   b. 5 to 10 rad—no increased risk of malformations seen.
   c. Greater than 25 rad—definite increased risk in malformations.

d. Greater than 100 rad—at least some degree of growth retardation in all exposed embryos, in addition to malformation risk.

e. Compare risk of radiation exposure to risks of abnormality endogenous to pregnancy (3%) or risks associated with other factors (e.g., maternal age, smoking, alcohol) (Mossman and Hill [see bibliography]) to put problem in perspective for counseling.

f. There is no threshold dosage of radiation for the risk of carcinogenesis, mutagenesis, and miscarriage.

Mechanical Teratogenesis

1. Mechanisms of mechanical teratogenesis include the following:
   a. Deformation: mechanical molding of normal tissue (e.g., uterine constraint due to oligohydramnios, uterine anomaly).
   b. Disruption: destruction of normal tissue (e.g., amniotic band syndrome)
2. Amniotic band syndrome is the most common of this class.
   a. Nonrecurrent cause of various, and usually multiple, defects.
   b. Defects are usually asymmetric, do not follow embryologic development sequence, and often are associated with annular constrictions or congenital amputations of limbs or digits.
   c. Torpin proposed sequence of events (Seeds, Cefalo, and Herberts [see bibliography]).

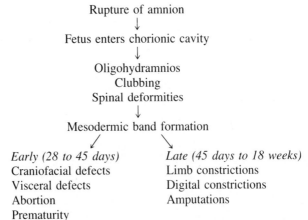

3. Must make accurate diagnosis to avoid erroneous recurrence-risk estimate.

MULTIFACTORIAL DISORDERS

These disorders are presumed to be caused by a combination of multiple genes (polygenic) and environmental factors. Most common anomalies fall into this category. Familial tendency is present but not as evident as in single-gene disorders.

1. Recurrence risk is 2% to 5% after one affected child.
2. Increasing recurrence risk with increased number of affected offspring or relatives.
3. Increased familial risk with increased severity of defect.

Common Multifactorial Disorders

1. Cleft lip/cleft palate—1/1000 births
2. Neural tube defect—1/1000 births
3. Congenital heart disease—6 to 8/1000 births

4. Orthopedic anomalies—club foot and hip dysplasia, scoliosis
5. Gastrointestinal anomalies—pyloric stenosis and Hirschsprung's disease
6. Renal anomalies

Remember that most of these defects may also result from mendelian, chromosomal, and teratogenic causes. Other causes should be considered before assigning a multifactorial etiology. For example, congenital heart disease may be drug induced (e.g., lithium), infectious (e.g., rubella), or chromosomal (e.g., Down syndrome), but it is usually multifactorial.

REVIEW
QUESTIONS

1. The effect of a potentially teratogenic agent depends upon:
   a. The dose given
   b. The gestational age at exposure
   c. The duration of exposure
   d. Maternal and fetal pharmacogenetics
   e. All of the above
2. What percent of birth defects are caused by chromosomal abnormalities?
   a. 0.5%
   b. 5%
   c. 15%
   d. 25%
   e. 65%
3. What percentage of liveborn and stillborn children, respectively, have chromosomal abnormalities?
   a. 0.5% and 5%
   b. 0.05% and 0.5%
   c. 5% and 15%
   d. 0.1% and 1%
   e. None of the above

ANSWERS

1. e
2. b
3. a

BIBLIOGRAPHY

Aselton P et al: First-trimester drug use and congenital disorders, Obstet Gynecol 65:451, 1985.
Briggs GG, Freeman RK, and Yaffe SJ: Drugs in pregnancy and lactation, ed 2, Baltimore, 1986, Williams & Wilkins.
Larsen JW, and Greendale K: Teratology, ACOG Tech Bull No 84, Washington, DC, Feb 1985, American College of Obstetricians and Gynecologists.
Mahony BS et al: The amniotic band syndrome antenatal sonographic diagnosis and potential pitfalls, Am J Obstet Gynecol 152:63, 1985.
Mole RH: Radiation effects on prenatal development and their radiological significance, Br J Radiol 52:89, 1979.
Mossman KL, and Hill LT: Radiation risks in pregnancy, Obstet Gynecol 60:237, 1982.
Seeds JW, Cefalo RC, and Herbert WNP: Amniotic band syndrome, Am J Obstet Gynecol 144:243, 1982.
Sever JL: TORCH tests and what they mean, Am J Obstet Gynecol 152:495, 1985.

Antenatal Fetal Assessment

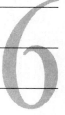

Jiri Sonek
Rosemary E. Reiss
Steven G. Gabbe

This chapter is divided into three sections; each describes major techniques in antenatal assessment of fetal status. Ultrasonography has become an integral part of obstetric practice throughout the entirety of gestation. It is described in the first section. Antenatal detection of abnormal fetal development is the focus of the second section, and assessment of fetal well-being in later pregnancy is reviewed in the third section.

ULTRASONOGRAPHY IN PREGNANCY

Ultrasonography's development has radically altered obstetric management. Ultrasonography may be used to diagnose congenital anomalies, guide invasive diagnostic or therapeutic procedures, measure blood flow, or assess fetal well-being. The discussion that follows is by no means exhaustive. Comprehensive discussions about the physics of ultrasound, scanning for fetal anomalies, and Doppler ultrasonography can be found in the texts referenced at the end of this chapter.

Overview of Real-Time Ultrasonography in Obstetrics
Equipment

Ultrasonographic units are composed of two parts: The transducer, which emits ultrasound wave energy and receives the reflected ultrasound energy (as echoes—hence, the common synonym, *echography*), and the video display terminal, which converts the reflected energy waves into a visual image on the screen. Real-time ultrasonography, in which the transducer continually sends and receives ultrasound waves, is most often used in obstetric examinations, producing a moving, or real-time, image of the fetus.

Transducers emit sound waves of frequencies varying from 2.5 to 7 MHz. Higher-frequency transducers (5 to 7 MHz) produce better resolution but penetrate tissue poorly, whereas lower-frequency transducers penetrate more deeply but sacrifice some image quality. Most obstetric scanning is done with 3.5 and 5 MHz transducers.

Transducers may be linear, curvilinear, or sector (pie-shaped). Transabdominal ultrasonography is most common, but transvaginal sonography is especially useful in early pregnancy.

Doppler ultrasonography may prove to be useful in assessing fetal, uterine, and placental blood flow. It is currently an investigational technique.

Basic ultrasonographic examination (level I)

Level I ultrasonography must include assessment of certain parameters to satisfy ACOG guidelines:
1. Fetal number
2. Fetal presentation
3. Documentation of fetal life
4. Placental localization
5. Amniotic fluid volume
6. Gestational dating
7. Detection and evaluation of maternal pelvic masses (best done in first trimester)
8. Survey of fetal anatomy for gross malformations (in second and third trimester)

Targeted ultrasonographic examination (level II)

Level II ultrasonography provides a thorough evaluation of the fetus for a patient who is suspected of carrying a physiologically or anatomically defective fetus because of her history, a clinical evaluation, or a prior ultrasonographic examination. Level II examination should be performed by an operator with expertise in scanning for anomalies.

Patient preparation for an ultrasonographic examination

Usually, no special preparation is needed. Bladder filling is useful in some cases:
1. Evaluation of nonpregnant patients.
2. Evaluation of a pregnancy that is less than 12 weeks, especially when looking for specific pregnancy abnormalities, such as an ectopic pregnancy.
3. Evaluation of the cervix and lower uterine segment (e.g., to evaluate for cervical incompetence). Note that excessive bladder filling can give a false impression of lower-uterine-segment funneling.
4. Evaluation for placenta previa needs to be done with a full bladder, as well as after voiding.

General caveats

1. Both the patient and the physician must be aware of the limitations of an ultrasonographic examination. These vary with gestational age, fetal position, maternal habitus, and other technical variables. Full evaluation of the fetus, placenta, amniotic fluid, uterus, and adnexa may be suboptimal or impossible because of unfavorable fetal position, maternal habitus, distortion of anatomy, or inadequate patient preparation.
2. A normal obstetric ultrasonogram does not guarantee normalcy of the pregnancy.
3. The ultrasonographic appearance of the pregnancy is greatly gestational-age dependent.
4. The accuracy of gestational-age estimation by ultrasonography decreases with advancing gestational age because ultrasonography estimates age by measuring size. The range of embryonic sizes is very narrow in early gestation, making estimation of age relatively precise. As pregnancy progresses, the range of normal fetal size broadens so that inference of age based on size becomes less reliable.
5. Detection of one abnormality on an obstetrical ultrasonogram should lead to a detailed search for associated anomalies. When abnormalities are found or if an ultrasonographic evaluation was inadequate, a follow-up ultrasonographic evaluation is always wise.
6. The only recognized risk of ultrasonography for both the mother and fetus is a scan performed by inadequately trained personnel.

First-Trimester Scanning
   Advantages
1. Estimation of gestational age is most accurate in the first trimester, provided the crown-rump length (CRL) can be measured.
2. Evaluation of the adnexa and uterine structure is easiest at this point in gestation.

   Disadvantages
1. Adequate evaluation of fetal structure is not possible. (Resolution is improving with the use of transvaginal sector probes.)
2. Fetal number in the first trimester does not always correspond to the fetal number in later trimesters (the "vanishing twin").
3. Location of the placenta in the first trimester does not always correspond to its location later in pregnancy.
4. Even severe fetal anomalies may not present as detectable abnormalities in the first trimester. Only occasionally does a lag in growth of the embryo or an abnormal gestational-sac size signal a problem.

   Findings in first-trimester scanning (up to 12 weeks gestational age)
1. Fetus (greater than 7 weeks estimated gestational age)
   a. Regular heart activity
   b. A well-defined fetal body
   c. Four limbs
   d. Biparietal diameter (BPD), occipitofrontal diameter, abdomen, femur, and humerus can often be distinguished from 10 weeks on.
   e. CRL measurement
      (1) Underestimation of CRL can occur if fetus is not in full extension.
      (2) Overestimation of CRL can occur if fetal limbs or the yolk sac are included in the measurement.
   f. At 12 weeks a diagnosis of anencephaly can be made.
2. Amniotic cavity (5 weeks—10 mm in size; 6 to 7 weeks—15-mm sac is present, surrounded by double line, which consists of decidua capsularis and decidua vera)
   a. Amniotic fluid is not influenced by fetal condition because fetal contribution is minimal in the first trimester.
   b. Yolk sac can usually be seen as a saclike echolucent projection at the lower portion of the fetal abdomen.
   c. The amnion can be differentiated at up to 10 to 11 weeks.
3. Trophoblast/placenta: In the presence of a normal-appearing gestation, the evaluation of placental location in the first trimester is of little use except when performing chorionic villus biopsy.
4. Adnexa
   a. Most common abnormal finding is corpus luteum cyst (corpus luteum of pregnancy). Cysts with diameters of more than 6 cm are very uncommon and should regress by 16 weeks.
   b. Most common true neoplasia of the ovary that complicates pregnancy is benign cystic teratoma (dermoid cyst).
   c. Malignant ovarian tumors comprise only 3% to 5% of the true ovarian neoplasms in pregnancy.
   d. Ectopic pregnancy (see 5, e. below).
5. Ultrasonographic findings of common early-pregnancy complications (all of these can be associated with bleeding):

a. Blighted ovum (anembryonic pregnancy). Gestational sac without evidence of fetus. (Note that this can be normal at 6½ to 8 weeks gestation, especially if patient's habitus does not permit an optimal view of the gestation.)
b. Missed abortion (early fetal death): gestational sac with embryo or fetal pole but no fetal heart activity.
c. Incomplete abortion (part of the gestation passed through the cervix with some tissue remaining in the uterus—usually associated with *a.* or *b.* above). Depending on the amount of tissue remaining, this can be cystic or homogeneous tissue density.
d. Hydatidiform mole and other gestational trophoblastic neoplasias. Depending on the amount of intrauterine bleeding, the appearance varies from classic multi-cystic ("snowstorm") appearance to homogeneous tissue density.
e. Ectopic pregnancy:
   (1) Absence of pregnancy in the uterus; may see pseudogestational sac.
   (2) Presence of an adnexal mass.
   (3) Fetal pole and fetal heart motion outside the uterus may or may not be seen. Now seen frequently with vaginal probes.

Second- and Third-Trimester Ultrasonographic Findings

Pelvic anatomy
Uterus

Fibroids
Müllerian fusion abnormalities

Cervix

Dilation
Length of cervix
Funneling may suggest incompetence

Adnexa

Masses
Solid
Cystic
Size
Regression or growth over time

Amniotic fluid*
Decreased (oligohydramnios)

No pocket is >1 cm in two perpendicular planes
Amniotic-fluid index (sum of 4 quadrant vertical measurement) is ≤4 cm

Excessive (polyhydramnios)

Largest pocket is ≥8 cm in two perpendicular places

Fetus
Viability

Heart-activity motion

Number

Twins, triplets, etc.
Dividing membrane
Single or double placenta
20% of first-trimester twins "resorb"

Position/presentation

Vertex
Breech
Oblique
Transverse

Placenta
Location

Previa: over cervix; partial/marginal; complete
Abruption: suggested, but not established by ultrasonography

Grade

1 ⎫
2 ⎬ see Fig. 6-1
3 ⎭

*Both diminished and excessive amniotic fluid are associated with poor pregnancy outcome.

f. Threatened abortion—vaginal bleeding with no passage of tissue and with the cervix closed. If apparently normal intrauterine gestation with fetal heart motion is demonstrated, the rate of pregnancy loss is less than 5%.

Second- and Third-Trimester Scanning
General principles

1. From 18 weeks gestation until term, the amount of information obtainable by ultrasonography (see box on opposite page) remains relatively constant, with the accuracy of gestational age estimation decreasing with advancing gestational age. The implications and the management decisions based on these findings, however, vary tremendously with gestational age.
2. Optimal time for a targeted ultrasonographic examination and fetal echocardiography is 18 to 22 weeks of gestation. The fetus is large enough for the detection of the vast majority of structural abnormalities, the option of pregnancy termination is still available, and there is ample time for additional confirmatory studies if necessary.
3. Certain congenital anomalies, such as duodenal atresia, microcephaly, achondroplasia, infantile polycystic kidney disease, and x-linked hydrocephaly, may not become apparent until after the customary time for targeted scanning. Some abnormalities may not develop until later in pregnancy (e.g., fetal ovarian cysts).
4. The diagnosis of placenta previa cannot by definition be made until 27 weeks gestation.

Ultrasound examinations use fetal size to estimate age; when age of the fetus is known, growth can be compared to standard tables.

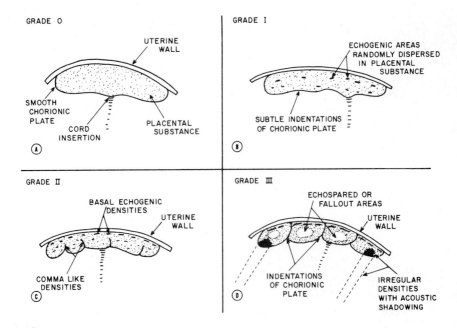

Fig. 6-1
Placental grading.
From Grannum P, Berkowitz R, and Hobbins J: Am J Obstet Gynecol 133:915, 1979.

Estimation of gestational age

1. Tables have been developed that correlate measurements of many fetal bony and soft tissue structures with gestational age.
2. By measuring several different structures, fetal age can be accurately estimated.
3. If only a single parameter is measured, it is possible to miss clues of fetal anomalies such as dwarfism or microcephaly.
4. Commonly used parameters for assignment of gestational age
   a. BPD
   b. Head circumference (HC)
   c. Femur length (FL)
   d. Humerus length
   e. Abdominal circumference (AC)
   f. CRL—first 12 weeks only

Fetal growth parameters

1. Estimated fetal weight (EFW) can be assessed by using nomograms that combine AC and either FL or BPD. The 10th percentile represents intrauterine growth retardation (IUGR) if dates are well established.
2. HC/AC greater than 95th percentile—suggests asymmetric IUGR.
3. FL/AC greater than or equal to .24—suggests IUGR.
4. FL/AC less than .20—suggests macrosomia.
5. EFW less than or equal to 10th percentile for population-adjusted growth curves—suggests IUGR.
6. EFW greater than or equal to 90th percentile for population-adjusted growth curves—suggests macrosomia

Ultrasound is also used to evaluate fetal structure. A detailed examination includes the following observations:

1. Shape of the head—defects in the fetal skull. "Lemon sign" is suggestive of spina bifida.
2. Size and configuration of the cerebral ventricular system, lateral ventricular width, hemisphere width, anterior horn, and posterior horn.
3. Shape of cerebellum—"banana sign" is suggestive of spina bifida.
4. Lips, nose.
5. Spine.
6. Four-chamber heart view, position of the heart within the chest, direction in which the apex is pointing. If any of these are abnormal, thoracic circumference and heart diameter should be obtained, and a fetal echocardiogram is indicated.
7. Examination of thoracic cavities, abdomen, head, and subcutaneous spaces for excessive fluid.
8. Size of stomach bubble and shape of stomach bubble ("double bubble").
9. Size and consistency of kidneys and size of the collecting system and the urinary bladder.
10. Cord insertion and abdominal-wall defects near the cord insertion.
11. Examination of ankles and feet.
12. Number of digits.
13. Number of vessels in the cord.
14. Placental grading, placental masses, and retroplacental or retromembranous clot.
15. Amount of amniotic fluid.

Figs. 6-2, 6-3, 6-4, and 6-5 show the ultrasonographic planes used to obtain the ultrasound images on following pages, labeled with letters A through E for Fig. 6-2, F through J for Fig. 6-3, and K through M for Fig. 6-4. Fig. 6-5 highlights other potential ultrasonographic findings.

Text continued on p. 78

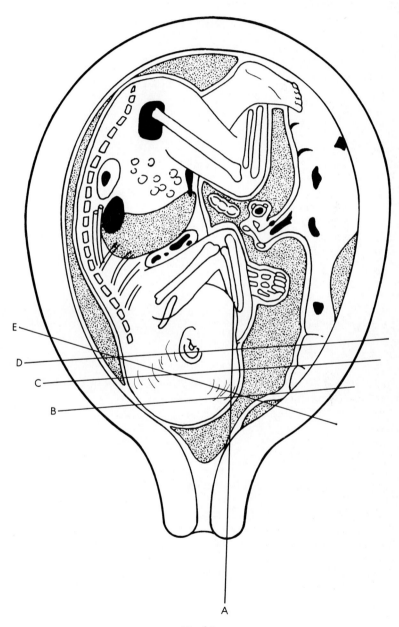

Fig. 6-2

Continued.

A

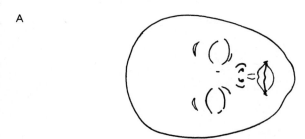

A. Facial Structures

A coronal section of the fetal face is useful in detecting facial clefts. Abnormalities that are detectable: (1) cleft lip/cleft palate, (2) proboscis, (3) arhinia, (4) epignathus, (5) Robin's anomalad, and (6) otocephaly.

B

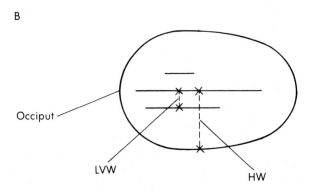

B. Lateral Ventricular Width *(LVW)*/Hemisphere Width *(HW)* Ratio

LVW/HW is used for detection of ventriculomegaly and fetal hydrocephalus. Tables for normal LVW/HW ratio exist. Bilateral indentations of the fetal skull in the frontal region ("lemon sign") before 24-weeks estimated gestational age (EGA) are suggestive of neural tube defect (NTD).

C

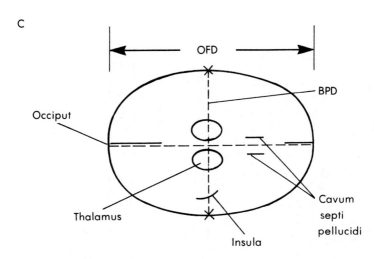

C. Biparietal Diameter *(BPD)*

Measure leading edge to leading edge. BPD is used for estimating gestational age. Tables for normal BPD exist: (1) 14 to 26 weeks ± 10 days, (2) 27 to 28 weeks ± 14 days, and (3) 29 to 42 weeks ± 21 days.

Occipitofrontal Diameter *(OFD)*

OFD is used for estimating cephalic index (CI).

$$CI = \frac{BPD}{OFD}$$

CI less than .75—*dolichocephaly;* CI greater than .85—*brachycephaly.*

$$\frac{OFD + BPD}{2} \times 3.14 = \text{Head circumference (HC)}$$

HC can be used for estimating gestational age in setting of abnormal CI.

Continued.

D

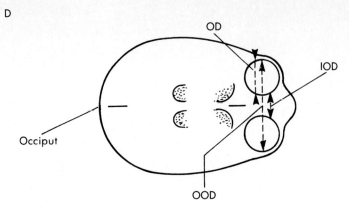

D. Outer Orbital Diameter (OOD), Interorbital Distance (IOD), and Ocular Diameter *(CD)*

OOD is used for estimating gestational age. An abnormal IOD suggests hypertelorism or hypotelorism. An abnormally small OD suggests microphthalmia.

E

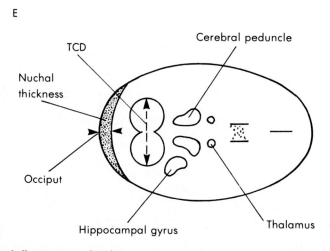

E. Transcerebellar Diameter *(TCD)*

TCD is used for estimating gestational age. It is thought to be spared to some degree in IUGR. Abnormal shape of cerebellar hemisphere ("banana" shape rather than round shape) is associated with NTDs.

Nuchal Thickness

Nuchal thickness of more than 5 mm in fetuses that are 15 to 20 weeks EGA has been associated with some chromosomal disorders (e.g., trisomy 21) and uncommon non-chromosomal disorders.

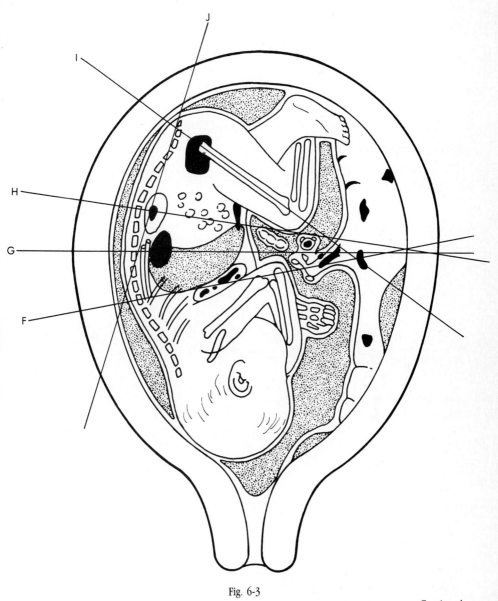

Fig. 6-3

Continued.

F

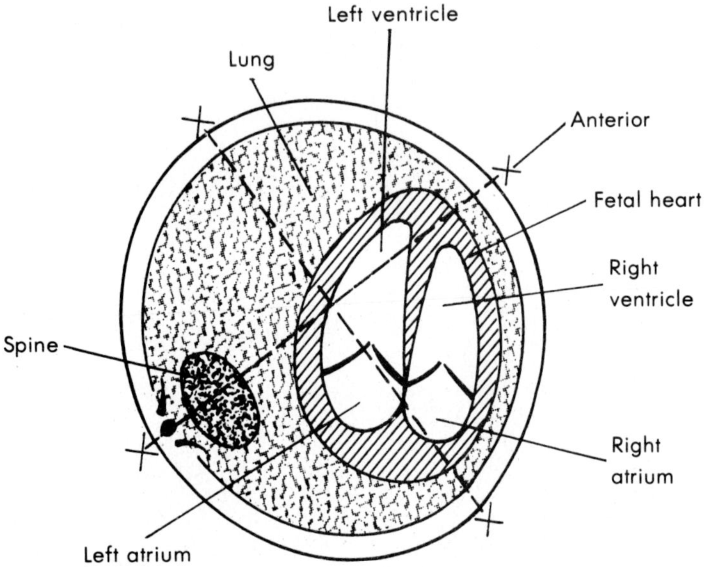

Left ventricle

Lung

Anterior

Fetal heart

Right ventricle

Spine

Right atrium

Left atrium

F. Four-Chamber Heart View

Cross section of fetal chest shows four-chamber view of fetal heart and the spine in cross section—used to assess cardiac anatomy and measure thoracic circumference. A normal four-chamber heart rules out most (80%) cardiac anomalies. Disorders of rhythm may be associated with cardiac structural defects. Absence of fetal heart motion is the sine qua non for the diagnosis of intrauterine fetal demise.

$$\text{Thoracic circumference (TC)} = \frac{D_1 + D_2}{2} \times 3.14$$

TC can be used for predicting the presence or absence of significant pulmonary hypoplasia, especially if used as an AC/TC ratio.

G

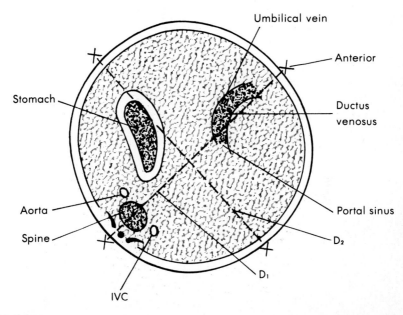

G. Fetal Abdomen

Cross section of the fetal abdomen at the level of the liver and stomach. This view shows the ductus venosus in the liver and is the plane used for measuring the abdominal circumference (AC).

$$AC = \frac{D_1 + D_2}{2} \times 3.14$$

AC can be used for estimating gestational age but is affected early in fetal growth disorders. Most useful for estimation of fetal weight.

Growth disorders (charts for normal fetuses exist) include:

1. HC/AC high—asymmetric IUGR
2. HC/AC low—macrosomia or microcephaly
3. FL/AC high—IUGR
4. FL/AC low—macrosomia
5. EFW low but HC/AC within normal limits—symmetric IUGR

Continued.

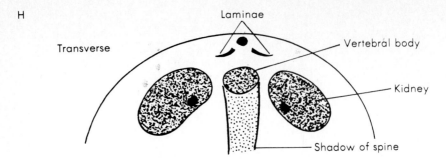

H. Fetal Abdomen

Cross section of the fetal abdomen at the level of the kidneys; note the shadow made by the echodense spine. This view has been compared to "eyeglasses over a nose." Evaluate spine for NTDs (open and closed), which are most frequent in lumbosacral region—look for separation of laminae and absence of skin covering (see *B.* and *E.* for associated intracranial abnormality). Evaluate kidney for size and consistency.

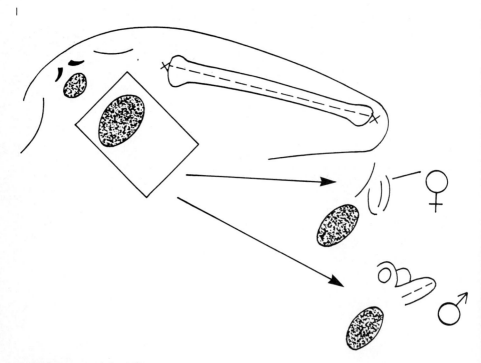

I. Fetal Femur and Genitalia

Femur length (FL) is used for gestational age estimation: (1) 14 to 19 weeks ± 6 days, (2) 20 to 29 weeks ± 14 days, and (3) 30 weeks to term ± 21 days. Gender determination is useful in sex-linked disorders and for determination of zygosity in multiple gestations.

J

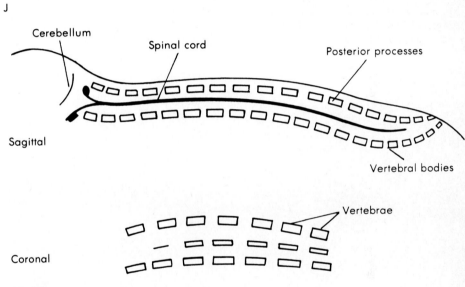

Cerebellum

Spinal cord

Posterior processes

Sagittal

Vertebral bodies

Coronal

Vertebrae

J. Spine

Longitudinal sagittal and coronal views of the fetal spine are used to detect NTDs.

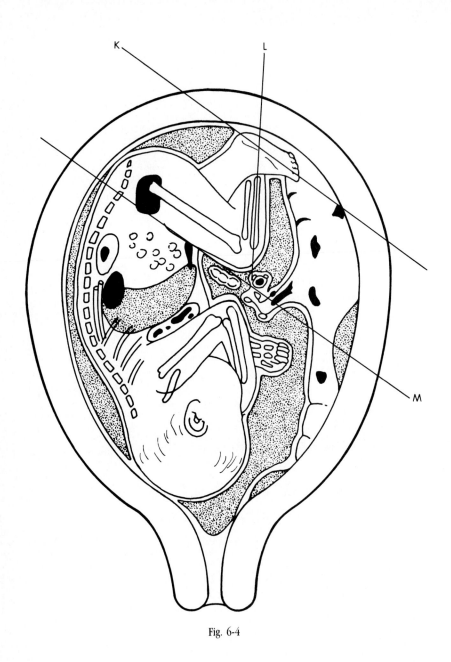

Fig. 6-4

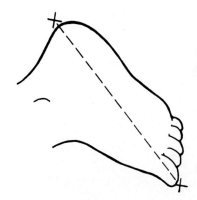

K. Fetal Foot

Gestational age estimation is obtained by foot measurement. Foot/femur ratio is useful in diagnosing skeletal dysplasia (foot size is relatively spared) and dwarfism in the fetus. Table exists.

Continued.

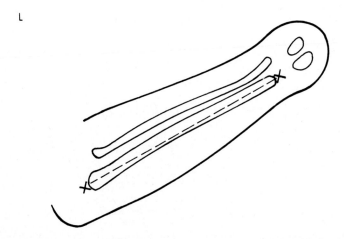

L. Fibula and Tibia

Gestational age estimation. Long-bone measurement useful in diagnosis of suspected skeletal dysplasia.

M

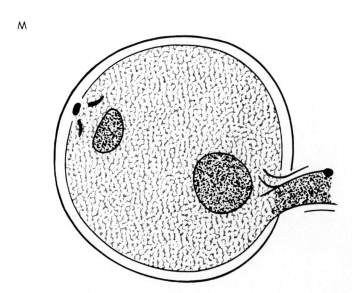

M. Umbilical Cord and Bladder

Oblique cross section of fetal abdomen shows umbilical cord entry and fetal bladder. Cord insertion is abnormal in presence of omphalocele. In gastroschisis, the abdominal defect is usually to the right of the cord insertion.

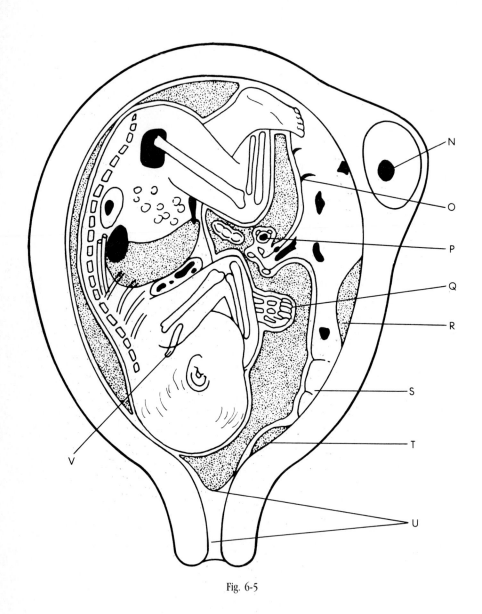

Fig. 6-5

N. Abnormalities of the Uterine Structures

Leiomyoma (pictured), disorders of müllerian fusion.

O. Placenta

Location and maturity of placenta can be noted.

P. Number of Vessels in Cord

Two arteries and one vein are normal. Two-vessel cord should lead to search for other anomalies.

Q. Count Digits

Excessive number of digits can be associated with other anomalies.

R. Retroplacental Clot

Retroplacental clot may be identified in abruptio placentae.

S. Grade III Placenta

Placenta shows well-developed lobules.

T. Retrochorionic Clot

Retrochorionic clot can be seen in abruptio placentae.

U. Lower Uterine Segment

Examination of lower uterine segment can suggest cervical incompetence (funneling). Cervix can be examined for dilatation and length. Presence of placenta previa is best detected with ultrasonography. *Placenta previa* is placenta covering the internal cervical os at more than 26 weeks EGA.

V. Clavicle Length

Clavicle length is helpful in estimating gestational age and cleidocranial dysplasia.

ANTENATAL DIAGNOSTIC TECHNIQUES

Since the introduction in the 1970s of amniocentesis for karyotyping, skill in making antenatal diagnosis of genetic diseases has increased. A wide array of inherited disorders are now amenable to diagnosis by either first-trimester chorionic villi sampling (CVS), amniocentesis (after 12 weeks gestation), or fetal-blood sampling from the umbilical cord. Amniocentesis and fetal-blood sampling continue to have applications in the third trimester, ranging from assessment of fetal pulmonary maturity to evaluation and treatment of isoimmunized pregnancies. The first step in antenatal diagnosis is to identify the appropriate population for testing.

Noninvasive Screening Techniques

Noninvasive techniques are applicable to any pregnant patient or patients who are seeking preconception counseling.

Medical history

1. Should include questioning regarding common birth defects (e.g., congenital cardiac defects, NTDs, facial clefting, urinary tract anomalies) and heritable disorders.
2. Should include detailed history of pregnancy wastage and prior evaluation.

Family history (both partners)

1. History of congenital defects.
2. History of metabolic and other heritable disorders.
3. History of mental retardation.
4. History of pregnancy losses (especially recurrent).
5. History of neonatal deaths.
6. Detailed pedigree should be obtained if any of the above are present (see Fig. 6-6).

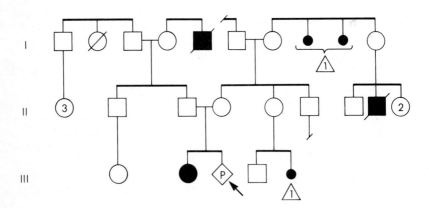

Fig. 6-6
Sample pedigree obtained at genetic counseling. ⬦₍ₚ₎, Fetus in current pregnancy; △, first-trimester abortion; □, male; ○, female. Shaded shapes indicate individuals affected by a genetic disorder.

Optional screening for parents of ethnic origin

1. Tay-Sachs disease: Ashkenazi Jews
2. Sickling disorders and β-thalassemia: Blacks and people of African, Mediterranean, Indian, or Pakistani origin.
3. α-Thalassemia: Southeast Asians
4. Cystic fibrosis: Caucasians—screen will be available soon.
5. Neural tube defects—Irish-English origin, MS-AFP.

Maternal serum α-fetoprotein (MS-AFP)

1. AFP is a fetal protein that is not synthesized by normal adult tissues.
2. AFP produced by the fetus enters both the amniotic fluid and maternal circulations in gestational age–dependent amounts.
3. By measuring AFP in maternal blood between 14 and 20 weeks gestation, populations at risk for carrying a fetus with congenital disorders can be identified.
   a. High MS-AFP: can be a marker for NTDs, abdominal-wall defects, and other disorders of incomplete fusion.
   b. Low MS-AFP: can be a marker for trisomy.
4. MS-AFP is only a screening tool: most abnormal MS-AFPs are not caused by fetal defects (see Fig. 6-7).

Amniocentesis
Indications for amniocentesis

1. Prenatal diagnosis of genetic disorders.
   a. Fetal karyotype.
   b. AFP assessment.
   c. Inherited metabolic disorders.
2. Assessment of pulmonary maturity.
   a. Lecithin/sphingomyelin ratio (L/S).
      (1) L/S greater than 2—2% incidence of respiratory distress syndrome (RDS).
      (2) L/S of 1.5 to 1.9—greater than or equal to 50% incidence of RDS.
      (3) L/S less than 1.5—75% incidence of RDS.
   b. Phosphatidylglycerol (PG): presence of PG—incidence of RDS virtually 0%.
   c. Note that a compromised neonate may develop RDS even with a reassuring lung-maturity profile.
   d. Shake test: depends on the ability of the pulmonary surfactant to generate a stable foam in the presence of ethanol. This is a screening procedure that yields useful information if mature and in the absence of blood and meconium.
   e. Foam stability test: same principle as *a*. above. The test kit contains test wells with predispensed volume of ethanol. Extremely sensitive as well as moderately specific. A useful screening test when L/S is not available.
   f. Optical density (OD) 650: turbidity believed to be dependent on the total amniotic-fluid phospholipid concentration. OD 650 greater than .15 correlates extremely well with absence of RDS. Contamination with blood and meconium invalidates the results.
3. Assessment of severity of isoimmunized pregnancies.

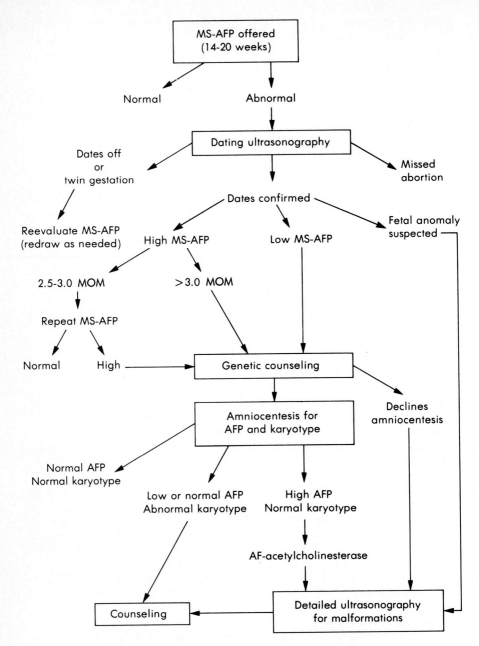

Fig. 6-7
Protocol for screening for anomalies and trisomies using MS-AFP.
MOM, Multiples of the median.

Amniocentesis technique

1. With direct ultrasonographic guidance, amniocentesis can be performed as early as 12 weeks gestation.
2. Fluid volume and sites of pockets are assessed by ultrasonography.
3. Skin cleansed with antiseptic solution.
4. Local anesthesia in maternal subcutaneous layer is optional.
5. 22-gauge spinal or Whitacre tip needle is introduced into fluid pocket under ultrasonographic guidance, using sterile technique.

Potential complications of amniocentesis

1. Premature rupture of membranes—1% to 2% of patients
2. Direct fetal injury—less than .1% of patients
3. Fetal bleeding from laceration of the umbilical cord or the placenta
4. Fetal-maternal bleeding—approximately 1% of patients
5. Premature labor—less than .1% of patients
6. Abruptio placentae—less than .1% of patients
7. Pregnancy loss
   a. Incidence of approximately 0.5% within 2 weeks after amniocentesis for procedures after 15 weeks gestation
   b. Complication rates for amniocentesis that is performed earlier than 15 weeks are still under study
   c. Complications in the third trimester are rare; premature rupture of membranes (PROM) most common
8. Hemorrhage (especially epigastric or uterine vessels)
9. Isoimmunization—protect woman with Rh-negative blood by giving her RhIg
10. Infection—less than .1% of patients

Chorionic villus sampling (CVS)

Prospective, multicenter, NIH-sponsored trials have determined procedure-related fetal loss rates from CVS to be no more than 1% to 2%. Placental mosaicism is a rare problem with CVS which may lead to the finding of a karyotype that does not reflect that of the fetus. If samples are not free of decidual contamination, the maternal karyotype may be inadvertently obtained.

Indications for CVS

1. Same as for genetic amniocentesis.
2. Usually done at 9 to 11 weeks of gestation.
3. Cannot obtain AFP measurements with CVS; measurement of maternal AFP should be postponed until at least 2 weeks after CVS.

CVS procedure

1. Transabdominal CVS
   a. Sterile conditions
   b. Local anesthesia
   c. Under ultrasonographic guidance, a 17-gauge spinal eedle is introduced transabdominally to the edge of the placenta. A 19- or 20-gauge spinal needle is then inserted through the first needle and passed into the placenta, taking care not to penetrate the amniotic cavity. The chorionic tissue is then aspirated with a syringe. The adequacy of this sample is ascertained under a dissecting microscope.

2. Transcervical CVS
   a. Negative cervical cultures for gonorrhea and chlamydia should be obtained before procedure.
   b. Same technique as abdominal CVS except the route of entry is the cervix. A Portex catheter of 1.5-mm diameter is passed into the placental substance and aspirated.

Cordocentesis

Direct cord puncture for blood studies is a new technique that offers many possibilities.

Indications for cordocentesis

1. Rapid karyotyping—can be obtained in 48 hours
   a. Delayed prenatal care . . . and an indication for karyotyping
   b. Anomalies discovered in late pregnancy if the karyotype would affect antepartum management (e.g., antenatal fetal therapy [medical or surgical] and antenatal testing or management of labor and delivery [cesarean section for distress])
   c. Failed amniocentesis
2. Fetal clotting disorders
   a. Immune thrombocytopenia (ITP) (to guide mode of delivery)
   b. Hemophilia (to identify affected fetus)
3. Hemolytic disease
   a. Fetal blood type
   b. Fetal hemoglobin and hematocrit
   c. *In utero* transfusion directly into a cord vessel
4. Nonimmune hydrops
   a. Fetal hemoglobin and hematocrit
   b. Karyotype
5. Severe IUGR
   a. Fetal acid-base status
   b. Karyotype
   c. Fetal glucose and calcium levels
   d. Tests for evidence of fetal infections
6. Suspected intrauterine infection
   a. Fetal IgM
   b. Isolation of organism
   c. Complete blood count and differential
   d. Liver enzymes
7. Congenital disorders with circulating markers not present in the amniotic fluid
   a. Hemoglobinopathies
   b. Hemophilia
   c. Immune deficiency diseases
   d. Other
8. Direct injection of pharmaceuticals into the fetal circulation (e.g., intravascular therapy for intractable supraventricular tachycardia [investigational at present]).

Cordocentesis procedure

1. Under direct ultrasonograpohic guidance, with or without a needle guide
   a. Cordocentesis usually is not performed before 17 weeks gestation
   b. Sterile conditions

   c. Local anesthesia
   d. Spinal needle—20- to 26-gauge (22-gauge most commonly used)
   e. Cord at puncture site needs to be relatively immobile
     (1) Cord insertion into the placenta (most common site)
     (2) Cord insertion into the fetus (should not be used if fetus is active)
   f. "Trapped" loop of cord, especially in setting of oligohydramnios

Complications of cordocentesis

1. Blood streaming from umbilical cord: common and self-limiting
2. Transient fetal bradycardia
3. Cord hematoma and ensuing fetal distress
4. Intrauterine infection

ANTENATAL FETAL TESTING

Whereas first- and second-trimester antenatal assessment is directed primarily at the diagnosis of fetal congenital abnormalities, the goal of third-trimester testing is to determine whether the intrauterine environment continues to be hospitable to the fetus. Whether the method is real-time ultrasonography, Doppler ultrasonography, or fetal heart–rate monitoring, testing is used to guide the timing of delivery of patients at risk for uteroplacental insufficiency. The goals of antenatal testing are to prevent *in utero* demise and perinatal morbidity while avoiding unnecessary iatrogenic prematurity. Both the regimen and the interpretation of tests must always be established in the context of the patient's risk factors and the gestational age of the fetus.

Indications for Antenatal Testing

1. Suspected IUGR
2. Maternal diabetes
3. Preterm preeclampsia
4. Prior unexplained stillbirth
5. Postdates
6. Rh isoimmunization
7. Maternal chronic hypertension
8. Presence of lupus anticoagulant or anticardiolipin antibodies
9. Other chronic maternal disease, especially when a compromised vasculature may be present
   a. Autoimmune disorders (SLE, ITP, scleroderma)
   b. Renal disease
   c. Hemoglobinopathies
   d. Cyanotic heart disease
10. Maternal perception of decreased fetal movement

Antenatal Testing Methods
Nonstress test (NST) (Figs. 6-8 and 6-9)

1. Rationale: In the healthy fetus with an intact central nervous system, 90% of gross fetal movements are associated with accelerations of fetal heart rate. This response can be blunted by hypoxia or acidosis, as well as by drugs (e.g., narcotics, barbiturates, and β-blockers), fetal sleep, and some congenital anomalies.
2. Technique
   a. Patient in semi-Fowler's or left lateral recumbent position.
   b. External fetal heart–rate monitor and tocodynamometer are applied.

- Baseline heart rate ——————————————————110 - 150 bpm
- (Baseline variability)————————————————5 - 15 bpm
- Accelerations
  — Amplitude ————————————————————≥ 15 bpm
  — Duration ——————————————————————≥ 15 sec
  — With fetal movement or contraction ——————2 in any 10 min

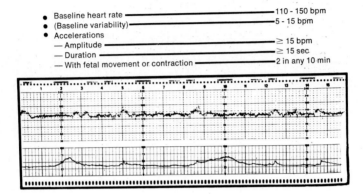

Fig. 6-8
Nonstress test tracing showing typical features of a normal or reactive tracing.

- Baseline heart rate ——————————————————110 - 150 bpm
- (Baseline variability)————————————————< 5 bpm
- Accelerations
  — Amplitude ————————————————————< 15 bpm
  — Duration ——————————————————————< 15 sec
  — With fetal movement or contraction ——————< 2 in any 10 min

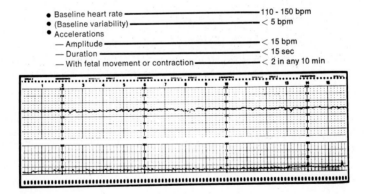

Fig. 6-9
Nonstress test tracing showing a nonreactive or worrisome tracing.

c. Patient presses button, which produces a mark on the uterine activity channel, when she feels a fetal movement.

d. Monitoring is continued until criteria for reactivity are met or for at least 40 minutes.

3. Interpretation
   a. Many criteria for reactivity have been proposed.
   b. Most commonly accepted standard requires 2 accelerations of 15 beats per minute that last at least 15 seconds in any 20-minute period.
   c. A test that lacks these accelerations is considered nonreactive and an indication for further evaluation.
   d. Tracing should also be reviewed for baseline variability and presence of decelerations, with or without contractions.

4. Advantages of NST over other techniques
   a. Well-adapted to outpatient setting.
   b. Inexpensive and rapid and therefore good for screening test.
   c. Has no contraindications.

5. Disadvantages
   a. High false-positive rate for nonreactive NST (75% to 90%)
   b. Slightly lower sensitivity to fetal compromise than contraction stress test (CST) or biophysical profile.

Contraction Stress Test (CST)

See Fig. 6-10.

1. Rationale: Uterine contractions decrease uterine blood flow and placental perfusion. If this decrease is sufficient to produce hypoxia in the fetus, a deceleration in fetal heart rate will result, beginning at the peak of the contraction and persisting after its conclusion (late deceleration). In a healthy fetoplacental unit, uterine contractions usually do not produce late decelerations; when there is underlying uteroplacental insufficiency, contractions, whether induced or spontaneous, will produce late decelerations.

2. Techniques of CST
   a. Oxytocin challenge test (OCT)
      (1) Patient placed in semi-Fowler's or left lateral recumbent position.
      (2) External fetal heart–rate monitor and tocodynamometer are applied.
      (3) Baseline tracing obtained for 15 minutes.
      (4) If less than 3 spontaneous contractions occur in 10 minutes, an intravenous oxytocin infusion is begun at 0.5 milliunit/min. This rate is increased until 3 contractions that last at least 40 seconds occur within 10 minutes.
   b. Nipple stimulation test
      (1) Technique is the same as for OCT except that unilateral nipple rolling is used in place of oxytocin infusion to induce adequate contractions.
      (2) Close monitoring of tracing is needed to avoid hyperstimulation.

3. Interpretation of CST (see Table 6-1)

4. Advantages of CST
   a. Provides earlier warning of fetal compromise than NST.
   b. Lower false-positive rate than NST, especially in early third trimester.

5. Disadvantages
   a. Contraindicated if patient at risk for preterm labor (e.g., twins, PROM, or incompetent cervix) or for bleeding (e.g., previa or abruptio).

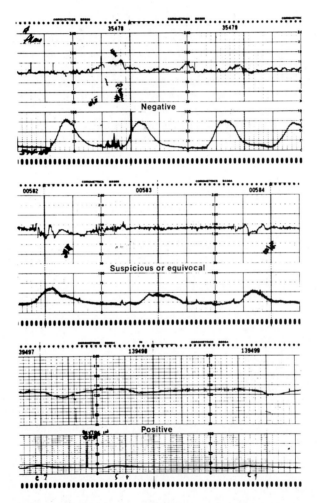

Fig. 6-10
Contraction stress test tracings showing normal (negative) worrisome (suspicious) and abnormal (positive) tracings.

Table 6-1   Interpretation of the contraction stress test

Interpretation	Description	Incidence (%)
Negative	No late decelerations appearing any-where on the tracing with adequate uterine contractions (3 in 10 min)	80
Positive	Late decelerations that are consistent and persistent are present with the majority (greater than 50%) of con-tractions without excessive uterine activity; if persistent late decelera-tions are seen before the frequency of contractions is adequate, test is interpreted as positive	3-5
Suspicious	Inconsistent late decelerations	5
Hyperstimulation	Uterine contractions closer than every 2 min or lasting more than 90 sec or 5 uterine contractions in 10 min; if no late decelerations are seen, test interpreted as negative	5
Unsatisfactory	Quality of the tracing is inadequate for interpretation, or adequate uterine activity cannot be achieved	5

From Gabbe SG et al: Obstetrics: normal and problem pregnancies, New York, 1986, Churchill Livingstone Inc.

    b. Requires observation on or adjacent to labor and delivery area with close nurs-ing supervision.
    c. Relatively expensive and time-consuming.

Biophysical profile

1. Rationale: Real-time ultrasonography can provide information about parameters that reflect fetal well-being in addition to fetal heart–rate patterns. The incorpora-tion of several markers of biophysical state into a scanning system can improve the positive and negative predictive value of testing.
2. Technique
    a. Perform NST.
    b. Observe fetus with real-time ultrasonography for up to 30 minutes to evaluate criteria in Table 6-2.
3. Interpretation
    a. Score of 8 to 10—normal test.
    b. Score of 6—suspect chronic asphyxia and repeat in 24 hours or perform CST.
    c. Score less than 6—strongly suspect chronic asphyxia, perform CST, or repeat test immediately, and if still less than 6, deliver fetus.
    d. With any score less than 10, oligohydramnios should be considered as an indi-cation for delivery unless PROM is present.

Table 6-2   Fetal biophysical profile score

Variable	Score 2 (Normal)	Score 0 (Abnormal)
Fetal breathing movements (FBM)	The presence of at least 30 sec of sustained FBM in 30 min of observation	Less than 30 sec of FBM in 30 min
Fetal movements	Three or more gross body movements in 30 min of observation; simultaneous limb and trunk movements are counted as a single movement	Two or less gross body movements in 30 min of observation
Fetal tone	At least one episode of motion of a limb from a position of flexion to extension and a rapid return to flexion	Fetus in a position of semi- or full-limb extension with no return to flexion with movement; absence of fetal movement is counted as absent tone
Fetal reactivity	The presence of two or more fetal heart–rate accelerations of at least 15 beats/min that last at least 15 sec and are associated with fetal movement in 40 min	No acceleration or less than two accelerations of the fetal heart rate in 40 min of observation
Qualitative amniotic-fluid volume	A pocket of amniotic fluid that measures at least 1 cm in two perpendicular planes	Largest pocket of amniotic fluid measures <1 cm in two perpendicular planes
Maximal score	10	—
Minimal score	—	0

Modified from Manning F et al: Am J Obstet Gynecol 140:289, 1981.

4. Advantages
   a. Can be performed in outpatient setting.
   b. Lower false-positive rate than NST alone.
   c. No contraindications.
   d. Can be used effectively in early third trimester.
5. Disadvantages
   a. Requires trained ultrasonographer and real-time ultrasonographic equipment in addition to fetal heart–rate monitor.
   b. More time consuming than NST alone.

Doppler measurement of blood flow in the fetal and placental circulations

1. Rationale: Doppler ultrasonography can be used to assess directly perfusion of the fetus and placenta. In pregnancies suspected of uteroplacental insufficiency, analysis of Doppler waveforms could allow identification of jeopardized fetuses before asphyxial fetal compromise has occurred.

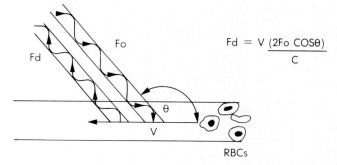

$$Fd = V\frac{(2Fo\ COS\theta)}{C}$$

Fig. 6-11
Fd equals the Doppler-shifted frequency, which is dependent on the angle of the ultrasonographic beam relative to the direction of blood flow (Θ), as well as on the velocity of flow. *Fo,* Frequency of the original sound; *Fd,* magnitude of the frequency shift; Θ, angle of the incidence of ultrasonographic beam and the velocity vector; *V,* velocity of flow; and *C,* speed of sound in tissue (1540 m/sec).

2. Principles
   a. Because of the principle of the Doppler shift, the velocity of a moving object (such as a red blood cell) can be determined by measuring the change in frequency in a sound wave reflected off that object (see Fig. 6-11).
   b. Doppler-shifted frequencies can be displayed as velocity (or amplitude of frequency shift) versus time. The shape of these waveforms (as well as peak velocities in some vessels) can be analyzed to yield information about blood flow and resistance in a given circulation.
   c. In vessels that are coiled (e.g., umbilical artery and uterine vessels), the angle between the Doppler beam and the vessel cannot be accurately measured, and therefore absolute velocity cannot be assessed. Angle-independent indices using ratios of peak-systolic to end-diastolic frequencies are instead used as indicators of resistance to flow. In general, reduction in end-diastolic flow indicates increased resistance (see Fig. 6-12).
3. Instrumentation
   a. Continuous-wave Doppler ultrasonography (sound is constantly emitted, and its reflection is constantly received):
      (1) Advantages: simple to operate, easily portable, low output intensity, will accommodate a very high intensity shift, and relatively inexpensive.
      (2) Disadvantages: path of the beam is not visualized and therefore cannot be measured, vessels must be identified by characteristic flow pattern because no relative image is pronounced, and range lacks specificity.
   b. Pulsed-wave (duplex) Doppler system (sound is intermittently emitted and received by the same crystals)
      (1) Advantages: depth specific (can be selected), the beam can be visualized by integrating it into a real-time ultrasonographic imaging system and therefore velocity of flow in fetal vessels can be assessed, and a wider range of fetal vessels can be studied.
      (2) Disadvantages: higher sound output intensity, depth at which the duplex system can be used is limited, larger and less mobile, and more expensive.

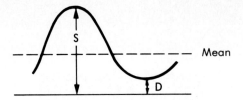

Fig. 6-12
Angle-independent indices of blood flow. Increases in these ratios above normal ranges suggest increased downstream resistance to forward blood flow.

$$\frac{S}{D} = \text{S/D ratio}$$

$$\frac{S-D}{S} = \text{Resistance index}$$

$$\frac{S-D}{\text{Mean}} = \text{Pulsatility index}$$

4. Vessels subject to examination
  a. Uterine or arcuate arteries
    (1) Normally forward flow is present throughout the cardiac cycle.
    (2) Systolic/diastolic (S/D) ratio normally less than 2.6 after 26 weeks. Abnormal values occur in IUGR and preeclampsia.
    (3) Persistence or development of a dicrotic notch in the third trimester is correlated with IUGR and preeclampsia.
    (4) There is debate about best site for measurement and effect of placental site.
    (5) Must be careful to distinguish from internal iliac vessel.
  b. Umbilical arteries (see Fig. 6-13)
    (1) Normally forward flow is present throughout the cardiac cycle. Should see nonpulsatile flow in adjacent umbilical vein.
    (2) S/D ratio decreases with advancing gestation.
    (3) S/D normally less than 3.0 after 30 weeks.
    (4) Decreased or absent end-diastolic flow correlates with IUGR, preeclampsia, and increased perinatal morbidity.
    (5) Doppler assessment of umbilical artery flow has been proposed as screening technique in high-risk pregnancies.
  c. Umbilical vein
    (1) Straight and nonpulsatile volume of flow in the umbilical vein can be measured. Accurate measurements require complex equipment that is currently available in few institutions.
    (2) Has been used to assess IUGR and isoimmunized pregnancies.
  d. Fetal descending aorta
    (1) End-diastolic flow sometimes normally absent.
    (2) Peak velocity of flow is decreased with fetal hypoxia.
  e. Carotid artery and cerebral blood flow
    (1) In fetal hypoxic states, blood flow to cerebral circulation increases (head-sparing), and therefore Pulsatility index (PI) decreases.
    (2) These changes may precede umbilical artery increase in S/D ratio or PI.

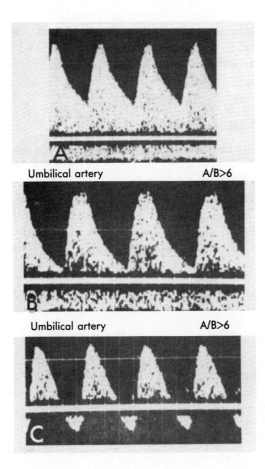

Fig. 6-13
Umbilical artery flow velocity-time waveforms in which the vertical dimension represents the Doppler-shifted sound frequencies *(Hz)* and the horizontal dimension represents time. Waveforms presented below the broad horizontal line represent flow in the direction opposite to that above the line. *A,* Normal umbilical artery flow velocities over umbilical vein flow velocities at 34 weeks gestation. *B,* Waveform characterized by a high A/B ratio indicative of high impedance with low end-diastolic velocities that approach the limits of the high-pass filter. *C,* Very abnormal waveform with reversal of the direction of flow in diastole as indicated by the segment of the arterial waveform in each cardiac cycle, which appears below the broad horizontal line. Umbilical vein flow velocities do not appear in *C.*
From Trudinger BJ et al: Br J Obstet Gynecol 93:171, 1986. © 1986; Blackwell Scientific Publications, Oxford, England.

5. Application
   a. The best role for Doppler protocols for assessment of fetal well-being remains to be determined. A prospective randomized study of the use of umbilical-artery Doppler ultrasonography in managing more than 300 high-risk pregnancies has suggested that it may reduce perinatal morbidity.
   b. At present, the results of Doppler studies should be seen as indications for increased surveillance (using other techniques of antenatal assessment) rather than as indications for delivery.

Protocols for Management

See Fig. 6-14.
1. Frequency of testing needed varies depending on risk factor and testing method used.
2. Most institutions use NST for screening with biophysical profile or CST for back-up.
3. If NST is used for primary screening, it should be performed at least twice weekly for patients with insulin-dependent diabetes, postdate pregnancy, and confirmed IUGR.
4. In general, testing frequency should be increased if patient is unstable (e.g., progressive hypertension or proteinuria, sickle-cell crisis).
5. Any protocol must be used cautiously and be tailored to the specific clinical situation.

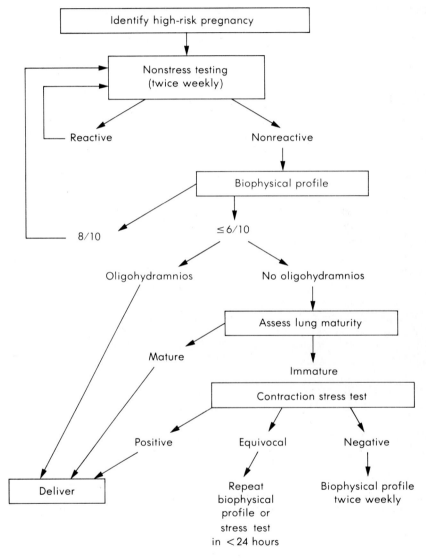

Fig. 6-14
Antenatal testing: an example of a protocol for management of IUGR.

REVIEW
QUESTIONS
True or False

1. The accuracy of gestational age estimation decreases with advancing gestational age.
2. Duodenal atresia, microcephaly, achondroplasia, infantile polycystic kidney disease, and x-linked aquaeductal stenosis may not be detected on a level II ultrasonogram at 18 to 22 weeks gestation.
3. IUGR may be detected by measuring the HC/AC and FL/AC ratios and by estimating the fetal weight.

Select the Best Answer

4. The method of fetal karyotyping that requires the longest time for processing of the fetal sample is:
   a. Amniocentesis
   b. Chorionic villus biopsy
   c. Cordocentesis
5. The antenatal fetal testing technique that is usually the least time-consuming and the least labor intensive is:
   a. Biophysical profile
   b. Nonstress test
   c. Contraction stress test
6. The following is an indication for delivery in most cases:
   a. Nonreactive nonstress test
   b. Biophysical profile of 6
   c. Positive contraction stress test
7. An increase in pulsatility index or an increase in the S/D ratio is always indicative of:
   a. IUGR
   b. Fetal compromise
   c. Increase in vascular resistance
   d. None of the above

ANSWERS

1. T
2. T
3. T
4. a
5. b
6. c
7. d

BIBLIOGRAPHY
Ultrasonography: Real-Time and Doppler

Arduini D et al: Fetal blood flow velocity waveforms as predictors of growth retardation, Obstet Gynecol 70(1):7, 1987.
Campbell S, Bewley S, and Cohen-Overbeek T: Investigation of the uteroplacental circulation by Doppler ultrasound, Semin Perinatol 11(4):362, 1987.
Romero R et al: Prenatal diagnosis of congenital anomalies, East Norwalk, Conn, 1988, Appleton & Lange.

Sanders RC, and James AE: Principles and practice of ultrasonography in obstetrics and gynecology, East Norwalk, Conn, 1988, Appleton-Century-Crofts.

Taylor KJW, Burns PN, and Wells PNT, editors.: Clinical applications of Doppler ultrasound, New York, 1988, Raven Press.

Trudinger BJ et al: Umbilical artery flow velocity waveforms in high-risk pregnancy, Lancet 1:188, 1987.

Trudinger BJ et al: Fetal umbilical artery flow velocity waveforms and placental resistance: clinical significance and pathologic correlation, Br J Obstet Gynecol 92:23, 1985.

Prenatal Diagnosis

Blakemore K: Prenatal diagnosis by chorionic villus sampling. Obstet Gynecol Clin North Am 15(2):179, 1988.

Daffos F, Capella-Parlovsky M, and Forestier F: Fetal blood sampling during pregnancy with use of a needle guided by ultrasound: a study of 606 consecutive cases, Am J Obstet Gynecol 153:655, 1985.

Grannum PA et al: *In utero* exchange transfusion by direct intravascular injection in severe erythroblastosis fetalis, N Engl J Med 314:1431, 1986.

Hanson FW et al: Amniocentesis before 15 weeks gestation: outcome, risks, and technical problems, Am J Obstet Gynecol 156:1524, 1987.

Nicolaides KH et al: Ultrasound-guided sampling of umbilical cord and placental blood to assess fetal well-being, Lancet 1:1065, 1986.

Assessment of Fetal Well-Being

Freeman R, Anderson G, and Dorchester W: A prospective multi-institutional study of antepartum fetal heart rate monitoring, Am J Obstet Gynecol 143:771, 1982.

Manning FA, Platt LD, and Sipos L: Antepartum fetal evaluation: development of a fetal biophysical profile, Am J Obstet Gynecol 136:787, 1980.

Platt LD et al: A prospective trial of the fetal biophysical profile versus the nonstress test in the management of high-risk pregnancies, Am J Obstet Gynecol 153:624, 1985.

Thacker SB, and Berkelman RL: Assessing the diagnostic accuracy and efficacy of selected antepartum fetal surveillance techniques, Obstet Gynecol Surv 41(3):121, 1986.

Medical Diseases During Pregnancy

7

Mark B. Landon
Philip Samuels

Managing medical conditions during pregnancy is a great challenge. The physician caring for a pregnant woman with a chronic or acute disease must be aware of the effect of pregnancy on the disease process and, similarly, the possible effect of the condition on pregnancy outcome. A knowledge of therapeutic options and their potential interactions with the growing fetus is also essential. The woman who has a chronic medical condition antecedent to pregnancy will often have an internist or family physician also involved in her care. Medical conditions beginning during pregnancy will first come to the attention of the obstetrician, whose task is to distinguish the normal physiologic changes of pregnancy from both serious medical illnesses and obstetric complications. Routine prenatal care is therefore more challenging than it might at first appear.

CARDIAC DISEASE

Cardiac disease complicates approximately 1% of all pregnancies and is a major nonobstetric cause of maternal mortality in the United States. The normal cardiovascular changes of pregnancy may impose a tremendous risk on women with certain types of heart disease. Fetal well-being may also be adversely affected if maternal cardiac condition deteriorates. Particularly, the delivery of poorly oxygenated blood to the fetus can limit growth and reduce viability.

Knowledge of the basic cardiac changes that occur during pregnancy is essential for understanding the cardiac diseases that complicate pregnancy (see Chapter 3).

Rheumatic heart disease remains the most common serious cardiac problem encountered in pregnancy, despite a declining incidence of rheumatic fever in the United States. For patients receiving primal care, the maternal mortality rate is less than 1%. Patients at greatest risk are those in whom severe congestive heart failure (CHF) or atrial dysrhythmias develop.

An increasing number of women with congenital heart disease are becoming pregnant. Improvements in surgical techniques and neonatal care have contributed to this phenomenon. However, the maternal mortality rate for patients with right-to-left shunting and increased pulmonary pressure approaches 50%.

Diagnosis of Cardiac Disease in Pregnancy

The physical changes of normal pregnancy may mimic cardiac disease. These include fatigue, dyspnea, orthopnea, and peripheral edema. Systolic outflow murmurs are

present in 90% of pregnant women. An S_3 is common. Underlying cardiac disease is suggested by the following:
1. Progressive limitation of physical activity resulting from progressive dyspnea.
2. Chest pain that accompanies exercise or increased activity.
3. Syncope preceded by palpitations or physical exertion.
4. A diastolic murmur.

Mitral Stenosis

1. The most common form of rheumatic heart disease in pregnancy is mitral stenosis.
2. Symptoms of pulmonary congestion may develop in 25% of pregnant women, with obstruction to the left arterial outflow followed by a rise in atrial pressure and pulmonary capillary wedge pressure. Symptomatic patients should undergo surgical correction before planning pregnancy.
3. Treatment includes limitation of activity, diuresis of fluid overload, and control of dysrhythmias, particularly atrial fibrillation. Refractory patients are treated with commissurotomy (3% mortality rate) or valve replacement.
4. Labor and delivery management includes the following guidelines:
    a. Significant disease requires invasive cardiac monitoring.
    b. Semi-Fowler's position.
    c. Oxygen therapy.
    d. Avoid tachycardia as it results in decreased cardiac output.
    e. Epidural anesthesia may reduce pain and alleviate tachycardia.
    f. Avoid hypotension; systemic resistance should be maintained with alpha-agonist, metaraminol, as the beta component of ephedrine results in tachycardia.
    g. Valsalva efforts shortened by forceps or vacuum extraction.
    h. Antibiotic prophylaxis.

Aortic Stenosis

1. Aortic stenosis is a rare complication of pregnancy because most patients become symptomatic in the fifth or sixth decade of life.
2. The mortality rate is as high as 17% in pregnant women.
3. Symptoms occur because of obstruction to left ventricular outflow and reduced cardiac output. A triad of angina, syncope, and dyspnea signals progressive disease.
4. Hypovolemia is poorly tolerated because of the need for an adequate end-diastolic volume in the face of increased left ventricle (LV) filling pressures and impedance to outflow. Regional anesthesia must be used with great caution because of this consideration.
5. Labor and delivery management includes the following:
    a. Tachycardia must be avoided because it decreases LV filling time.
    b. Invasive cardiac monitoring for labor in symptomatic patients.
    c. Antibiotic prophylaxis is recommended.

Mitral Regurgitation

1. Mitral inefficiency occurs as a sequela of rheumatic fever or endocarditis or may be found in women with idiopathic hypertrophic subaortic stenosis (IHSS) or mitral valve prolapse (MVP) (see below).
2. Symptoms of fatigue and dyspnea occur when diminished ventricular output produces pulmonary congestion. Hemodynamic changes of pregnancy are well tolerated in patients with mild disease.

3. Typical decrescendo systolic murmur is diminished with the fall in peripheral vascular resistance, which reduces regurgitant flow across the mitral valve.
4. Labor and delivery management includes the following:
   a. Central monitoring to guide fluid and drug therapy in symptomatic patients.
   b. Epidural anesthesia is recommended to decrease sympathetic activity, which may increase systemic resistance and hence mitral regurgitation.
   c. Antibiotic prophylaxis is recommended.

Aortic Regurgitation

1. Aortic regurgitation may occur because of rheumatic fever, congenital bicuspid valve, collagen vascular disease, or Marfan's syndrome (see below). In this condition, progressive LV dilation results from a state of chronic volume overload.
2. Valve replacement is often recommended; heterograft valve replacement is preferred in women likely to become pregnant because they do not require anticoagulation.
3. Pregnancy is complicated by failure in less than 10% of cases. Digitalis, diuretics, and restriction of activity can be used if failure occurs.
4. Labor and delivery management includes the following:
   a. Afterload reduction with phentolamine or sodium nitroprusside is advisable if vascular resistance remains high.
   b. Epidural anesthesia is recommended to decrease systemic resistance.
   c. Bradycardia should be avoided because duration of ventricular diastole is increased, along with regurgitation.

Ventricular Septal Defect

1. Women with small ventricular septal defects (VSDs) tolerate pregnancy well if their baseline pulmonary vascular resistance is normal, but patients with large VSDs may experience increased shunting (left to right) with the increased blood volume of pregnancy.
2. Labor and delivery management includes the following:
   a. Continuous epidural anesthesia is recommended to decrease systemic resistance and thereby decrease the degree of left-to-right shunting.
   b. Women with pulmonary hypertension will exhibit increased right-to-left shunting with a fall in pO_2 if systemic resistance is markedly reduced. Cyanosis with a good cardiac output signals this process.
   c. Monitoring with Swan-Ganz catheter is indicated if significant disease is present or if cyanosis develops.

Atrial Septal Defect

1. Atrial septal defect (ASD) is the most common congenital heart lesion in adults. The interatrial shunting is generally well tolerated by pregnant women unless pulmonary hypertension develops.
2. In advanced cases, shunting increases during pregnancy and atrial distension worsens. Atrial dysrhythmias and right-sided failure may occur.
3. Labor and delivery management includes the following:
   a. Invasive cardiac monitoring is indicated only for women with right-sided failure or dysrhythmias.
   b. Prophylactic antibiotics are probably not necessary in patients without complications.

Patent Ductus Arteriosus

1. Most women with patent ductus arteriosus (PDA) have had it corrected during childhood. Small PDAs usually have a benign course during reproductive years.
2. Large PDAs are associated with intrauterine growth retardation (IUGR) and respiratory infections. Mortality is increased for such women during pregnancy, and pregnancy termination may be indicated if significant right-to-left shunting is present.

Tetralogy of Fallot

1. Tetralogy of Fallot consists of:
   a. Right ventricular outflow obstruction.
   b. VSD.
   c. Right ventricular hypertrophy.
   d. An overriding aorta.
2. Right-to-left shunting is often present, resulting in cyanosis.
3. Pregnancy outlook is good for patients with corrected lesions (78% live birth rate), although IUGR is common; 40% of women with uncorrected lesions experience failure during pregnancy.
4. Labor and delivery management includes the following:
   a. Invasive monitoring is indicated to permit prompt recognition of failure.
   b. Regional anesthesia should be used with caution because of potential for hypotension, which may limit the ability of the right ventricle to perfuse the pulmonary bed.

Eisenmenger Syndrome

1. Eisenmenger syndrome describes a condition in which right-to-left or bidirectional shunting occurs at the atrial or ventricular level, combined with pulmonary hypertension.
2. Maternal mortality is high (12% to 70%), and fetal mortality approaches 50%; termination is strongly recommended.
3. Labor and delivery management includes the following:
   a. Monitoring with Swan-Ganz catheter is essential.
   b. Avoid central hypovolemia.
   c. Epidural anesthesia should be used with extreme caution, as right-to-left shunting may worsen. Therefore, PaO_2 must be followed closely.

Coarctation of the Aorta

1. Significant outflow obstruction may be exacerbated during pregnancy because tachycardia may not maintain an adequate output.
2. Maternal death is rare because most lesions are corrected surgically before pregnancy.
3. Antihypertensive therapy is offered to reduce the risk of aortic dissection.
4. Labor and delivery management includes the following:
   a. Hypotension should be avoided.
   b. Antibiotic prophylaxis is indicated.

Marfan's Syndrome

1. Marfan's syndrome is marked by joint deformities, arachnodactyly, and ocular lens dislocation, as well as cardiac features.

2. Cardiac manifestations include the following:
   a. Weakness of aortic root and wall, presenting a risk for aortic dissection.
   b. MVP.
3. An aortic root diameter greater than 40 mm as measured sonographically is a contraindication to pregnancy. Maternal mortality rates approach 50% in Marfan's syndrome. Termination of pregnancy is recommended.
4. Treatment involves therapy for hypertension and beta-blockade to reduce contractile force transmitted to aortic wall.
5. Labor and delivery management includes the following:
   a. Epidural anesthesia is well tolerated.
   b. Avoid hypertension if general anesthesia is necessary.
   c. Antibiotic prophylaxis is indicated.

Mitral Valve Prolapse

1. MVP is the most common congenital heart lesion in women of childbearing age, but most affected women have uneventful pregnancies.
2. Antibiotic prophylaxis is indicated if:
   a. Mitral regurgitation is present.
   b. Placenta is removed manually.
3. Prophylaxis for other women with MVP with routine vaginal delivery remains controversial.

Peripartum Cardiomyopathy

1. Peripartum cardiomyopathy is defined as CHF with cardiomyopathy during the last month of pregnancy or the first 5 months postpartum. Etiology remains unknown, with autoimmune, viral (coxsackie B, influenza), and genetic influences suggested.
2. Symptoms are left-sided failure and dilated hypocontractile ventricles.
3. Treatment includes bed rest, sodium restriction, digitalis, and diuretic therapy. Anticoagulation may be necessary to prevent thrombi.
4. Persistent cardiomegaly has a 5-year mortality rate exceeding 50%.

PULMONARY DISEASE
Tuberculosis

Pulmonary infection is caused by the acid-fast bacillus, *Mycobacterium tuberculosis*. Despite its declining frequency of occurrence in the United States, tuberculosis (TB) should be considered in immigrants.
1. Diagnosis
   a. Subcutaneous purified preterm derivative (PPD) skin testing is a screening test.
   b. The PPD detects only 80% of those with reactivation of TB.
   c. Patients who have received the bacille Calmette-Guérin (BCG) vaccine will display a positive PPD test.
   d. Chest radiograph (with abdominal shield) is indicated if a previous negative skin test becomes positive, the patient has respiratory or constitutional symptoms, and history of BCG vaccine administration is in doubt in women with a positive PPD.
   e. Definitive diagnosis rests on sputum culture.
2. Treatment
   a. With adequate treatment, TB appears to have no adverse effect on pregnancy, and pregnancy does not alter the natural history of the disease.

b. Preferred chemotherapeutic treatment regimen for pregnancy (18 to 24 months) includes isoniazid, 300 mg/day, and ethambutol, 15 mg/kg/day.
c. Isoniazid prophylaxis for those with recent skin test conversions should be delayed until the postpartum period.
d. Offspring of women with active TB have up to a 50% chance of developing the disease during the first year of life. Daily isoniazid prophylaxis or BCG vaccine administration may be undertaken.

Sarcoidosis

Sarcoidosis is a multisystem granulomatous disease with hallmark histologic findings of noncaseating granulomas.
1. Diagnosis
   a. Symmetric bilateral hilar adenopathy on chest radiographs is evident. Advanced cases demonstrate interstitial disease.
   b. Definitive diagnosis can be made by lymph node biopsy.
2. Course of the disease
   a. Two-thirds of patients improve spontaneously within 2 to 3 years of diagnosis.
   b. Pregnancy has no long-term effect on the disease course. Many patients improve with gestation. Minor relapses during the postpartum period are common.
3. Treatment
   a. Identify renal, hepatic, or myocardial involvement.
   b. Perform pulmonary function tests early in pregnancy and near term.
   c. Glucocorticoid therapy is indicated if progressive deterioration of pulmonary function occurs. The usual starting dose is prednisone, 60 mg/day.

Pneumonia

The most common bacterial pneumonia seen during pregnancy is pneumococcal pneumonia (*Streptococcus pneumoniae*). The other common pneumonia is caused by *Mycoplasma pneumoniae*. Symptoms include cough, fever, and pleuritic pain. Tachypnea and purulent sputum are seen with pneumococcal disease.
1. Diagnosis
   a. A chest radiograph will show lobar consolidation in pneumococcal disease and a fluffy infiltrate in mycoplasma infection.
   b. Sputum and/or blood cultures should be run.
2. Treatment
   a. For pneumococcal disease, 600,000 units of aqueous penicillin G administered intravenously 4 times daily is the treatment of choice. After defervescence, oral penicillin 4 times daily for 10 to 14 days may be administered.
   b. For mycoplasma pneumonia, oral erythromycin, 500 mg administered 4 times daily for 14 days is the choice during pregnancy.

Asthma

Asthma is the most common obstructive pulmonary disease in pregnancy, observed in 0.4% to 1.3% of pregnant women. During pregnancy, 49% of women will show no change in disease severity, whereas 29% will improve and 22% will deteriorate. The risk of perinatal morbidity and mortality is minimally increased in the treated asthmatic patient.
1. Management goals
   a. Reduce the number of asthmatic episodes.
   b. Prevent severe attacks (status asthmaticus).
   c. Ensure adequate fetal oxygenation.

2. Pharmacologic therapy
   a. Theophyllines (bronchial smooth-muscle relaxant), including aminophylline, keep blood levels at 10 to 20 mg/ml.
   b. β-Mimetics (bronchial smooth-muscle relaxant), including terbutaline, can be used, 2.5 to 5.0 mg 4 times daily.
   c. Corticosteroids are indicated if patients cannot be adequately managed with theophylline preparations and β-mimetics. Systemic steroids are used when corticosteroid aerosols are ineffective.
   d. Treatment of status asthmaticus requires supplemental oxygen therapy, subcutaneous epinephrine or terbutaline; IV aminophylline, and parenteral steroids if response is inadequate to the previous measures. If the patient is hypoxic despite the above measures, endotracheal intubation may be necessary.

Pulmonary Embolus

Pulmonary embolus (PE) complicates .09 to 0.7 of every 1000 pregnancies. Untreated PE has a 12.8% mortality rate in pregnant women. Most PEs arise from thrombophlebitis of the deep femoral and pelvic veins. Incidence of deep venous thromboembolism during pregnancy is 0.4 to 1.0 per 1000 women.
1. Clinical presentation
   a. Chest pain may be apparent, as well as occasional dyspnea and pleural friction rub.
   b. Arterial blood gas *may* reveal hypoxemia.
   c. Massive PE is accompanied by hypotension and cardiovascular collapse.
2. Diagnosis
   a. Pulmonary perfusion and ventilation scans are helpful if the chest radiograph is normal. Fetal radiation exposure is minimal and well worth the risk because PE and its treatment are serious and complicated.
   b. If ventilation/perfusion scan is equivocal or if the chest radiograph is abnormal, selective pulmonary angiography is indicated.
3. Treatment
   a. Anticoagulation with heparin is the treatment of choice because heparin does not cross the placenta.
   b. Partial thromboplastin time is adjusted to be 1½ to 2 times normal. The heparin dose necessary to achieve this may be increased in pregnancy because of the normal rise in coagulation factor levels and increased blood volume.
   c. Oral anticoagulants are contraindicated. Coumadin crosses the placenta and is a known teratogen.

RENAL DISEASE
Renal Physiology in Pregnancy

1. Glomerular filtration rate (GFR) increases about 50% over baseline values early in pregnancy.
2. Renal plasma flow (RPF) also increases greatly during gestation.
3. The increase in GFR is greater than RPF values (elevated filtration fraction), which leads to a fall in serum blood urea nitrogen (BUN) and creatinine.

Urinary Tract Infection

1. Asymptomatic bacteriuria (ASB)
   a. ASB is defined as a colony count greater than 100,000 colonies/ml of a single organism on a "clean catch" specimen.

  b. Untreated asymptomatic bacteriuria will lead to UTI in 40% of untreated pregnant women. All pregnant women should be screened for ASB on their first prenatal visit.
  c. *Escherichia coli* is the most common organism found in ASB. Treatment consists of administering one of the following agents: nitrofurantoin, ampicillin, cephalosporins, or short-acting sulfa drugs (avoid sulfa drugs near term as they may displace bilirubin). Treatment period is 10 to 14 days, followed by a reculture.
  d. Patients with recurrent UTI should receive antibiotic suppression for the remainder of their pregnancy. An IVP postpartum may demonstrate upper tract abnormalities in these women.
2. Acute pyelonephritis
  a. Acute pyelonephritis is found in 1% to 2% of all pregnancies, and it has a strong association with preterm labor. The right side is more commonly affected.
  b. Treatment should be on an inpatient basis, with the patient receiving IV antibiotic therapy. Empiric therapy is instituted pending culture results (usually a broad-spectrum penicillin—ampicillin or cephalosporin). IV therapy should be continued until defervescence occurs and flank pain disappears, followed by oral antibiotics for 2 to 3 weeks. Urine cultures are then obtained periodically, and antibiotic suppression is recommended.

Urolithiasis

The prevalence of urolithiasis is 0.03% (same as in nonpregnant state).
1. Symptoms include colicky pain, recurrent UTI, and hematuria.
2. Diagnosis is made by a limited IVP study with abdominal shield.
3. Treatment consists of hydration and analgesia because most pregnant patients pass their stones. Surgery is rarely necessary.

Acute Glomerulonephritis

Acute glomerulonephritis occurs with a frequency of 1 per 40,000 pregnancies. Poststreptococcal glomerulonephritis is a rare cause of this illness in adults.
1. Symptoms include periorbital edema and hematuria, and the disease can be difficult to distinguish from preeclampsia.
2. Diagnosis rests on the urinary sediment and laboratory findings.
  a. RBC casts.
  b. Proteinuria.
  c. Azotemia.
  d. Antistreptolysin titer elevation if it is poststreptococcal glomerulonephritis.
  e. Renal biopsy is customarily deferred until after delivery, but may be performed in pregnancy in rare instances.
3. Treatment includes careful control of blood pressure, attention to fluid status, sodium restriction, and close following of serum K^+.

Chronic Renal Disease

1. Diagnosis of chronic renal disease may be difficult in late pregnancy because findings may mimic preeclampsia. They include the following:
  a. Reduced creatinine clearance (< 120 ml/minute).
  b. Proteinuria (> 300 mg/24 hours).

      c. RBCs or casts in urine sediment.
  2. Effect of pregnancy on renal disease
      a. A moderate decline in creatinine clearance may be seen in late gestation. Patients with markedly reduced clearance may not improve following pregnancy.
      b. Worsening proteinuria is common as gestation advances.
      c. The incidence of pyelonephritis increases in pregnant women with chronic renal disease.
      d. Severe hypertension and superimposed preeclampsia are the most serious complications.
  3. Pregnancy outcome. More than 85% of patients will have a successful pregnancy if adequate renal function is maintained, but IUGR, stillbirth, and preterm birth are increased in this population (20% to 50%).
  4. Treatment
      a. Frequently assess renal function and blood pressure.
      b. Control of hypertension is essential.
      c. Fetal assessment includes serial ultrasonography and fetal heart rate testing beginning at 28 weeks gestation.
      d. Delivery is indicated in cases of uncontrollable hypertension, significant superimposed preeclampsia, or worsening renal disease or if fetal wellbeing is in question.

Hemodialysis

  1. Most women on chronic hemodialysis experience oligomenorrhea and exhibit reduced fertility. Nevertheless, successful pregnancy has been reported in such patients, although preterm birth and preeclampsia are common.
  2. Treatment
      a. Meticulous control of blood pressure.
      b. Careful monitoring of fluid status and avoidance of hypotension during dialysis.
      c. Appropriate diet therapy.
      d. Correction of anemia.

Transplant Recipients

  1. Patients with allografts should wait 2 to 5 years before becoming pregnant. Evidence of allograft rejection is a contraindication to pregnancy.
  2. Immunosuppressive therapy (e.g., prednisone, azathioprine) should be *continued* during pregnancy.
  3. Preeclampsia is observed in 30% of patients. Preterm birth occurs in approximately 50% of cases.
  4. Fetal surveillance is mandatory (i.e., serial ultrasonography, heartrate testing, and daily fetal movement counting).

Hemolytic Uremic Syndrome

Hemolytic uremic syndrome (HUS) is a rare idiopathic disorder revealing hemolysis and renal failure during the postpartum period.
  1. Prodromal symptoms include vomiting, diarrhea, and a flulike illness.
  2. Disseminated intravascular coagulation usually accompanies renal failure. Mortality rates in excess of 50% have been reported.
  3. Treatment is generally supportive, with heparin, prostacyclin, and antithrombin III–concentrate infusions being therapeutic options.

ENDOCRINE DISEASES
Diabetes Mellitus

Fetal and neonatal mortality rates in diabetes mellitus have been reduced from approximately 65% before the discovery of insulin to 2% to 5% at this time. Excluding major congenital malformations, the perinatal mortality rate for insulin-dependent women receiving optimal care is nearly equivalent to that observed in women with normal pregnancies.

1. Carbohydrate metabolism during pregnancy
   a. Early in pregnancy, rises in maternal estrogen and progesterone levels lead to B-cell hyperplasia and increased insulin secretion.
   b. Relative maternal fasting hypoglycemia accompanies an increased peripheral utilization of glucose.
   c. Increased human placental lactogen (HPL) levels stimulate lipolysis in adipose tissue. HPL is partly responsible for the diabetogenic state of pregnancy. In normal pregnant women, glucose homeostasis is maintained by increased insulin secretion to counteract the decreased sensitivity to insulin at the cellular level.
   d. Glucose crosses the placenta by carrier-mediated–facilitated diffusion. Insulin and other protein hormones do not cross the placenta. Fetal blood glucose levels usually remain 20 to 30 mg/dl lower than maternal levels.
   e. Persistently elevated levels of maternal glucose lead to fetal hyperglycemia and result in fetal B-cell hyperplasia and hyperinsulinemia. Excessive growth, or *macrosomia*, may result (Pedersen's hypothesis). Fetal hyperglycemia and hyperinsulinemia may contribute to an increased risk of stillbirth and to neonatal morbidities such as respiratory distress syndrome, hypoglycemia, hyperbilirubinemia, hypocalcemia, polycythemia, and cardiomegaly.
2. Maternal classification of diabetes mellitus (see Table 7-1).
3. Detection of diabetes in pregnancy
   a. Of all cases of diabetes detected during pregnancy, 90% represent gestational diabetes. These women have significant risk for developing overt diabetes in later life.
   b. *All* pregnant women should be screened for gestational diabetes. Reliance on risk factors (e.g., age, previous stillbirth, or previous large infant) will detect only 50% of cases. Screening is performed at 24 to 28 weeks gestation with a 50 g oral glucose load, followed by a plasma glucose determination 1 hour later. An abnormal screening value (135 to 140 mg/dl) necessitates a diagnostic 3-hour oral glucose tolerance test (see Table 7-2).
4. Treatment of insulin-dependent patients

Table 7-1 White classification of diabetes in pregnancy

Class	Age of Onset (Years)		Duration (Years)	Vascular Disease	Insulin
A	Any		Any	None	Diet only
B	Over 20	or	<10	None	+
C	10 to 19	or	10 to 19	None	+
D	<10	or	>20	Benign retinopathy	+
F	Any		Any	Nephropathy	+
R	Any		Any	Proliferative retinopathy	+
H	Any		Any	Heart disease	+

    a. Self glucose monitoring, with frequent glucose assessments (fasting, prepran-
dial, and postprandial). Maintain fasting levels at < 100 mg/dl and postprandial
levels (2 hours) at less than 120 mg/dl.

    b. Multiple insulin injection regimens will be employed by most patients to
achieve these goals.

    c. Evaluate ophthalmologic and renal status at least once each trimester.

    d. Fetal surveillance consists of the following:

      (1) MS-AFP at 16 to 18 weeks gestation because neural tube defects are com-
mon.

      (2) Sonography at 18 to 20 weeks gestation to rule out anomalies.

      (3) Fetal echocardiography because cardiac anomalies are common.

      (4) Serial sonography to assess growth.

      (5) Fetal heartrate testing or biophysical profiles during the third trimester, and
daily fetal movement counting in women with insulin-dependent diabetes.

5. Timing and mode of delivery

    a. Elective delivery is often planned at 38 weeks, after ensuring fetal lung maturity
by amniocentesis.

    b. Preterm delivery is indicated for suspected fetal jeopardy, worsening maternal
vascular disease, or preeclampsia.

    c. Cesarean rates are declining for women with insulin-dependent diabetes. An ar-
rest pattern occurring in labor should alert the obstetrician to the possibility of
CPD and/or fetal macrosomia.

    d. Euglycemia should be maintained throughout labor. Continuous insulin infusion
and frequent glucose testing is mandatory.

6. Management of gestational diabetes

    a. Dietary therapy of 2000 to 2500 calories per day without concentrated sweets.

    b. Insulin therapy is reserved for fasting hyperglycemia (>105 mg/dl) and/or post-
prandial hyperglycemia (>120 mg/dl after 2 hours).

    c. Patients with a history of stillbirth or preeclampsia or those requiring insulin
should undergo fetal testing as for women with insulin-dependent diabetes.

    d. Ultrasound assessment of fetal size before delivery is recommended.

Thyroid Disease

1. Hyperthyroidism complicates 0.2% of pregnancies. Although pregnancy does not
worsen the disease, uncontrolled disease does increase neonatal morbidity resulting
from preterm birth and low birth weight. Approximately 1% of offspring of women
with Graves' disease demonstrate hyperthyroidism through placental passage of
thyroid-stimulating immune globulin.

Table 7-2   Detection of gestational diabetes—upper limits of normalcy

Test	Plasma (mg/dl)
50 g 1 hour screening	135-140
Oral GTT* (diagnostic)	—
Fasting	105
1 hour	190
2 hours	165
3 hours	145

*Diagnosis of gestational diabetes is made when two values are met or exceeded. Class A diabetes is
characterized by a normal fasting glucose.

a. Graves' disease is the most common cause of hyperthyroidism, resulting in a diffuse glandular enlargement. Toxic nodular goiter, thyrotoxicosis factitia, and gestational trophoblastic disease are less common causes.

b. Normal symptoms of pregnancy may be confused with hyperthyroidism (e.g., heat intolerance, nervousness, and mild tachycardia). Resting tachycardia (>100 beats/minute) or weight loss should suggest possible hyperthyroidism. Ophthalmologic signs such as exophthalmus and lid lag are helpful diagnostic clues.

c. Laboratory diagnosis consists of an elevated free thyroxine index (FT_4I). As T_4 increases with normal pregnancy, FT_4 I must be calculated.

d. Treatment includes:

   (1) Medical therapy consisting of administering propylthiouracil (PTU) or methimazole is the first line of therapy. PTU is preferred because methimazole has been associated with aplasia cutis of the scalp of newborns.

   (2) Surgery is indicated only in cases refractory to medical therapy.

   (3) Thyroid function should be assessed every 2 weeks, with adjustments in dosage of PTU being made.

   (4) PTU crosses the placenta and may cause fetal hypothyroidism. Prompt therapy in the newborn period probably prevents neurologic sequelae.

e. Thyroid storm is an uncommon endocrinologic emergency. It is seen in undiagnosed and partially treated patients. It may result in cardiovascular collapse. Hyperpyrexia ($>102°$ F), tachycardia, and agitation are symptoms. Treatment consists of propranolol administration, vigorous fluid replacement, antipyretics, and antithyroid medication (i.e., sodium iodide or oral saturated solution of potassium iodide followed by PTU therapy).

2. Hypothyroidism is rare in pregnancy because most hypothyroid women are infertile. The effect on pregnancy is debated. Early reports suggested an increased frequency of fetal malformations, but more recent studies do not support these findings. The diagnosis is made in the presence of low FT_4I and an elevated TSH level. Hypothyroidism treatment begins with 0.05 to 0.1 mg/day of L-thyroxine (synthroid), with the dose increased to a maximum of 0.2 mg/day. Therapy is guided by following TSH levels, which may take weeks to return to baseline.

Hyperparathyroidism

Hyperparathyroidism is rarely encountered in pregnancy, although detection may increase with automated serum calcium determinations. It is associated with increased perinatal morbidity and mortality. Stillbirth is increased, as are neonatal deaths (2%) from tetany, which occurs in 15% of cases. Neonatal tetany results from fetal hypercalcemia and subsequent fetal parathyroid suppression.

1. Diagnosis. Symptoms, including fatigue, muscle weakness, constipation, abdominal pain, bone pain, fractures, and nephrolithiasis, signify progressive disease. Laboratory diagnosis consists of elevated serum calcium and reduced serum phosphate levels. Marked phosphaturia may be present. PTH levels, which are increased in normal pregnancy, are elevated out of proportion to serum calcium levels.

2. Treatment. Medical therapy employing oral phosphate may be attempted in mild cases, particularly if delivery can be accomplished. Surgical therapy is indicated if marked hypercalcemia and progressive symptoms are present.

Hypoparathyroidism

Hypoparathyroidism is also an uncommon disorder, resulting from inadvertent parathyroidectomy or as an autoimmune process. The principal concern in pregnancy is inadequate transfer of calcium to the fetus, causing subsequent secondary hyperparathyroidism in the fetus (bone demineralization).

1. The diagnosis is established by the presence of hypocalcemia, hyperphosphatemia, previous easy surgery, irritability, and tetany (Trousseau's sign, or carpopedal spasm).
2. Treatment is with supplemental calcium, 1 to 4 g daily, and with 100,000 to 150,000 vitamin D IU or calcitrol, 2 to 3 mg/day.

Prolactin-producing Adenomas

1. Microadenomas (<1 cm). Pregnancy is becoming more common in women with prolactinomas with the use of ovulation induction and prolactin suppression by bromocriptine. Most women with microadenomas have uneventful pregnancies, but 5% will experience headache and visual disturbance. Bromocriptine therapy is indicated if these symptoms appear. Transphenoidal surgery is rarely necessary. Breastfeeding is not contraindicated in these women.
2. Macroadenomas (>1 cm). In women with macroadenomas, definitive therapy (surgery or radiation) is preferred before attempting pregnancy because more than a third of these women will experience symptoms during pregnancy. Visual field and ophthalmologic exams should be performed at least once each trimester. Symptoms are treated primarily with bromocriptine. If fetal maturity is established in a symptomatic patient, delivery should be accomplished.

Diabetes Insipidus

Diabetes insipidus, a rare disorder of inadequate antidiuretic (vasopressin) production by the protein pituitary gland, rarely complicates pregnancy. Massive polyuria and dilute urine (specific gravity of less than 1.005) are characteristic findings. Polyuria and urinary hyposmolarity continue despite water restriction. Diabetes insipidus may worsen during pregnancy because of the increased GFR. Treatment consists of intranasal 1-deamino-8-D-arginine vasopressin (DDAVP) administration.

Pituitary Insufficiency

Sheehan's syndrome is postpartum ischemic necrosis of the anterior pituitary and is typically observed following severe postpartum hemorrhage and hypotensive shock. Delayed diagnosis is extremely common. Failure to lactate is often an early finding. Progression of the disease leads to loss of axillary and pubic hair, oligomenorrhea, or amenorrhea and senile vaginal atrophy. Hypothyroidism is present with advanced disease. Treatment consists of replacing the multiple deficient hormones, and patients may conceive with replacement hormonal therapy (87% live birth rate).

Cushing's Syndrome

Characterized by excess glucocorticoid production, Cushing's syndrome is usually secondary to excess adrenocorticotropic hormone (ACTH) production by a pituitary adenoma. Other causes include adrenal tumor, neoplastic ectopic ACTH production, nodular adrenal hyperplasia, and exogenous corticosteroid therapy. Clinical features may initially be difficult to distinguish from those of normal pregnancy (e.g., weakness, weight gain, edema, striae, hypertension, and impaired glucose tolerance). Early-onset hypertension, easy bruising, and proximal myopathy suggest Cushing's syndrome. Pregnancy in women with Cushing's syndrome is marked by a high rate of preterm delivery and stillbirths in pregnancies not terminated.

The diagnosis is established by laboratory assays. Elevated serum cortisol with failure to suppress with dexamethasone indicates Cushing's syndrome. Pregnant individuals may fail to suppress with the 1 mg (low dose) suppression test. Identifying the source of hormone production is necessary before treatment can begin. Pituitary disease is treated surgically. An abdominal CT to rule out adrenal tumor is indicated if the patient fails to suppress cortisol with the high-dose (8 mg) dexamethasone test.

Adrenal Insufficiency

Adrenal insufficiency may be primary (Addison's disease) or secondary to pituitary disease or exogenous adrenal suppression.
1. Presentation and diagnosis. Fatigue, weakness, anorexia, hypotension, hypoglycemia, and skin hyperpigmentation are common initial complaints. The diagnosis is confirmed by decreased plasma cortisol levels and failure to stimulate cortisol production with cosyntropin (synthetic ACTH) administration.
2. Treatment. Glucocorticoid replacement with prednisone and mineralocorticoid replacement with fludrocortisone acetate constitute treatment. Dosages may need to be adjusted during pregnancy, labor, and delivery.

Pheochromocytoma

Pheochromocytoma, arises from adrenal medulla or sympathetic nervous tissue and may be malignant in 10% of cases. Pheochromocytoma may manifest as a hypertensive crisis with cerebral hemorrhage or severe congestive failure. The diagnosis is not established until postmortem in 30% of cases.
1. Symptoms. Symptoms mimic severe preeclampsia. Paroxysmal hypertension onset occurring before 20 weeks gestation and lack of significant proteinuria may be helpful in the differential diagnosis. Definitive diagnosis is made by laboratory measurement of catecholamines and metabolites (vanillylmandelic acid) in a 24-hour urine collection. A phentolamine (L-adrenergic blocker) test should not be performed during pregnancy because it may provoke severe hypotension.
2. Treatment.
   a. Localize tumor by CT scan.
   b. Prompt surgical excision.
   c. Before surgery, patient is stabilized on alpha-blockers. Beta-blockade is reserved for treating arrhythmias.
   d. Cesarean section is preferred in untreated cases. Adrenal exploration may be performed.

HEMATOLOGIC DISEASE
Iron Deficiency Anemia

Approximately 75% of all anemias during pregnancy are secondary to iron deficiency.
1. Diagnosis
   a. Serum iron of less than 60 mg/dl.
   b. Less than 16% saturation of transferrin.
   c. Increased total iron-binding capacity (may also be seen in normal pregnancy).
   d. Significantly reduced ferritin level.
   e. Hypochromia and microcytosis on peripheral smear.

2. Treatment. Treatment begins with oral ferrous sulfate, 325 mg 3 times daily. The reticulocyte count should rise about 2 weeks after therapy is begun. Other iron forms are more expensive and less well absorbed. Parenteral iron therapy has risks of adverse reactions and is only rarely indicated.

Folate Deficiency

The most common cause of megaloblastic anemia during pregnancy is folate deficiency. The daily folate requirement (50 mg) rises threefold to fourfold with gestation.
1. Diagnosis
   a. Decreased serum folate level.
   b. Hypersegmentation of neutrophils.
   c. Megaloblastosis—seldom seen before third trimester.
2. Treatment. Oral folate, 1 mg/day, is usually sufficient, but women having hemoglobinopathies, receiving phenytoin therapy, or carrying twins may require additional folate.

Hemoglobinopathies

1. Hemoglobin S. One of twelve black Americans carries the sickle cell gene (Hb AS). Sickle cell (HbSS) disease occurs in approximately 1 in 700 black Americans.
   a. Perinatal outcome. The rate of spontaneous abortion may be as high as 25%. Perinatal mortality is severalfold greater than that in the normal population. Stillbirth, IUGR, and maternal preeclampsia are all increased in women with HbSS disease.
   b. Maternal morbidity. Painful vasoocclusive episodes involving multiple organs are the hallmark of HbSS disease. The extremities, joints, and abdominal viscera are most commonly affected. Analgesia, oxygen, and hydration are the standard treatment. Crises appear to be more common during gestation. An increased risk for UTI, pneumonia, and pulmonary thrombosis and infarction is present.
   c. Treatment. Folate and iron supplementation are given as needed. The role of prophylactic transfusions and exchange transfusions remains controversial. Some studies have demonstrated a reduction in fetal growth retardation, preterm birth, and maternal morbidity with prophylactic transfusions. Fetal surveillance, consisting of serial sonography to assess growth and antepartum fetal heartrate testing, are recommended.
2. Hemoglobin SC. This combination of hemoglobins S and C occurs in 1 of 833 adult blacks in the United States. Women with Hb SC suffer less morbidity than do Hb S patients during pregnancy. However, a crisis may first appear during gestation. An increased incidence of miscarriage and preeclampsia is observed in these women. Prenatal care is as outlined for women with Hb S disease.
3. Thalassemia. A defect in the rate of globin chain synthesis is the cause of thalassemia. β-thalassemia is the most common disorder in which minimal suppression to absence of β-chain synthesis may occur. Asymptomatic heterozygotes are detected by increased Hb A_2 levels and microcytosis. Thalassemia intermedia patients exhibit hepatosplenomegaly and often require transfusions during pregnancy. Homozygotes (thalassemia major) are dependent on transfusions and demonstrate hepatosplenomegaly. The few patients that reach childbearing age often suffer from heart failure and require transfusion therapy during pregnancy. Antepartum fetal surveillance is essential.

Immune Thrombocytopenic Purpura

Thrombocytopenia results from peripheral destruction and sequestration of platelets, which results from antiplatelet antibody production. Immune thrombocytopenic purpura (ITP) may be the harbinger of SLE (see below) or other autoimmune diseases.

1. Pregnancy concerns
    a. Fetal platelet count may be lowered by transplacental passage of antiplatelet IgG. Fetal counts below $50,000/mm^3$ are associated with intracranial hemorrhage during labor and delivery.
    b. Maternal platelet count is a poor predictor of fetal platelet count. Elevated maternal circulating antiplatelet IgG levels may signify an increased risk for fetal thrombocytopenia.
    c. Fetal platelet count may be assessed with scalp platelet count in early labor or with cordocentesis. A count exceeding 50,000 allows for attempted vaginal delivery. Elective cesarean section is performed if neither of the above procedures can be accomplished.
    d. Thrombocytopenia may not be evident in the newborn until 4 to 6 days of life.
2. Treatment
    a. Glucocorticoid therapy, which prevents antibody binding, is instituted for maternal thrombocytopenia (defined as a platelet count below $100,000/mm^3$).
    b. Splenectomy is considered in patients who fail steroid therapy. These patients continue to produce antibody, posing a risk to the fetus.
    c. Cytotoxic agents may be used if the above fails.
    d. Immunoglobulin infusion may be attempted as a temporary measure to raise maternal counts enough to perform cesarean section.
    e. Platelet transfusions are indicated for severe bleeding with counts of $50,000/mm^3$ or immediately before cesarean section in thrombocytopenic mothers.

von Willebrand's Disease

von Willebrand's disease, an inherited disorder of coagulation occurring in 1 of every 1000 people, is marked by a decrease in the von Willebrand's portion of the factor VIII complex. It is usually inherited as an autosomal dominant trait.

1. Diagnosis and presentation. Clinical manifestations include menorrhagia, easy bruising, gingival bleeding, and epistaxis. Patients may first manifest postoperative or postpartum hemorrhage. Postpartum hemorrhage may be delayed as factor VIII-C levels return to normal. Diagnosis is made by a prolonged bleeding time. The partial thromboplastin time (PTT) may be normal or abnormal.
2. Treatment
    a. If factor VIII-C level is greater than 50% normal and if normal bleeding time is present, there is little risk of excessive bleeding during vaginal delivery.
    b. For women who require delivery by cesarean section, factor VIII-C level should be 80% of normal with a normal bleeding time.
    c. If the above criteria are not met, cryoprecipitate should be given before delivery.

AUTOIMMUNE DISEASES
Systemic Lupus Erythematosus

SLE, a chronic autoimmune disease affecting multiple organs, is characterized by exacerbations, and remission occurs most often in women of childbearing age.

1. Clinical manifestations
    a. Skin lesions consisting of malar butterfly rash, alopecia, or discoid lesions are found in 80% of patients. Photosensitivity is common.

   b. Arthralgia with some arthritis is observed in 90% of patients.

   c. Nephritis and neuropsychiatric features are seen in 50% of patients.

2. Laboratory diagnosis

   a. Significant titers of antinuclear antibodys (ANAs) are found in 90% of patients.

   b. Antibodies against DNA are seen in more than 70% of patients.

   c. Extractable nuclear antibodies include anti-RNP, anti-Sm, anti-SS-A (Ro) and anti-SS-B (La). Anti-SS-A and Anti-SS-B are found in 25% and 12% of patients, respectively. These antibodies have been associated with fetal and neonatal heart block.

3. Effect of pregnancy on SLE

   a. Pregnancy does not alter the long-term prognosis of women with SLE.

   b. Worsening disease may develop during pregnancy and puerperium.

   c. Patients should be advised against conception when disease is active. A 6-month disease-free interval is recommended.

4. Effect of SLE on pregnancy

   a. Spontaneous abortion increases 23% to 40%.

   b. Second-trimester losses are common and may be observed in women with only serologic evidence of SLE or the lupus anticoagulant. The lupus anticoagulant is associated with placental infarction. It is present in 15% of women with SLE and is also seen in the absence of lupus. Treatment includes steroid therapy and low doses of aspirin.

   c. Preterm birth occurs in 16% to 37% because of spontaneous preterm labor and obstetric intervention for suspected fetal compromise or maternal complications.

   d. IUGR occurs as a result of vasculitis of decidual and placental vessels.

   e. Stillbirth is often seen (12% to 30%) when lupus nephropathy, lupus anticoagulant, or active disease occur during pregnancy.

5. Treatment during pregnancy

   a. Check for lupus anticoagulant before conception. Treatment with low doses of aspirin and prednisone is indicated in women with the lupus anticoagulant.

   b. Assess baseline renal function and platelet count. Follow these parameters monthly.

   c. Early in pregnancy, check for anti-SS-A and anti-SS-B antibodies (associated with congenital heart block and neonatal cutaneous lupus).

   d. Early sonography to ensure dating serial sonography to assess fetal growth.

   e. Begin antepartum fetal heartrate testing at 28 weeks gestation.

   f. Timing of delivery is individualized according to maternal and fetal condition.

   g. Administer peripartum steroids to prevent postpartum flare of the disease.

Rheumatoid Arthritis

Women are affected two to three times more commonly than men with rheumatoid arthritis, which results in inflammation of synovial membranes.

1. Clinical manifestations

   a. Articular swelling of the metacarpophalangeal joint. Proximal interphalangeal and wrist joints are also involved.

   b. Extraarticular manifestations include rheumatoid nodules, pericarditis, myocarditis, endocarditis, and skin vasculitis. Kidneys are rarely involved.

2. Laboratory findings include rheumatoid factors IgM and IgG directed against IgG. ANA is detectable in 20% percent of patients.

3. Effect of pregnancy on rheumatoid arthritis. Most patients improve during pregnancy; however, postpartum exacerbation is observed in up to 90% of patients.

4. Effect of rheumatoid arthritis on pregnancy. No adverse effect on pregnancy if dis-

ease is limited to joint involvement, but there may be a theoretic risk of IUGR if vasculitis is present.

5. Treatment
    a. Aspirin remains the mainstay therapy. Therapeutic drug level is 15 to 20 mg/dl, requiring ingestion of 3.6 to 4.0 g daily in divided doses. The risks of aspirin therapy during pregnancy include prolonged gestation, increased blood loss at delivery, and newborn clotting disorder.
    b. Gold therapy is not recommended during pregnancy.
    c. Immunosuppressives may be required in severe cases.

Scleroderma/Progressive Systemic Sclerosis

Scleroderma is a collagen vascular disease of unknown etiology resulting in tight, bound-down skin, sclerodactyly, and Raynaud's phenomenon. Gastrointestinal viscera, pulmonary, and renal involvement may be seen in progressive systemic sclerosis (PSS).

1. Laboratory diagnosis
    a. Speckled pattern of ANA is seen in 50% of patients.
    b. Anti-Scl-70 (an extractable unclear antibody) is seen in 40% of patients.
2. Effect of pregnancy on scleroderma/PSS
    a. In women without visceral involvement, 39% experience no change, 30% worsen, and 22% improve.
    b. The disease course in women with PSS is poorly documented.
3. Effect of scleroderma on pregnancy. Preterm birth and stillbirth are increased.
4. Treatment. If visceral involvement is present, termination should be considered. If only skin involvement is present, follow expectantly with knowledge that renal or cardiac involvement may be fatal.

Myasthenia Gravis

An autoimmune disease affecting the motor endplate of skeletal muscles, myasthenia gravis is most common in females of reproductive age. This prevalence is 1/25,000 with a female-to-male ratio of 2:1, and the peak incidence is between ages 20 and 30.

1. Clinical manifestations
    a. Easy fatigability of skeletal muscles with ocular/extraocular muscles often affected, causing ptosis and diplopia.
    b. A total of 60% of patients have an enlarged thymus and 8% have a malignant thymoma. Thymectomy improves symptoms in 40% of patients.
2. Diagnosis
    a. Edrophonium (short-acting acetylcholinesterase [AChE] inhibitor) infusion results in rapid improvement if myasthenia gravis is present.
    b. Serum antibodies against acetylcholine (ACh) receptors are present.
3. Effect of pregnancy on myasthenia gravis. Of these patients, 32% display no change, whereas 41% have more frequent exacerbations and 27% undergo remission during pregnancy. Postpartum exacerbations may be severe.
4. Effect of myasthenia on pregnancy
    a. Preterm labor and delivery are increased (25% to 60%).
    b. Neonatal myasthenia is seen in 10% to 20% of newborns. Onset is within 48 hours of birth and may last weeks. The disease probably results from transplacental passage of IgG directed against ACh receptors.
5. Management
    a. Most patients continue on AChE inhibitors or glucocorticoid therapy, with dosage adjustments often needed.

b. Prolonged second stage of labor may occur because of inefficient expulsive efforts.

c. Epidural anesthesia using amide agents is preferred. Esters may be poorly metabolized in patients receiving AChE inhibitors.

d. Nondepolarizing muscle blockers should be used with caution if general anesthesia is necessary.

e. Magnesium sulfate is contraindicated as it interferes with myoneural transmission.

f. Aminoglycosides and β-mimetics are used with caution as they may precipitate myasthenic crisis. Preterm labor is therefore difficult to treat in women with myasthenia.

GASTROINTESTINAL DISEASE
Peptic Ulcer Disease

Symptoms and complications of peptic ulcer disease seems to decrease during gestation. Improvement in the disease may result from (1) progesterone-induced decreases in gastric acid output, (2) progesterone-induced increases in gastric mucus production, and (3) placental histaminase activity.

1. Diagnosis. Dyspepsia during pregnancy is frequently ascribed to gastroesophageal reflux. This disorder generally responds to antacid therapy and position change. Patients with peptic ulcer disease frequently respond to this regimen as well. In pregnant patients who fail to respond to these measures, panendoscopic examination of the stomach is performed. Barium swallow (upper GI tract) is avoided in pregnancy.

2. Treatment

   a. Primary therapy is antacids and diet. Avoidance of caffeine, salicylates, and ethanol is stressed.

   b. Cimetidine is the secondary therapy chosen in pregnancy. Experience is limited with histamine blockade during gestation.

   c. Bleeding, perforation, and obstruction are treated as in nonpregnant patients.

Acute Pancreatitis

Pancreatitis is found in 1/1000 to 3000 pregnancies. Before the early 1970s, maternal mortality was great with this condition; however, prompt diagnosis is now usual, so maternal death is uncommon. Pancreatitis may be more common during pregnancy because of an increased risk of cholelithiasis and ineffective emptying of the gallbladder.

1. Clinical presentation

   a. The disease is more common in the third trimester and puerperium.

   b. Epigastric pain radiating to the glands or shoulders along with tenderness should prompt laboratory investigation.

   c. Nausea, vomiting, fever, and leukocytosis are often present.

2. Diagnosis

   a. Elevated serum amylase is the hallmark of the disease but may also be seen with cholecystis, intestinal obstruction, peptic ulcer disease, hepatic trauma, and ruptured ectopic pregnancy.

   b. Amylase/creatinine clearance ratio may be useful in pregnancy when serum amylase can be lowered.

3. Treatment

   a. Keep patient NPO.

   b. Provide nasogastric suction.

   c. Administer fluids and electrolytes, including calcium if necessary.

   d. Provide total parenteral nutrition for advanced cases.

   e. Surgery (drainage) is indicated only if the above measures fail.

Inflammatory Bowel Disease

Inflammatory bowel disease, ulcerative colitis, and Crohn's disease (or regional enteritis) are idiopathic disorders with a peak incidence in the reproductive age group. Ulcerative colitis is primarily a disease of the colon or rectum marked by bloody stools, diarrhea, and crampy abdominal pain. Crohn's disease is more subacute, with symptoms of fever, diarrhea, and abdominal pain. Crohn's disease may be found in any location of the GI tract, including the anus, and may also involve the perineum.

1. Ulcerative colitis
   a. Ulcerative colitis has little effect on fertility.
   b. Effect on pregnancy depends on whether the patient is disease-free at conception. For those free of disease symptoms, nearly 90% will achieve term pregnancies, and 30% to 50% will remain disease-free during pregnancy. Women with active disease at conception tend to experience exacerbations during gestation or the postpartum period (75%).
2. Crohn's disease
   a. Patients with large-bowel disease may be subfertile.
   b. Live birth rates exceed 85%, with most pregnancies reaching term, but active Crohn's disease may increase the risk of first-trimester miscarriage.
   c. Disease first occurring during pregnancy carries with it a greatly increased risk of preterm birth, as with any intraperitoneal inflammatory condition.
   d. Women who conceive while in remission tend to remain disease-free (84%), whereas women with active disease at conception experience remission in only 35% of pregnancies.
3. Treatment
   a. Frequent antepartum visits to assess weight gain and disease activity and to provide nutritional counseling are necessary.
   b. Initial therapy for diarrhea includes narcotics. Chronic use should be avoided because it may incite toxic megacolon in patients with ulcerative colitis.
   c. Sulfasalazine and steroid therapy are used if simple measures fail. Sulfasalazine is a weak bilirubin displacer, so it is safe during the third trimester.
   d. Patients with severe dehydration may require hospitalization. Total parenteral nutrition may be necessary in some patients.
   e. Surgery is reserved for perforation or obstruction. Elective surgery (colectomy in patients with ulcerative colitis) is best accomplished following pregnancy.

HEPATOBILIARY DISEASES
Intrahepatic Cholestasis of Pregnancy

Intrahepatic cholestasis of pregnancy is usually characterized by pruritus and mild jaundice during the last trimester. It tends to recur in subsequent pregnancies and may follow oral contraceptive use in susceptible individuals.

1. Clinical manifestations
   a. Pruritus is intense and is often worse at night.
   b. Jaundice follows pruritus in 50% of patients.
   c. Symptoms abate within 48 hours of delivery.
   d. Differential diagnosis includes hepatitis and biliary tract disease. In contrast to these entities, fever and abdominal pain are absent.
2. Laboratory diagnosis

  a. Alkaline phosphatase is increased to 5 to 10 times normal.
  b. Bilirubin is mildly elevated (most is direct fraction).
  c. Serum transaminase levels are normal or mildly elevated.
  d. Serum cholesterol and triglyceride levels are mildly elevated.
  e. Serum bile acids are increased at least 10 times normal.
3. Perinatal outcome. Risk of preterm birth and stillbirth may be elevated; antepartum fetal heartrate testing is therefore recommended.
4. Management
  a. Cholestyramine resin is administered to reduce reabsorption of bile acids.
  b. Antihistamines are of little value in controlling pruritus.
  c. Vitamin K should be administered if the prothrombin time (PT) is prolonged (cholestyramine may inhibit vitamin K absorption).
  d. Phenobarbital may be added (induces hepatic microsomal enzymes, thereby increasing bile salt secretion).

Acute Fatty Liver of Pregnancy

Acute fatty liver, an extremely rare idiopathic condition, results in severe hepatic dysfunction usually during the final month of pregnancy. In the past, maternal mortality rates approached 85%. However, early recognition and prompt delivery have led to survival rates exceeding 70% in recent years.
1. Clinical manifestations
  a. Unrelenting vomiting, severe abdominal pain, and headache are present.
  b. Tenderness is present in the right upper quadrant, and the liver is not palpable.
  c. Jaundice is apparent.
  d. Somnolence and coma signify advanced disease.
2. Laboratory abnormalities
  a. Serum transaminases are elevated but remain below 300 IU/L.
  b. Bilirubin is elevated but rarely above 5 mg/dl.
  c. PT and PTT are prolonged secondary to DIC.
  d. Renal failure is often present.
  e. Hypoglycemia is often profound.
  f. Liver biopsy reveals pericentral microvesicular fatty change.
3. Management
  a. Prompt delivery is indicated once the diagnosis is established, by induction or by cesarean section if the cervix is unfavorable.
  b. Correct coagulopathy with fresh-frozen plasma or cryoprecipitate.
  c. Dextrose should be provided if hypoglycemia is present.

Viral Hepatitis

Hepatitis B is primarily a blood-borne disease, although infection may be transmitted through various body secretions. Thus it is potentially a sexually transmitted disease. Mother-to-infant transmission is a major mode of spread of this infection throughout the world.
1. Clinical manifestations
  a. As many as 75% of infections are asymptomatic.
  b. The incubation period is 30 to 180 days.
  c. Prodromal symptoms may include flulike symptoms, fatigue, nausea and vomiting, arthralgias, and skin rash and may occur in 15% of cases.
  d. Pruritus, reflux upper quadrant pain, and dark urine are followed by the icteric stage.

2. Diagnosis
   a. Differential diagnosis includes acute fatty liver, severe preeclampsia, and chole-static jaundice.
   b. Serologic testing establishes the diagnosis. Presence of the hepatitis B surface antigen (HbsAg) indicates active infection and potential infectivity. The e anti-gen (HbeAg) is associated with great potential for infectivity. Chronic carriers display HbsAg on 2 tests performed 6 months apart. The presence of high anti-body titers to the core antigen may help determine if early infection is present rather than a chronic carrier state.
   c. Serum transaminases are markedly elevated in acute hepatitis. Bilirubin levels may be significantly elevated as well, and the PT may be prolonged.
3. Treatment. In the absence of severe dehydration or coagulopathy, infected individ-uals can be managed as outpatients with nutritional and supportive care.
4. Prevention of disease
   a. Hepatitis B immunoglobulin (HBIg) should be administered if significant expo-sure to HbsAG-positive blood has occurred. Its use is not contraindicated in pregnancy.
   b. Hepatitis vaccine may be administered to at-risk pregnant women. This gener-ally consists of hospital and health care workers.
   c. Women with the following risk factors of HbsAG should be screened early in pregnancy. Some have recommended routine screening for hepatitis for all preg-nant women.
      (1) Asian descent/immigrant.
      (2) Haitian or African origin.
      (3) Unknown liver disease.
      (4) Hemodialysis workers.
      (5) Workers with close contact with mentally retarded persons.
      (6) History of blood transfusions.

NEUROLOGIC DISEASES
Seizure Disorders

Seizure disorders are the most common major neurologic problem complicating preg-nancy, with a frequency of 0.15% of all pregnancies.
1. Effect of pregnancy on epilepsy. Early studies suggested seizure activity increased in 45% percent of women, but these data antedate techniques for measuring anti-convulsant levels. Drug dosages usually need to be increased as the blood volume expands during pregnancy to keep serum drug levels in the therapeutic range.
2. Effect of epilepsy on pregnancy.
   a. Anomalies. Untreated epileptic mothers may have an increased risk of fetal mal-formations; for treated epileptic mothers, the risk of infants with birth defects is increased 8% to 9%. It is unclear whether that risk inherently results from the disorder itself or from the drugs used to treat it. Phenytoin (Dilantin) is a known teratogen. The hydantoin syndrome consists of microcephaly, mild to moderate retardation, growth delay, facial clefts, limb abnormalities, distal phalangeal and nail hypoplasia, and congenital heart disease. The complete syndrome is present in a minority of affected infants. Sonographic prenatal diagnosis is rec-ommended for women using phenytoin during pregnancy. Valproic acid carries with it a 3% risk of neural tube defects. Alpha-fetoprotein analysis and sonog-raphy can establish this diagnosis. Trimethadione, an anticonvulsant, is a potent teratogen used to treat petit mal seizures. A syndrome of IUGR, microcephaly, and facial dysmorphisms has been described with its use.

b. Coagulopathy. Phenytoin, phenobarbital, and primidone may also cause neonatal coagulopathy (suppresses fetal synthesis of vitamin K–dependent factors).
3. Treatment of epilepsy during pregnancy.
  a. Careful monitoring of drug levels is necessary. With expansion of plasma volume, anticonvulsant levels may fall. However, free drug, versus bound drug, is biologically active. Free-drug levels may actually increase as total levels decrease, particularly if serum albumin is depressed. Supplemental folate may be necessary in patients taking phenytoin because it interferes with GI absorption of folate.
  b. Consider withdrawal of antiseizure medication in patients who have been disease-free for many years.
  c. Tonic-clonic seizures should be treated with phenobarbital if possible; it is the oldest, best studied anticonvulsant. If a patient is being successfully treated with phenytoin and has had poor seizure control on other medication, she should remain on this medication.
  d. Detailed sonography to assess fetal anatomy and growth is recommended.
  e. All infants born to women receiving anticonvulsants should receive intramuscular vitamin K after birth to prevent coagulopathy.

Migraine

Migraine may affect as many as 15% to 20% of pregnant women. Classic migraine headaches are accompanied by photosensitivity and nausea. Migraine symptoms tend to improve during pregnancy, with nearly 80% of women reporting amelioration of their headaches.

Supportive therapy consists of aspirin, and, if migraine is severe, narcotics are recommended. Antiemetics may be necessary in some cases. Propranolol may also be used in severe cases as prophylactics for migraine.

Carpal Tunnel Syndrome

Carpal tunnel syndrome, or compression of the median nerve within the retinaculum flexorum, may result from weight gain and fluid accumulation during pregnancy. It is a common neurologic complication of pregnancy. Clinical manifestations include pain, numbness, and tingling in the distribution of the median nerve in the hand and wrist. In severe cases, weakness and decreased motor function may occur.
1. Supportive and conservative therapies are usually adequate. Splints may be placed on the dorsum of the hand to maximize the space of the carpal tunnel. Local injections of steroids are used in severe cases. Diuretics provide only temporary relief. The condition remits spontaneously in most cases within a few weeks of delivery, although recovery may take longer in lactating women.
2. Surgical decompression is performed in cases of deteriorating muscle tone and motor function.

Multiple Sclerosis

Multiple sclerosis (MS) is an idiopathic demyelinating disease that affects men and women equally. The disease is characterized by exacerbations and remission. Less than a third of patients show steady progression of disease.

Clinical manifestations include weakness of one or both of the lower extremities, visual complaints, and loss of coordination. The diagnosis is made by finding an elevated IgG in cerebrospinal fluid. However, this is a nonspecific finding. There is no specific therapy, although steroids are helpful if optic neuritis develops.

Pregnancy does not appear to increase the chance of disease activation, although most flares occur during the puerperium. There is no increase in perinatal mortality. Maternal urinary retention may occur postpartum, and UTIs are most frequent throughout pregnancy.

Cerebrovascular Disease

1. Arterial occlusion. The incidence of cerebral arterial occlusion during pregnancy is 1/20,000 live births. Mortality rates are increased several fold in pregnant women. Hemiplegia and dysphasia are frequent findings of middle cerebral artery occlusion. Predisposing factors such as preeclampsia, chronic hypertension, or puerperal hypotension are present in a third of patients. Physical and rehabilitative therapy are begun as soon as possible.
2. Cortical vein thrombosis. This disorder occurs most often during the postpartum period (1 in 10,000 pregnancies) and may be attributable to a hypercoagulable state. Clinical manifestations include headache, lethargy, and vomiting. Hemiplegia is gradual in onset, and seizure activity is common. The diagnosis is made by cerebral CT scan. Phenytoin is give to prevent convulsions.
3. Subarachnoid hemorrhage. The rate of subarachnoid hemorrhage is 1/10,000 pregnancies, with berry aneurysms or arteriovenous (A-V) malformations being the usual origin. A-V malformations tend to bleed before 20 weeks gestation, whereas berry aneurysms often bleed later in pregnancy. Pregnancy increases the risk of bleeding from an untreated A-V malformation, with a maternal mortality rate of 33%.
   a. Management in pregnancy is the same as for nonpregnant individuals and is surgical whenever possible. Surgery under hypothermia may be performed during pregnancy. Patients treated successfully may deliver vaginally. Epidural anesthesia is recommended, with decreased Valsalva efforts.
   b. In women with untreated or inoperable lesions, there is controversy about the safest mode of delivery. Although conclusive evidence of benefit is lacking, cesarean section is often recommended for these patients.

Pseudotumor Cerebri

Pseudotumor cerebri is more common in pregnant women than in nonpregnant women. The origin is unknown, although increased cerebrospinal fluid (CSF) prolactin levels have been demonstrated in affected individuals. Decreased CSF production may be related to this observation. Pregnancy outcome is unaffected by this illness.

Clinical manifestations include headaches in 95%, diplopia in 15%, and papilledema in 100% of patients. Elevated CSF pressure and absence of mass on CT scan confirm the diagnosis.

The objectives of therapy are relief from pain and preservation of vision, as for nonpregnant patients. Visual fields should be carefully followed. Acetazolamide diuresis will reduce CSF production in many patients and can be used during pregnancy. Prednisone may be added if necessary. Surgical approaches for visual deterioration are used in severe cases. Vaginal delivery with epidural anesthesia and a shortened second stage of labor is recommended. Cesarean section may be performed for obstetric indications. The recurrence risk in subsequent pregnancy is 10% to 12%.

MALIGNANT DISEASES

Cancer complicates approximately 1 in 1000 pregnancies, whereas slightly less than 1% of women found to have cancer will be pregnant at the time of diagnosis. Malignancy coexisting with pregnancy raises great concerns about therapy and its risks to the mother and fetus. In general, pregnancy does not seem to adversely affect maternal cancer, yet delayed diagnosis can clearly influence the stage of the disease and thus survival. The following section outlines the more common nongynecologic malignancies found in pregnant women.

Breast Cancer

Approximately 15% of breast malignancies occur in women under the age of 41, with 2% to 3% diagnosed during pregnancy. The outlook for the gravid patient with breast cancer is not much different from that for nonpregnant individuals. Pregnancy appears to decrease the risk of breast neoplasia. Multiparous women, particularly those who have breast-fed, have a lower incidence of breast cancer than do nulliparous women.

1. Detection and diagnosis
   a. Breast examination should be performed at initial visit, and women should be educated regarding breast self-examination during pregnancy.
   b. Masses with or without unilateral discharge require prompt evaluation. Mammography is of limited value during pregnancy because of increased density of the breast.
   c. Fine-needle aspiration for cytologic study is the primary diagnosis procedure during pregnancy. An equivocal cytologic diagnosis requires excision of the tumor under local anesthesia.
2. Prognosis
   a. The 5-year (82%) and 10-year (71%) survival rates for women without nodal disease are similar to those observed in nonpregnant women.
   b. Prognosis depends on the stage of disease at the time of diagnosis. During pregnancy, 62% to 85% of women have positive axillary nodes at the time of diagnosis. Delay in diagnosis probably increases the proportion of women found to have advanced disease.
3. Treatment
   a. Mastectomy is often used to treat early disease, regardless of gestational age. The risk of miscarriage is less than 1%.
   b. Patients who are candidates for wide local excision and axillary node samplings followed by radiation are often advised to terminate pregnancy because fetal radiation exposure may be excessive.
   c. There is no benefit to prophylactic abortion or oophorectomy.
   d. Systemic chemotherapy may be undertaken during later pregnancy with minimal risks, but treatment during the first trimester with certain cytotoxic drugs may be harmful to the fetus.
4. Subsequent pregnancy. Although pregnancy does not affect survival, women without nodal disease should wait 2 to 3 years before contemplating pregnancy. Patients with nodal disease should wait at least 5 years before considering pregnancy. A full metastatic workup should be undertaken in these women before pregnancy because of the difficulty in detecting recurrences during pregnancy.

Hodgkin's Disease

Hodgkin's disease complicates approximately 1 in 6000 pregnancies. Fertility is probably unaffected by early disease, and spontaneous abortion and stillbirth rates are no higher than those in the general population. Preterm birth is not increased, and pregnancy does not appear to have an adverse effect on the course of disease. Transplacental dissemination has rarely been reported.

1. Diagnosis. Hodgkin's disease often manifests as an enlarged cervical or axillary lymph node. Systemic symptoms consist of fever, night sweats, and weight loss. The diagnosis is established by biopsy and histologic examination of suspicious nodes.
2. Staging. Minimal staging during pregnancy includes chest radiograph, liver function tests, bone marrow biopsy, complete blood cell count, and urinalysis. A chest CT scan may be necessary to evaluate nodal disease in the thorax. A complete staging laparotomy carries a risk of preterm labor and is therefore best avoided after 24 to 26 weeks gestation. Modified lymphangiography or magnetic resonance imaging (MRI) may be undertaken.
3. Treatment. Early-stage disease is treated with radiation, but disseminated disease or bulky masses probably require chemotherapy (i.e., with nitrogen mustard, vincristine, procarbazine, and prednisone). When subdiaphragmatic disease occurs in pregnancy, abdominal shielding and fetal dosimetry are recommended. Pregnancy termination is an option for those with disease discovered during the first half of gestation. Chemotherapeutic regimens are used with caution, yet many successful pregnancies have occurred following MOPP chemotherapy. Advanced disease should be treated aggressively, with early delivery performed if necessary.
4. Subsequent pregnancy. Following treatment, pregnancy should not be attempted for at least 2 years to facilitate appropriate follow-up care. Fertility may be greatly reduced by radiation and/or chemotherapy. Patients receiving both therapies have a significantly lower chance of retaining normal ovulatory function. Age is an important determinant of the likelihood of subsequent fertility.

Acute Leukemia

Acute leukemia occurs in fewer than 1 in 75,000 pregnancies. Intensive chemotherapy in older patients has been primarily effective in achieving remissions so that a third of patients with acute lymphocytic leukemia appear to be long-term disease-free survivors after 4 to 5 years.

1. Diagnosis. Symptoms include fatigue, fever, infection, and easy bleeding with petechiae. Leukemia is suggested by an elevated WBC, but some patients may be leukopenic. Diagnosis is confirmed by bone marrow biopsy and aspirate. Acute myelocytic leukemia accounts for 50% of acute leukemia found in pregnancy. There is no evidence that pregnancy has a deleterious effect on the course of leukemia. Fetal survival approaches 90%.
2. Therapy. Exposure to chemotherapeutic agents during the first trimester, particularly folate antagonists, is associated with a significant risk for malformations, but there are several reports of successful pregnancies in mothers treated aggressively with combined chemotherapy. Exposure to single drugs or combination therapy during the second and third trimesters generally has not been associated with fetal malformation.

Chronic Leukemia

Chronic leukemia accounts for 50% of cases of leukemia during pregnancy, with most being chronic myelogenous leukemia (CML). The diagnosis is again made by leukocytosis and bone marrow aspiration. Granulocyte counts average 200,000/dl, and thrombocytosis and normochromic normocytic anemia are common. Pregnancy does not adversely affect CML, but, not surprisingly, chemotherapy increases the likelihood of preterm birth and low birthweight. An attempt should be made to limit chemotherapy to the second and third trimesters.

Melanoma

One to ten percent of all melanomas are discovered during gestation. Melanoma is the most common tumor to metastasize to the placenta, although this is a rare phenomenon. Melanoma occurring during pregnancy occurs in less favorable locations (e.g., the trunk) and is found in a more advanced stage than that found in nonpregnant women. The vulva is the site of 7% of melanomas. Fair-skinned women are at greatest risk. Any suspicious change in a preexisting mole warrants biopsy.

When the stage of the disease and primary site are considered, prognosis is not worsened by pregnancy. Advanced metastatic disease carries with it a bleak prognosis and is treated with combined chemotherapy employing nitrosoureas. Abortion should be considered if metastatic disease is found before 20 weeks gestation. Pregnancy should be avoided for several years in treated patients and may be inadvisable if nodal metastases have been detected.

REVIEW QUESTIONS

Key: a, 1,2,3 correct   d, 4
      b, 1,3 correct   e, all correct
      c, 2,4 correct

1. Cardiac output during pregnancy:
   1. Increases 30-50% over baseline by 20-24 weeks gestation.
   2. Falls in the supine position in early pregnancy due to venacaval compression by the uterus.
   3. Increases 20 percent during labor and delivery.
   4. Is decreased in twin gestation.
   5. Is increased with epidural anesthesia during labor.
2. Mitral stenosis during pregnancy:
   1. Is the most common form of rheumatic heart disease in pregnancy.
   2. Is complicated by congestive heart failure in 25% of cases.
   3. May be treated with commisurotomy or valve replacement in patients refractory to medical therapy.
   4. Is an indication for primary cesarean section.
   5. Is often a result of mitral valve prolapse in young women.
3. Active tuberculosis during pregnancy:
   1. Is present if the PPD skin test is positive.
   2. Is treated with isoniazid if the PPD test becomes positive.
   3. Is often seen in patients that have received BCG vaccine.
   4. Represents a high risk condition for disease in the offspring of women with active disease.
   5. Should be treated after pregnancy is completed.
4. The following statements are true concerning urinary tract infection in pregnancy:
   1. All pregnant women should be screened for asymptomatic bacteriuria on their first prenatal visit.
   2. Untreated asymptomatic bacteriuria will progress to pyelonephritis in 40% of untreated women.
   3. *E. coli* is the most common organism found in aymptomatic bacteruria.
   4. Patients with recurrent UTI should undergo an IVP during pregnancy.
   5. Asymptomatic bacteriuria is defined as a colony count greater than 50,000 colonies/ml of a single organism.
5. These statements are true concerning carbohydrate metabolism in pregnancy:
   1. Increased insulin secretion is evident by the end of the first trimester.

2. Relative maternal fasting hypoglycemia is present.
3. Human placental lactogen (LPL) stimulates lipolysis in adepose tissue thereby. sparing glucose as a fuel.
4. Glucose crosses the placenta by carrier-medicated facilitated diffusion.
5. Postprandial hyperglycemia is most common in the third trimester.

6. Gestational diabetes mellitus:
   1. Carries with it a risk for overt diabetes in later life.
   2. Is diagnosed by the 50 gram oral glucose screen.
   3. Represents 90% of the cases of diabetes in pregnancy.
   4. Is generally managed with multiple injections of insulin.
   5. Is present if a patient has been treated with oral hypoglycemic agents prior to pregnancy.

7. Hyperthyroidism secondary to Graves disease:
   1. Is the most common etiology for hyperthyroidism during pregnancy.
   2. Should be controlled in order to lower the risk of preterm birth and low birthweight.
   3. Is a risk for hypothyroidism in the fetus if maternal thiouracil therapy is employed.
   4. Is diagnosed if total T_4 levels are elevated.
   5. Should be treated with thyroidectomy because propylthiouracil may cross the placenta.

8. The following statements are true concerning ITP during pregancy:
   1. Disease usually worsens in early pregnancy.
   2. Maternal platelet count is a poor predictor of fetal platelet count.
   3. Delivery should be by cesarean section.
   4. Glucocorticoids are used to treat maternal thrombocytopenia.
   5. Continuous immunoglobulin therapy throughout pregnancy may be helpful.

9. The following medical conditions may predispose to preterm birth:
   1. Systemic lupus erythematosus.
   2. Myasthenia gravis.
   3. Crohn's disease.
   4. Breast cancer.
   5. Epilepsy.

10. Acute fatty liver of pregnancy:
    1. Usually occurs during the final month of pregnancy.
    2. May produce symptomatic hypoglycemia.
    3. May lead to renal failure.
    4. Rarely produces jaundice.
    5. Is often a secondary complication of viral hepatitis.

ANSWERS

1. b	4. b	7. a
2. a	5. e	8. c
3. d	6. b	9. a
		10. a

BIBLIOGRAPHY

Burrow GN, and Ferris TF: Medical complications during pregnancy, ed 3, Philadelphia, 1988, WB Saunders Co.

Hollingsworth DR, and Resnik, R: Medical counseling before pregnancy, New York, 1988, Churchill & Livingstone.

Lindheimer MD, and Barron WM: Medical disorders during pregnancy: a symposium issue devoted to this topic, Clin Perinatol 12:481, 1985.

Samuels P, and Landon MB: Medical complications. In Gabbe SC, Niebyl JR, and Simpson JL, editors: Obstetrics: normal and problem pregnancies, New York, 1986, Churchill & Livingstone.

Premature Birth

8

Jay D. Iams

DEFINITIONS

Premature birth, which is defined by gestational age (regardless of birth weight), is a birth before 37 menstrual weeks of gestation (i.e., more than 21 days before the estimated due date).

Low birth weight, on the other hand, is defined by weight (regardless of gestational age); a weight of less than 2500 g constitutes low birth weight, and weight less than 1500 g is called *very low birth weight.*

Intrauterine growth retardation (IUGR) is defined as weight less than the 10th percentile for the gestational age at birth.

An infant may therefore be one, two, or all three of the above. For example, an infant weighing 2600 g at birth at 34 weeks gestation would be premature but would not have low birth weight or growth retardation. An infant weighing 1499 g at 31 weeks gestation would not be growth retarded but would be premature (also called *preterm*) and have very low birth weight. These distinctions are clinically important because the consequences of prematurity differ from those of IUGR, although there is certainly some overlap.

IMPORTANCE OF LOW BIRTH WEIGHT AND PREMATURITY

Among infants without congenital anomalies, more than 75% of all *perinatal* (defined as the time period between 20 weeks gestation and 28 days of neonatal life) morbidity and mortality is due to complications of prematurity and low birth weight.

Morbidity of Prematurity

1. Pulmonary
   a. Respiratory distress syndrome (RDS)
   b. Bronchopulmonary dysplasia
   c. Pneumothorax and interstitial emphysema
2. Cardiovascular
   a. Hypotension
   b. Persistent fetal circulation
   c. Patent ductus arteriosus
   d. Sudden infant death syndrome
3. Central nervous system
   a. Intracranial hemorrhage
   b. Apnea/bradycardia
   c. Vision/hearing problems
4. Gastrointestinal
   a. Necrotizing enterocolitis

    b. Inadequate nutrition
5. Metabolic
    a. Hypothermia
    b. Hypoglycemia
    c. Hypocalcemia
    d. Jaundice
6. Infectious
    a. Generalized sepsis
    b. Increased susceptibility to:
       (1) Herpes simplex
       (2) Group B streptococcus
       (3) Listeria monocytogenes
7. Psychosocial
    a. Poor parent/child attachment
       (1) Subsequent child abuse

There has been little recent progress in reducing the prevalence of premature birth in the United States, which is currently about 10% of all births, nor in reducing the prevalence of low birth weight, which is currently about 7% to 8% of all births. Recent improvements in perinatal and neonatal survival have occurred rather as a result of better neonatal care for preterm infants.

EPIDEMIOLOGY OF LOW BIRTH WEIGHT

The epidemiology of births less than 2500 g varies throughout the world. In underdeveloped nations, the majority of births of infants less than 2500 g is due to IUGR, with a minority caused by prematurity. The ratio is reversed in more affluent countries like the United States, where two thirds of infants with low birth weight are preterm and one third are growth retarded (Fig. 8-1).

Spontaneous Versus Indicated Preterm Birth

An *indicated* preterm birth is one in which the intrauterine environment is more hazardous to the fetus than the risks of prematurity. These comprise about 30% of all preterm births and are caused by maternal or fetal disorders such as:
1. Hypertension
2. Diabetes
3. Isoimmunization
4. IUGR
5. Abruptio placentae or placenta previa

A *spontaneous* preterm birth is one in which the intrauterine fetal environment is presumed to be favorable until spontaneous preterm labor or preterm premature rupture of membranes. (A word of explanation is in order here about the confusing nomenclature of ruptured membranes: *Premature* rupture of the membranes (PROM) refers to rupture of the amniotic sac before the onset of labor at any gestational age. It is therefore necessary to add the seemingly redundant word *preterm* to *premature rupture of membranes* when this occurs before 37 weeks gestation.)

Spontaneous preterm births account for approximately 70% of preterm deliveries in the United States.

Etiology of Spontaneous Preterm Births

The cause(s) of spontaneous preterm delivery is at present incompletely understood, but it appears to be the result of premature initiation of the processes leading to normal

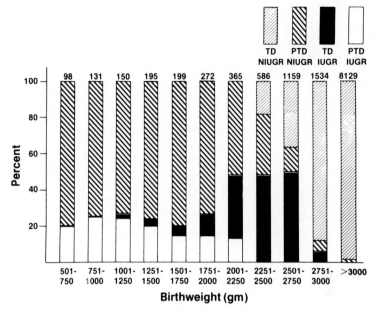

Fig. 8-1
The percentages of infants in various birth-weight categories classified as term and not growth re-
tarded *(TD NIUGR)*, preterm and not growth retarded *(PTD NIUGR)*, term and growth retarded *(TD
IUGR)*, and preterm and growth retarded *(PTD IUGR)*.
From Goldenberg RL, et al: Am J Obstet Gynecol 152:980, 1985.

labor at term. This may occur because of inflammatory or infectious stimuli to prostaglandin production by the decidua, with subsequent development of labor. These or
other stimuli may lead in some cases to enzymatic degradation of the amnion, leading
to rupture and then to labor. The interrelated nature of preterm labor and preterm
PROM is suggested by the similar, if not entirely identical, epidemiology attending
each condition, as the following summarizes.

Epidemiology of spontaneous preterm births

1. Demographic risks
   a. Low socioeconomic status (SES)
      (1) Preterm PROM more common with very low SES
      (2) Preterm labor more common than preterm PROM in private patients
   b. Maternal age less than 18
   c. Low education (not a high-school graduate)
   d. Unmarried/limited social support
   e. Black women, independent of SES, have a two to three times greater risk
2. Obstetrical history
   a. Prior preterm/low birth weight delivery—threefold to sixfold increase in risk
      (to 25% to 50% chance of premature birth)
   b. Prior second trimester loss or abortion or cervical cerclage
   c. History of first trimester abortion does *not* carry much risk of subsequent pre-
      term birth *unless* cervix is injured

3. Medical history
   a. Anemia—hematocrit less than 34%
   b. Urinary tract infection, especially pyelonephritis
   c. Uterine malformation
      (1) Diethylstilbestrol exposure
      (2) Müllerian duct fusion anomaly (septate, bicornuate)
      (3) Large uterine fibroids
      (4) Cervical dilation
   d. Vaginal infection—vaginosis, chlamydia, possibly others
4. Behavioral
   a. Smoking—very common among women with preterm births
   b. Inadequate prenatal care
   c. Stress
   d. Poor nutrition
5. Current pregnancy risks
   a. Multiple gestation—33% to 50% of twins and 75% or more of triplets will be delivered preterm
   b. Premature cervical dilation
      (1) Risk of preterm birth is approximately 20% to 25% if the internal cervical os is dilated more than 1 cm before 34 weeks
   c. Bleeding may be a cause of indicated preterm birth, as in placenta previa or abruptio placentae; women who have unexplained bleeding after 14 weeks gestation also have a greater risk of spontaneous prematurity (about 33%)

PREVENTION OF PREMATURITY/LOW BIRTH WEIGHT

Prevention of prematurity is a difficult and elusive goal. Prevention of indicated preterm births will require improved prevention, diagnosis, and therapy of the multiple medical and obstetrical disorders that currently conclude with a necessary premature delivery. Improvements in spontaneous preterm birth rates will require diverse strategies aimed at eliminating both medical and social risk factors and at improved care of patients with preterm labor once it occurs.

Strategies to Prevent Prematurity

1. Prepregnancy
   a. Promote *planned* pregnancy
   b. Eliminate/modify medical risks
      (1) Anemia
      (2) Smoking
      (3) Nutritional deficits
      (4) Cervicovaginal infections
      (5) Urinary tract infection
   c. Avoid unnecessary cervical trauma
   d. Educate the public, especially reproductive-age females, about the hazards of preterm birth
2. During pregnancy
   a. Education for all pregnant women about the medical and social risks associated with preterm birth
   b. Increased awareness of the early warning symptoms of preterm labor:
      (1) Contractions at a rate of more than four an hour, with or without pain
      (2) Pelvic pressure

(3) Increased vaginal discharge

(4) Menstrual-like cramps or backache

c. Frequent contact with high-risk women—a large and contradictory literature exists on this subject, but most studies show some benefit

d. Prophylactic medication

(1) Progesterone and β-mimetic drugs have been used in this way, but there is no evidence of benefit

e. Prophylactic cerclage

(1) This procedure has been proposed for use in women without cervical incompetence who have increased risk for preterm birth; it has not been found effective in these patients

f. Prophylactic antibiotics

(1) Increased evidence linking infection to prematurity has led to interest in using prophylactic antibiotics.

g. Increased rest—the "chicken soup" of obstetrics, recommended for most pregnancy problems

Some or all of the above have been combined into prematurity prevention programs in large clinics, states, or even entire nations (such as France). Most, but not all, have found some decrease in the prevalence of prematurity; more data is necessary.

MANAGEMENT OF PRETERM LABOR
Diagnosis

To make the diagnosis of preterm labor, all of the following must be present:

1. Gestational age greater than 20 weeks and less than 37 weeks

2. Uterine contractions occurring at a rate of more than six an hour, despite bedrest and hydration

3. Change in the dilation, effacement, position, length, or consistency of the cervix between one examination and the next

Initial evaluation

1. Place patient in lateral recumbent position and give oral or IV fluids while obtaining history

2. Monitor contractions and fetal heart with a continuous fetal monitor

3. Look for contraindications to arrest of labor: Is this an indicated preterm birth?

a. Maternal contraindications

(1) Heart disease—β-mimetic drugs hazardous

(2) Hypertension, especially if acute

(3) Hyperglycemia—poorly controlled diabetes is a contraindication to β-mimetics

(4) Hemorrhage—a matter of degree; spotting associated with preterm labor is not a contraindication, but significant vaginal bleeding from any cause does contraindicate tocolysis

(5) Hyperthyroidism

b. Fetal contraindications

(1) Fetal demise or lethal anomaly

(2) Uncorrectable fetal distress

(3) IUGR in the presence of fetal pulmonary maturity

(4) Ruptured membranes or suspected amnionitis

4. Ultrasonographic evaluation

a. Fetal presentation and weight (possible IUGR)

    b. Placental location
    c. Amniotic fluid volume
    d. Fetal anomaly screen
5. Laboratory evaluation
    a. Complete blood cell count—anemia, occult infection
    b. Urinalysis and culture
    c. Vaginal group B streptococcus culture—this potential pathogen is found in the vagina of 15% to 30% of normal women, but in more than 40% of women with preterm labor and preterm PROM; intrapartum antibiotics can eliminate it in most cases
    d. Evaluation of blood glucose, electrolytes, and creatinine because tocolytics can lead to metabolic derangements
    e. Electrocardiogram, if any suspicion of heart disease
    f. C-reactive protein analysis: if greater than 0.8, then 80% chance of delivery in less than 7 days; if less than 0.8, then 80% chance of continuing pregnancy for more than 7 days
6. Role of amniocentesis
    a. To identify subclinical infection, which is seen in 20% to 25% of patients with preterm labor, especially if white blood cell count is greater than 15,000 or if contractions persist despite treatment
    b. To evaluate fetal pulmonary maturity if dates are uncertain and estimates overlap term/preterm or if IUGR or fetal compromise is suspected

The goal of therapy for premature labor is delivery at term, when morbidity and mortality are lowest. Treatment once begun should therefore continue until 36 to 37 weeks, unless the intrauterine environment becomes hazardous to the infant (e.g., preterm PROM or IUGR) or significant side effects occur.

Choice of Tocolytic

β-Sympathomimetic agents

β-Sympathomimetic agents (see Table 8-1) act by stimulating the β-2 receptor in the myometrial muscle cell, leading to a decrease in free intracellular calcium, which is in turn necessary for muscle contraction. Complications and side effects are associated with β-1 and β-2 receptor stimulation elsewhere in the body, producing tachycardia, widened pulse pressure, hyperglycemia, and hypokalemia in most patients. Ritodrine has been approved specifically for use as a tocolytic. Terbutaline, which is marketed as a bronchodilator for use by persons with asthma, has an abundant literature to guide its use as a tocolytic, but it is not specifically approved by the FDA for this purpose.

Magnesium sulfate

Magnesium sulfate (see Table 8-1) acts by directly competing with calcium in its role in muscle contraction. It has a long history of safe use as an anticonvulsant in pregnant women with severe preeclampsia.

Other agents

A number of other drugs have labor-arresting (tocolytic) properties, including the antiprostaglandin drug, indomethacin; the calcium channel blockers, nifedipine, nicardipine, and diltiazem; and diazoxide, an antihypertensive. None have been sufficiently evaluated to recommend for use at present.

Table 8-1   Tocolytic choices

Agent	Dose and Route of Administration	Side Effects/Comments
Ritodrine	50-350 μg/min IV; start at 50 μg/min; increase by 50 μg/min every 20 min, until labor stops or side effects occur, to a maximum of 350 μg/min; once contractions cease, hold infusion rate for 60 min, then decrease by 50 μg/min until lowest effective dose; sustain this rate for 12 hr; oral ritodrine 20 μg every 2 hr × 24 hr, then every 4 hr	Only FDA-approved agent **Maternal Side Effects** Tachycardia—decrease rate if maternal pulse is 120-130; arrhythmia—decrease rate and get ECG, serum K+; chest pain—stop infusion and check ECG and serum K+; hyperglycemia—usually requires no treatment in non-diabetics; hypokalemia—no treatment unless arrhythmia is also present; pulmonary edema—see text under Complications of Therapy **Neonatal Side Effects** Rate unless IV infusion continued to within few hours of delivery—hypoglycemia, hypocalcemic ileus
Terbutaline	0.25 mg SQ every 1-3 hr; useful before transfer to tertiary center; oral dose 2.5-5.0 mg every 2-4 hr	**Maternal and Neonatal Side Effects** Maternal and neonatal side effects same as ritodrine; not FDA approved, but has abundant support in literature; can use larger doses than for preeclampsia with relative safety because patients with preterm labor rarely have impaired renal function
Magnesium sulfate	4-6 g loading dose followed by 2-4 g/hr infusion; intravenous magnesium sulfate usually followed by oral β-mimetic, but some favor oral magnesium gluconate 1 g po q 4 hr	**Maternal Side Effects** Nausea, vomiting, flushing, respiratory depression, pulmonary edema; diarrhea with oral magnesium **Neonatal Side Effects** Hypotonia, respiratory depression, hypocalcemia

Complications of therapy

Tocolytic drugs are potent agents with abundant potential for serious side effects and complications. The relative youth and good health of most women with premature labor allow them to tolerate these drugs in most instances, but complaints of side effects should never be ignored. Complications, particularly pulmonary edema, are more likely in the following situations:
1. Multiple gestation
2. Maternal anemia (hematocrit less than 34%)
3. Occult amnionitis or abruption
4. Unrecognized/undiagnosed heart disease
5. Combination therapy with multiple tocolytics
6. Prolonged (more than 24 hours) infusion of parenteral drugs
7. Concurrent administration of steroids
8. Maternal age of more than 30 years

Follow-up of successful tocolysis

The duration of hospitalization required for the patient with preterm labor is governed by a number of factors:
1. Status of the cervix
2. Associated medical problems (e.g., anemia, group B streptococcus colonization, urinary tract infection)
3. Home support and patient compliance
Those with advanced cervical dilation or effacement (greater than 2-cm dilation and/or greater than 80% effaced) or with intractable medical or social problems may need to remain in the hospital until minimal fetal morbidity/mortality is assured, which is usually at 34 weeks.

Use of Steroids

Glucocorticoids (betamethasone, dexamethasone, hydrocortisone) given to the mother within 7 days of a preterm delivery have been shown to reduce the frequency and severity of neonatal RDS, which is also called *hyaline membrane disease*. This disorder is caused by an absolute or relative deficiency of surfactant in the lung of the newborn premature infant. The process of fetal lung maturation is accelerated in some, but not all, fetuses whose mothers receive these drugs. Maternal complications from the short, 24-hour course of steroid therapy are very uncommon; only fear of unanticipated fetal/newborn/childhood sequelae brings some caution to their use. Steroids act in a general way to promote maturation at the expense of growth. Although no untoward effects have been seen in adolescents treated with betamethasone as fetuses, the use of steroids is currently considered to be indicated only when an unavoidable preterm delivery is imminent. Wide differences of opinion about what constitutes *unavoidable* and *imminent* exist among both obstetricians and pediatricians. Betamethasone is the agent in widest use, at a dose of 12 mg IM, q 12 hours × 2 doses. It is important to remember that the premature neonate may suffer significant morbidity because of immature organs other than the lungs; steroids therefore are not a "magic bullet" for averting the consequences of premature delivery.

MANAGEMENT OF PREMATURELY RUPTURED MEMBRANES

Premature rupture of membranes (PROM) is defined as rupture of the amniotic sac before the onset of labor, regardless of gestational age. It may therefore occur at term as well as preterm, but management differs according to gestational age.

The incidence is 5% to 15% of all deliveries and 30% to 40% of all deliveries before 37 weeks.

Diagnosis

1. A history of watery vaginal discharge or perineal wetness; may be either a sudden gush or persistent wetness
2. Pelvic examination with a sterile speculum, showing pooled amniotic fluid in the posterior vaginal vault
3. Confirmed by laboratory results showing characteristic fern pattern of dried fluid on a slide and pH of the fluid in the vagina (Nitrazine test) greater than 7.0
4. Ultrasonography may also confirm, or even suggest, the diagnosis, showing decreased or absent fluid in the uterus

Once the diagnosis is confirmed, the first and most important task is assessment of the gestational age. This is the first step in weighing the relative risks of continuing the pregnancy versus delivery of the infant. Management of PROM is summarized in the box below.

PROM Management Summary

1. Make a firm diagnosis
2. Establish gestational age
   a. More than 37 weeks:
      (1) Deliver if any of the following:
         (a) Ripe cervix
         (b) Abnormal fetal heart–rate tracing
         (c) Meconium-stained fluid
         (d) Any question of infection
            • Any history of herpes or group B streptococcus
         (e) Abnormal presentation (e.g., breech)
         (f) Maternal/fetal disease or anomaly
      (2) May wait for labor if cervix is unripe and *none* of the above are present
   b. Less than 37 weeks:
      (1) Deliver if any of the following:
         (a) Mature fetal pulmonary status: phosphatidylglycerol present or L/S $\geq$ 2:1
         (b) Abnormal fetal heart–rate tracing
         (c) Intrauterine infection suspected
            • Less evidence of infection required to choose delivery as gestational age approaches term; more evidence required for the extremely preterm infant
      (2) May wait for labor/infection/pulmonary maturity if none of the above are present
      (3) Alternate strategies:
         (a) Steroids, with or without immediate delivery — benefit is debatable; PROM may itself hasten lung maturity and may be associated with more infection — this is controversial
         (b) Tocolytics — no evidence of prolongation in random prospective trials; minimal, if any, benefit
         (c) Antibiotics — classic teaching is no benefit, but there are some recent studies to the contrary

PROM Before 37 Weeks

Rupture of the membranes without labor before 37 weeks is preterm PROM. Because the gestational age is less than 37 weeks, there are potential risks associated with both continued intrauterine and extrauterine existence for the fetus. This is especially so for pregnancies of less than 34 weeks. Therefore management of this situation becomes a continuous process of weighing the risks of delivery versus expectant management.

When preterm PROM occurs, the majority of women will go into spontaneous labor within 48 hours, and 80% will labor and deliver within 7 days of the time of rupture. Preterm labor and delivery are therefore the most frequent complications of preterm PROM. The risks of preterm delivery have been listed at the beginning of this chapter. The risk of RDS throughout pregnancy is shown in Table 8-2.

Risks of continuing the pregnancy include:

1. Infection
   a. About 10% (range 5% to 40%) of women with preterm PROM will develop amnionitis or intrauterine infection before delivery
   b. Of those mothers who become infected, about 5% will deliver infected infants
   c. The rate of perinatal mortality caused by amnionitis and neonatal sepsis in recent series is 0% to 13%
   d. Factors affecting the prevalence of infection in this situation include colonization with aggressive perinatal pathogens (e.g., group B streptococcus), SES, and residual fluid volume in the uterus
   e. Methods to detect amnionitis are not ideal and include serial uterine examinations, white blood cell counts, and observation of fever or fetal tachycardia. Amniocentesis is helpful but not always possible with ruptured membranes. Biophysical profile scoring may be helpful in some cases.
2. Other risks
   a. Cord prolapse—more common if the presentation of the fetus is breech
   b. Pulmonary hypoplasia—may occur in cases of prolonged preterm PROM, especially when gestational age is less than 25 weeks because the absence of amniotic fluid leads to inadequate fetal pulmonary development
   c. Abruptio placentae—also more common in cases of preterm PROM that occur before 25 weeks gestation

PROM After 37 Weeks

When membrane rupture without labor complicates pregnancy at term, there is presumably no advantage to the fetus in continuing the pregnancy. Traditional obstetric

Table 8-2   Frequency of respiratory distress syndrome

Gestational Age (weeks)	Chance of RDS (%)
Less than 28	62
29-30	61
31-32	41
33-34	24
35	6.5
36	3.4
37 or more	0.5

Source: March of Dimes Multicenter Prematurity Prevention Trial Data.

teaching has therefore favored the prompt induction of labor when PROM occurs at term because of the association of increased rates of newborn infection with increasing rupture-to-delivery intervals. The rates of newborn infection accompanying PROM at term are less than commonly thought; they were less than 3% to 4% in recent series. On the maternal side, induction of labor with PROM at term has been shown to produce rates of cesarean section as high as 50% because of failed induction.

These statistics have led to a reassessment of the traditional policy of routine induction. When the cervix is known to be "ripe" (i.e., ready for labor), prompt induction remains the best policy. If there is any evidence of fetal compromise (e.g., meconium-stained fluid or decelerations of the fetal heart rate on continuous monitoring), induction should be undertaken without regard to the status of the cervix. However, when the cervix is known to be long, closed, and firm, a policy of judicious observation may be followed as long as there is no evidence of fetal compromise. Recent series evaluating this approach have shown a decreased rate of cesarean delivery without an increase in neonatal infection.

REVIEW
QUESTIONS

More than one correct answer is possible.
1. In what percentage of premature births does a hostile intrauterine environment favor premature delivery?
   a. 20%
   b. 30%
   c. 40%
   d. 50%
   e. 60%
2. Which of the following are associated with preterm delivery?
   a. Black race
   b. Anemia
   c. Cigarette smoking
   d. Urinary tract infection
   e. All of the above
3. Contraindications to tocolytic drugs include:
   a. Maternal herpes
   b. Maternal heart disease
   c. Fetus with cleft palate
   d. Severe preeclampsia
   e. All of the above
4. Potential risks in prematurely ruptured membranes include:
   a. Cord prolapse
   b. Preterm birth
   c. Maternal and neonatal infection
   d. Pulmonary hypoplasia
   e. All of the above

ANSWERS

1. b
2. e
3. b, d
4. e

BIBLIOGRAPHY

Goldenberg RL et al: Low birthweight, intrauterine growth retardation, and preterm delivery, Am J Obstet Gynecol 152:980, 1985.

Iams JD: Premature rupture of the membranes. In Charles D, and Glover DD, editors: Current therapy in obstetrics, Toronto, 1988, BC Decker Inc.

Iams JD, editor: Preterm labor: a symposium, Clin Obstet Gynecol 31:519, 1988.

Main D, and Main E: Preterm birth. In Gabbe SG, Niebyl JR, and Simpson JL, editors: Obstetrics: normal and problem pregnancies, New York, 1986, Churchill Livingstone Inc.

McGregor JA: Prevention of preterm births: new initiatives based on microbial host interactions, Obstet Gynecol Surv 43:1, 1988.

Incompetent Cervix

Steven G. Gabbe
Jay D. Iams

Repetitive second-trimester pregnancy loss suggests the diagnosis of an incompetent cervix. *Incompetent cervix* is classically defined as repetitive second-trimester loss in the absence of any associated uterine activity, bleeding, or fluid leakage. The incidence is up to 1% of all pregnancies, and 20% or more of all second-trimester deliveries.

Etiology of the Incompetent Cervix

1. Patients with premature cervical dilation present with changes that mimic the normal biophysical and biochemical alterations in the cervix at term but are premature.
   a. At term, decreased collagen cross-links with increased dissociation and disorganization of collagen.
   b. Decreased hydroxyproline with loss of collagen.
   c. Increased glycosaminoglycans.
   d. No increase in relaxin in patients with incompetent cervix.
2. Abnormal cervical structure.
   a. Uterine cervix is basically fibrous, containing 10% to 15% smooth muscle.
   b. In the incompetent cervix, cervical smooth muscle exceeds 20%.
3. Association of cervical incompetence with uterine malformations.
   a. Failure of the circular muscle fibers at the internal os to act as a sphincter.
4. Association of cervical incompetence and diethylstilbestrol (DES) exposure.
   a. More common in patients with cervicovaginal DES effect.
5. Association of cervical trauma and cervical incompetence.
   a. Obstetrical trauma: spontaneous lacerations, operative forceps deliveries, or precipitous labor.
   b. Cone biopsy, especially a conization of the cervix that removes a large volume of tissue.
   c. Cervical amputation.
   d. Cervical dilation (e.g., D & C or see box on p. 138).
6. Association of cervical incompetence with multiple gestations.
   a. May be physiologic because of overdistension.

DIAGNOSIS
Clinical Presentation in Pregnancy

1. Classical presentation: gradual, painless dilation and effacement of the cervix, with bulging and later rupture of the membranes.
2. Early symptoms: vaginal or lower abdominal pressure with a watery or mucoid discharge that is occasionally bloody, urinary frequency, and a lump in the vagina.

Risk Factors for Cervical Trauma
With Therapeutic Abortion

Patients under 17 years of age
Laminaria not used
Inexperienced operator
General anesthesia
Second-trimester procedure

---

3. Short labors with delivery of an immature fetus.
4. Repeats at an earlier gestational age in successive pregnancies. First delivery may be beyond 30 weeks.
5. Premature rupture of the membranes at 18 to 26 weeks, with a cervix that is minimally dilated and/or effaced.
6. May present as labor with or without amnionitis or as amnionitis alone if amnion is exposed to vaginal milieu for prolonged time.

Causes of Second-Trimester Pregnancy Loss

Incompetent cervix
Müllerian abnormalities
Chromosomal abnormalities
Chronic uterine infections
Endocrine disorders: thyroid disease and diabetes
Immunologic factors
Collagen vascular disease

Diagnosis in Nonpregnant Individuals

1. Past history is critical. There are multiple causes of second-trimester losses or deliveries (see box above).
   a. Diagnosis by history of premature labor versus cervical incompetence. May be difficult to distinguish.
   b. Increased index of suspicion and surveillance of women with a history of delivery before 26 weeks caused by labor, premature rupture of fetal membranes (PROM), or amnionitis.
2. Physical examination.
   a. Passage of no. 8 Hegar's dilator during the luteal phase.
   b. Dilation of the cervical canal (3 to 7 mm) on hysterosalpingogram.
   c. Determination of cervical elastance using an intracervical balloon.
   None of the above tests establish or rule out cervical incompetence because an apparently normal cervix may become incompetent, and a cervix that appears defective may retain the pregnancy.

Contraindications to Cerclage

Ruptured membranes
Uterine bleeding
Uterine contractions not easily arrested
Chorioamnionitis
Cervical dilation greater than 4 cm
Lethal fetal malformation

MANAGEMENT OF PREGNANCY
Diagnostic Evaluation in the Pregnant Patient with Suggestive History

1. Frequent vaginal examinations during the period from 14 to 26 weeks.
2. Ultrasonography.
   a. May detect bulging of the membranes into a partially dilated cervix.
   b. May detect shortened cervical length.
3. Patient education: observation of changes in cervical discharge or pressure by the patient may permit timely intervention.

Treatment Once Diagnosis is Established

1. Preoperative evaluation.
   a. Elective cerclage, performed at 14 to 18 weeks gestation.
   b. Ultrasonography should be performed to document fetal viability.
   c. Cultures for gonorrhea and group B β-hemolytic streptococcus.
   d. Progestins and antibiotic therapy have no documented effectiveness but are commonly given, especially in cerclages placed after 20 weeks.
2. Selection of operative procedures.
   a. *Shirodkar procedure:* repair of cervical incompetence during pregnancy using a fascia lata band or surgical tape.
   b. *McDonald procedure:* pursestring cerclage that could easily be performed during pregnancy.
   c. The McDonald pursestring suture is as effective as the Shirodkar procedure, with less maternal morbidity, and it is therefore favored.
   d. *Benson and Durfee procedure:* transabdominal cerclage for patients with extensive cervical lacerations or a short or amputated cervix in which a vaginal approach is impossible.
   e. Cerclage should not be performed if any of the contraindications noted in box above are present.
3. Complications of cerclage.
   a. Infection: risks of chorioamnionitis or premature rupture of the membranes before 32 weeks are increased 2 to 3 times if cerclage is performed after 18 weeks rather than at 14 weeks.
   b. The incidence of premature rupture of the membranes is increased 15% to 30% if cerclage is placed in women with advanced cervical dilation and bulging membranes. Cerclage should be removed immediately if rupture of the membranes occurs because of the risk of sepsis.
   c. Premature labor.
   d. Suture displacement (3%).
   e. Cervical stenosis requiring cesarean section (2% to 5%).

    f. Cervical laceration during parturition (5% to 10%).

    g. Increased incidence of elective cesarean section after Shirodkar procedure.

    h. Hemorrhage in early labor.

    i. Uterine rupture if cerclage is not removed early in labor.

    j. Fistula formation occurs, especially with Shirodkar procedure. It is less common with McDonald procedure.

4. Postoperative care.

    a. Decreased physical and sexual activity.

    b. Frequent pelvic examinations.

    c. Eliminate vaginal infections.

    d. Elective removal of the cerclage at 37 weeks gestation.

5. Success after cervical cerclage.

    a. Fetal survival before cerclage is 20% to 25%.

    b. Fetal survival after elective cerclage is 80% to 90%.

    c. Fetal survival after emergency cerclage is 50%.

6. Nonoperative treatment of cervical incompetence.

    a. Pessary.

    b. Plastic cervical cuff.

    c. Strict bed rest in steep Trendelenburg's position.

    d. None of the above are associated with a high rate of success.

REVIEW
QUESTIONS

1. All of the following have been associated with second-trimester loss *except:*

    a. Müllerian abnormalities.

    b. Elective termination of a first-trimester pregnancy.

    c. Chromosomal abnormalities.

    d. History of DES exposure in utero.

2. The diagnosis of cervical incompetence is best made by:

    a. Identification of dilation of the cervical canal on hysterosalpingogram.

    b. Demonstration of decreased cervical elastance using an intracervical balloon.

    c. Recognition of a characteristic history of painless second-trimester loss.

    d. Passage of a no. 8 Hegar's dilator during the luteal phase.

3. When performing an elective McDonald cerclage at 14-weeks gestation, which of the following should be part of the treatment protocol?

    a. 100 mg of intramuscular progesterone preoperatively.

    b. Intravenous ampicillin on call to the operating room.

    c. Intravenous infusion of ritodrine.

    d. Ultrasonographic documentation of fetal viability.

ANSWERS

1. b

2. c

3. d

BIBLIOGRAPHY

Cousins L: Cervical incompetence, 1980: a time for reappraisal, Clin Obstet Gynecol 23:467, 1980.

Harger JF: Cervical cerclage: patient selection, morbidity, and success rates, Clin Perinatol 10:321, 1983.

Parisi VM: Cervical incompetence and preterm labor, Clin Obstet Gynecol 31:585, 1988.

Bleeding in Late Pregnancy 10

Jay D. Iams

Bleeding in the second half of pregnancy occurs in 3% to 4% of women and may result from various causes, some serious and others trivial. Prompt and thorough evaluation is required in all cases because the serious and trivial causes cannot easily be distinguished by history alone.

INITIAL EVALUATION

1. History
   a. Amount and character—a large amount of bright red blood is obviously serious, but small amounts of dark blood may also indicate a serious cause, such as abruptio placenta. Thin, watery bleeding suggests ruptured membranes or a cervical lesion.
   b. Contractions—the classic teaching, that placenta previa is painless and unaccompanied by contractions, whereas abruptio placenta is associated with a tender, irritable uterus, is useful but by no means an absolute. Contractions often accompany placenta previa, especially with low-lying or marginal previas.
   c. Recent trauma—abruptio placenta should always be considered when bleeding occurs following trauma to the pregnant abdomen. A Kleihauer-Betke test of maternal blood seeking fetal cells in the maternal circulation should be performed; if positive it predicts an increased chance of abruptio placenta.
   d. Coitus—bleeding may be precipitated by coitus with placenta previa or with lesions of the cervix.
2. Ultrasound
   a. An ultrasound should be performed promptly while the history is being taken because finding the placenta located away from the cervix will easily exclude placenta previa from further consideration in many cases. Similarly, a central placenta previa is usually a straightforward finding.
   b. Ultrasound findings in marginal placenta previa and low-lying placentas are less clear-cut. Repeated exams with variable degrees of bladder filling may be necessary to localize the placenta accurately in these cases.
   c. Ultrasound may aid in confirming a diagnosis of placental abruption if a clear retroplacental echolucency is seen in a patient with the classic presentation of painful vaginal bleeding. However, ultrasound cannot be used to exclude abruptio placenta, nor should all retroplacental echolucent areas seen on sonography be termed abruptio placentas.
   d. Ultrasound assessment of the size, presentation, and well-being of the infant are always important to know in women with bleeding in late pregnancy.

3. Physical examination
   a. Vital signs may be relatively normal even with significant blood loss because pregnant women have an increased blood volume. The presence of tachycardia, tachypnea, or hypotension or postural effect on blood pressure all indicate a very significant hemorrhage likely to require replacement.
   b. Digital examination should be deferred until the placenta has been localized with ultrasound. Although speculum exam may be performed cautiously in women with placenta previa to visually assess the degree of cervical dilation, digital examination of the patient with placenta previa is contraindicated unless performed in an operative delivery room with adequate personnel and blood replacement available should immediate cesarean section be required.
   c. Speculum examination is useful for the following:
      (1) Evaluating cervix for polyps, cervicitis friability, and cancerous lesions.
      (2) Obtaining blood for Apt test (to distinguish maternal from fetal bleeding).
      (3) Obtaining blood fluid for fern test and phosphatidyl glycerol if ruptured membranes are suspected.
   d. Uterine activity and fetal heart rate monitors should be applied immediately.
4. Laboratory assessment
   a. Tests requested depend on the amount of bleeding and suspected diagnosis. Get immediate CBC and coagulation studies on all patients.
   b. Women with placenta previa or suspected abruptio placenta, regardless of the amount of bleeding, and those with significant bleeding of uncertain origin will need the following:
      (1) Type and cross-match four units.
      (2) Fibrinogen, platelets, PT, PTT, and fibrin-split products.
      (3) "Wall clot"—the bedside test for hypofibrinogenemia. If clot fails to form in 5 to 6 minutes, or if it lyses within 30 minutes, then the fibrinogen is probably below 150 mg/dl.

PLACENTA PREVIA

1. Definition and classification—implantation of the placenta overlying the cervical os; may be central, partial, or marginal, (Fig. 10-1).
2. Incidence—1/200 births.
3. Etiology
   a. Uncertain but presumed defect in decidua.
   b. More common with previous cesarean and with increased parity.
4. Presentation
   a. Painless vaginal bleeding—70% to 80%.
   b. Bleeding with contractions—20%; more common with partial/marginal placentas.
   c. Ultrasound finding without bleeding—10%; many will migrate away from cervix in third trimester.
5. Diagnosis
   a. Ultrasound (Fig. 10-2).
      (1) 95% or greater accuracy in diagnosis of placenta previa.
      (2) Difficult with posterior low-lying placenta.
      (3) Vaginal ultrasound may assist when transabdominal sonography is doubtful.
   b. Digital exam may be performed only under "double set-up" conditions to assess possibility of vaginal delivery with partial or marginal placenta previa.

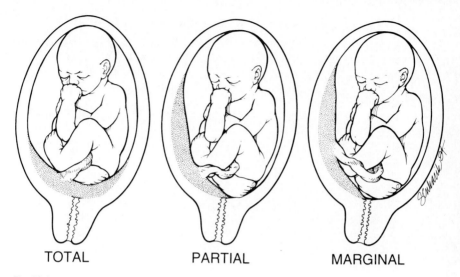

TOTAL   PARTIAL   MARGINAL

Fig. 10-1
Three variations of placenta previa. From Gabbe SG. Nieby I. Jr, and Simpson JL, eds: Obstetrics:
Normal and problem pregnancies, New York, 1986 Churchill Livingstone, 1 oc p. 495.

6. Management
   a. Expectant
      (1) Most bleeding episodes will cease spontaneously, and principal cause of
          perinatal mortality is prematurity.
      (2) Manage with blood replacement and hospital bedrest.
      (3) Deliver under following conditions:
          (a) Fetal maturity—do amniocentesis at 34 to 37 weeks gestation depend-
              ing on frequency and severity of bleeding.
          (b) Persistent hemorrhage—a judgment decision.
          (c) Labor—tocolytics generally not used (see below).
          (d) Infection or fetal distress.
   b. Aggressive expectant
      (1) Tocolysis—some centers use prophylatic and occasionally therapeutic toco-
          lytics (IV magnesium and/or oral β-mimetics) based on the theory that con-
          tractions cause or exacerbate bleeding.
      (2) Cerclage—one recent report of aggressive management with cerclage
          showed surprisingly good results. More study is needed.
   c. Management of delivery
      (1) Central and partial placenta previa—cesarean section.
      (2) Marginal/partial placenta previa—often cesarean, but may allow selected
          patients a trial of labor if fetal vertex will tamponade the placental edge.
      (3) Prepare patient for possibility of hysterectomy because of excessive bleed-
          ing or placenta accreta (¼ of women with a previous cesarean and a pla-
          centa previa will have placenta accreta).

ABRUPTIO PLACENTA

1. Definition—complete or partial separation of the normally implanted placenta before delivery of the fetus.

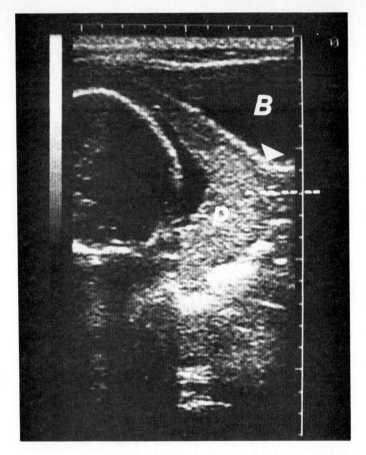

Fig. 10-2
Central previa. Here the placenta (p) is seen to lie directly over the internal os of the cervix. The bladder (B) angle *(solid triangle)* indicates the position of the internal os, and the dashed line shows the probable location of the endocervical canal.

2. Incidence—0.5% to 2.5%.
3. Etiology—diverse associated factors.
   a. Maternal hypertension—most common.
   b. Increasing parity.
   c. History of previous placental abruption.
   d. Trauma.
   e. Sudden decompression of an overdistended uterus.
4. Presentation
   a. Abdominal pain, uterine contractions, and vaginal bleeding are most common.
   b. External blood loss may not correlate with clinical picture because hemorrhage may be concealed.
   c. Coagulopathy—occurs with placental abruption large enough to result in fetal death. If a patient has a history typical of abruptio placenta and a coagulopathy, deliver fetus expeditiously.

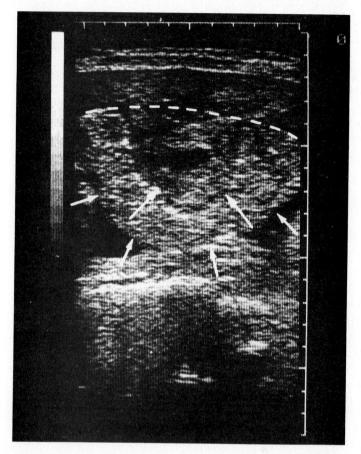

Fig. 10-3
Abruptio placentae. This scan of the placenta of a fetus demonstrating some decelerations illustrates a fresh, echogenic blood clot elevating the central portion of the placenta. The clot *(long arrows)* may be differentiated by texture from the placenta *(small arrows)*. The uterine margin is indicated by the dashed line. Delivery of this placenta shortly after this sonogram confirmed the composition of the central area as a blood clot.

    d. May be difficult to distinguish from premature labor with persistent uterine contractions.

5. Diagnosis
    a. Easily made in the most severe cases, with vaginal bleeding, increased uterine tone and tenderness, and fetal distress in a patient with hypertension.
    b. Conversely, can never be entirely excluded from consideration in any woman with either vaginal bleeding or abdominal pain in the second half of pregnancy.
    c. Ultrasound can suggest, but cannot exclude the diagnosis, which is more appropriately made on clinical grounds. An ultrasound image of a placental abruption is shown in Fig. 10-3. A similar picture may be seen with a degenerating fibroid beneath the placenta.

6. Management
   a. Dead fetus.
      (1) Large-bore IV, fluid replacement, blood and coagulation replacement if necessary, amniotomy, and vaginal delivery.
      (2) Central venous or balloon flotation catheter if vital signs unstable, once coagulopathy corrected.
      (3) Repeated assessment of coagulation, hemolysis, and urine output.
   b. Live fetus.
      (1) Abruptio placenta diagnosis certain.
         (a) Large-bore IV and fluid, blood, and coagulation replacement.
         (b) Amniotomy, with augmentation of labor if necessary.
         (c) Continuous internal fetal monitor.
         (d) Repeated assessment of coagulation, hemoglobin, and urine output.
      (2) Abruptio placenta diagnosis uncertain.
         (a) At term, may want to deliver rather than risk prolonging pregnancy.
         (b) Preterm, may employ tocolytics for presumed preterm labor with vaginal bleeding. Reassess uterine tenderness, ultrasound, fetal status, and coagulation frequently, especially if contractions are difficult to stop with tocolytics or if bleeding continues.

OTHER CAUSES OF BLEEDING

1. Preterm labor and PROM.
   a. Both preterm labor and PROM may present as bleeding, usually modest in amount, but may be greater with low-lying placenta.
   b. The marginal or low-lying placenta often presents with bleeding and contractions; ultrasound may show a clot at the placental edge near the cervix. Arrest of contractions may lead to cessation of bleeding.
2. Cervicitis/vaginitis—cervicovaginal infections (e.g., trichomonas) may lead to bleeding.
3. Cervical cancer—profuse watery discharge with occasional blood requires colposcopy even if Pap smear is normal.
4. Vasa previa.
   a. Fetal vessels traversing the membranes before reaching the placenta without the protection of Wharton's jelly are referred to as a *velamentous cord insertion*.
   b. When these vessels cross the cervix, this is called a vasaprevia. These vessels may rupture, producing fetal bleeding and exsanguination.
      (1) Fetal mortality of 50% or more.
      (2) Apt test will distinguish maternal from fetal blood.

REVIEW QUESTIONS

a = 1, 2, 3
b = 1 and 3
c = 2 and 4
d = 4 only
e = all

1. A 34-year-old pregnant woman presents at 32 weeks gestation with vaginal spotting, abdominal pain, and uterine contractions. Diagnostic possibilities include:
   1. Placental abruption
   2. Premature labor

    3. Placenta previa

    4. Cervicitis

2. Appropriate evaluation of the woman in question 1 should include:

    1. Digital examination of the cervix

    2. Ultrasound to locate the placenta

    3. Ultrasound to rule out abruptio placenta

    4. Sterile speculum examination to check for ruptured membranes

3. Initial evaluation of this patient reveals that the uterus is contracting regularly, the placenta is located in the fundus of the uterus and is normal in appearance, the hemoglobin is 12.0 g/dl, and the baby is dead. Which of the following statements are true?

    1. The normal hemoglobin and placental appearance make abruption **unlikely.** The patient has not had enough bleeding to cause fetal death. The patient is probably in preterm labor following fetal demise of uncertain etiology.

    2. This clinical presentation associated with fetal demise makes abruption very **likely.** The normal hemoglobin is not surprising in acute obstetric hemorrhage.

    3. Appropriate management includes prompt cesarean delivery to spare the patient labor with fetal demise. Careful collection of cultures for viral infection and blood for chromosomes at the time of section is important to evaluate the cause of death.

    4. Appropriate management includes starting a large bore IV, drawing blood for a "wall clot," cross matching the patient's blood type, and rupturing the membranes if possible to facilitate labor. Abruption that is severe enough to result in demise is usually associated with significant coagulopathy, and the patient should be delivered soon.

4. A 24-year-old woman calls to report vaginal spotting following coitus at 25 weeks gestation. This is her first pregnancy, and her general health is good. Diagnostic possibilities include:

    1. She is normal; the cervix is quite vascular in pregnancy, and bleeding occurs easily with intercourse.

    2. She may have a placenta previa. Placenta previa may be completely asymptomatic until the third trimester. An ultrasound should be done as soon as possible.

    3. She may have ruptured membranes without realizing it. PROM is often accompanied by bleeding. A sterile speculum examination should be done as soon as possible.

    4. She may have cervicitis due to *Chlamydia* or *Trichomonas*. A wet prep examination of vaginal secretions should be done.

5. A 30-year-old woman is pregnant for the fourth time. Her first three births were delivered by cesarean section; the first was for cephalopelvic disproportion, and the next two were elective repeat cesareans. She presents at 30 weeks with bright red vaginal bleeding associated with a low-lying anterior placenta that appears to encroach upon the cervical os. Which of the following statements are true?

    1. She should be treated with a cervical cerclage to prolong the pregnancy.

    2. The placenta will probably not "migrate" away from the lower anterior uterine wall, because this woman's partial previa is probably due to a defect in placental implantation caused by her multiple prior cesarean deliveries.

    3. She should be evaluated with weekly nonstress tests for fetal well-being.

    4. She should be prepared for the possibility of hysterectomy because of placenta accreta, which may occur in 25% of women with this presentation.

ANSWERS

1. a
2. c
3. c
4. e
5. c

BIBLIOGRAPHY

Benedetti TJ: Obstetric hemorrhage. In Gabbe SG, Niebyl JR, and Simpson JL, editors: Obstetrics: normal and problem pregnancies, New York, 1986, Churchill Livingston Inc.

Cotton DB, Ead J, Paul R, and Quilligan, EJ: The conservative aggressive management of placenta previa, Am J Obstet Gynecol 17:687, 1980.

Hurd WW, et al: Selective management of abruptio placenta: a prospective study, Obstet Gynecol 61:467, 1983.

Knab DR: Abruptio placenta: an assessment of the time and method of delivery, Obstet Gynecol 52:625, 1978.

McShane PM, Heyl PS, and Epstein MF: Maternal and perinatal morbidity resulting from placenta previa, Obstet Gynecol 65:176, 1985.

Isoimmunization in Pregnancy and Nonimmune Hydrops Fetalis

11

Jiri Sonek
Richard O'Shaughnessy

Erythroblastosis fetalis is a result of an isoimmune process in which maternal antibodies cause the destruction of fetal red cells. The antibodies interact with antigens on the fetal erythrocytes and activate the fetal immune mechanism against the erythrocytes. The outcome of this interaction varies from essentially no adverse effect on the fetus to severe anemia and fetal death. This variability is caused not only by the individual biologic variability of both the fetus and the mother but also by the type of antigen and antibody involved. With the current use of the rhesus immune globulin (RhIg), the incidence of isoimmune hydrops fetalis caused by anti-D sensitization is decreasing. Consequently, the relative incidence of hydrops caused by irregular antibodies and nonimmune causes is increasing. The rare problem with the alloimmunization that affects fetal platelets, resulting in fetal thrombocytopenia, is discussed in this chapter as well.

ABO incompatibility is the most common cause of sensitization in the human pregnancy. The consequences to the fetus from this disease, however, are minimal. Most of the discussion in this chapter is directed toward the issue of rhesus (Rh) (D antigen) sensitization, which is a less common cause of sensitization but is the most common cause of fetal hemolytic disease.

ISOIMMUNIZATION IN PREGNANCY

The mechanism of isoimmunization in pregnancy is immune system–mediated destruction of fetal and neonatal erythrocytes. In rare instances, this mechanism operates to affect the fetal and neonatal platelets.

HEMOLYTIC DISEASE

1. Causes
   a. Rh and ABO incompatibility—98% of cases.
   b. Minor erythrocyte antigens—2% of cases.

Rh Incompatibility

1. Genetics of the Rh antigen.
   a. Three genetic loci on the short arm of chromosome no. 1 with two possible alleles.
      (1) Fisher-Race nomenclature (most commonly used in obstetrics): CDE, cde, CDe, Cde, cDe, cDE, cdE, CdE.

2. D^u antigen is an incomplete D antigen. A mother with a pure D^u phenotype does not require RhIg administration. A mixed-field D^u positivity, however, may be caused by hemorrhage from an Rh-positive (Rh+) fetus into an Rh-negative (Rh-) mother.

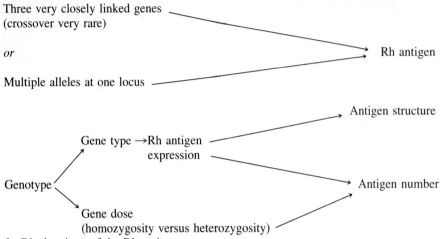

3. Biochemistry of the Rh antigen.

$$\text{Molecular weight} = 7 \times 10^3 - 10 \times 10^3$$

   a. The antigen is positioned in the lipid phase of the membrane and distributed in a nonrandom fashion.
4. Function of the Rh antigen.
   a. Rh- cells have increased osmotic fragility and an abnormal shape. The function of the Rh antigen, however, is not known. Unlike the A and B blood types, the Rh antigen is confined to the erythrocyte.
   b. The vast majority of Rh isoimmunization is caused by the D antigen. The Cc and Ee antigens are considered minor antigens.

Conditions necessary for Rh isoimmunization to occur

1. The fetus must be Rh+ and the mother must be Rh- (Rh incompatibility).
2. A sufficient number of fetal erythrocytes must enter the maternal circulation, or prior exposure to the Rh antigen must have occurred. The antigenic load necessary to induce an immune response is highly variable.
3. In addition to the above, the maternal ability to produce an anti-D antibody is necessary.

Population statistics

1. White population.
   a. Ten percent of pregnancies in whites are Rh incompatible.
   b. Overall Rh positivity—85%.
   c. Heterozygous Rh+ males (Dd)—60%.
   d. Homozygous Rh+ males (DD)—40%.
   e. Homozygous Rh- woman (dd) has a 50% chance to have an Rh-incompatible pregnancy if she mates with a heterozygous Rh+ male and a 100% chance of incompatibility if she mates with a homozygous Rh+ male (Rh- men excluded).

	D	d
d	dD	dd
d	dD	dd

$(.5)(.6)+(.4)(1.0) = .7$
70% incompatibility

	D	D
d	dD	dD
d	dD	dD

f. In the white population of Rh− mothers (Rh− men included):

$$(.85)(.70) = .6$$
60% incompatibility

g. With no prophylaxis, 20% of Rh-incompatible gravidas become sensitized:

$$(.6)(.2) = .12$$

h. Theoretically, 12% of white Rh-incompatible gravidas become sensitized with no prophylaxis.
2. Five percent of pregnancies in blacks are Rh incompatible.
3. One percent of pregnancies in Orientals are Rh incompatible.

Rates of sensitization (no prophylaxis)

1. Before delivery—very rare (1% to 2%).
2. After delivery—more common (15% to 20%).

Critical volume of fetal blood required for sensitization

The critical volume of fetal blood required for sensitization to occur may be as low as .1 ml. There is great individual variability, and in some, even very large volumes are nonimmunogenic.

Other pregnancy-related events that may result in sensitization

1. Ectopic pregnancy (especially if ruptured).
2. Elective pregnancy termination after 6 weeks of gestation.
3. Spontaneous abortion.
4. Amniocentesis, cordocentesis, or chorionic villus biopsy.
5. Abdominal trauma in pregnancy.
6. Abruptio placentae.
7. Fetal-maternal hemorrhage in an uncomplicated pregnancy—this occurs in more than 30% of normal pregnancies but is usually not sufficient to produce sensitization.*

Determinants of maternal immune response

1. Maternal immunocompetence.
2. Fetal antigenic expression of the Rh antigen and other erythrocyte antigens.

The use of RhIg

1. Proposed mechanism of action.
    a. Increased clearance of antibody-coated cells.
    b. Masking of the Rh antigens by the exogenous antibodies.
    c. Suppression of B lymphocytes by mediator substances produced by T cells. The production of these substances is in turn stimulated by the T-cell recognition of the antibody-coated Rh antigens.

*"Grandmother theory"—birth of an Rh− female to an Rh+ mother is not considered to be a cause of Rh sensitization in the offspring. Although maternal cells are measurable in the newborn, the immune response does not occur.

2. Postpartum administration.
   a. 300 g of RhIg reliably prevents sensitization with 30 ml of Rh+ blood (approximately 20 μg per cc of fetal cells).
   b. If given within 72 hours after delivery, the rate of sensitization is decreased to approximately 1%. It is possible that administration of RhIg weeks after delivery still has some protective effect.
3. Antepartum adminstration.
   a. Usual time of administration is at approximately 28 weeks of gestation. (The chances of sensitization occurring before 28 weeks are very small [less than 1%].)
   b. Postulated duration of protection is approximately 12 weeks.
   c. Antepartum sensitization with antepartum RhIg—.2%.

RhIg

1. Halflife of RhIg is 25 days.
2. Administration of 20 μg consistently prevents sensitization with 1 cc of fetal cells (1 cc of fetal cells equals approximately 2 cc of fetal blood because the hematocrit of the fetus is approximately 50%).

RhIg*	Volume of fetal cells covered by RhIg†
300 μg	15 cc
↓ 25 days	↓
150 μg	7.5 cc
↓ 25 days	↓
75 μg	3.75 cc
↓ 25 days	↓
37.5 μg	1.88 cc
↓ 25 days	↓
18.8 μg	.94 cc

*Total number of days: 100 (14 weeks).
†Number of cc's theoretically covered by term by 28-week RhIg: 1.

3. RhIg for 28 weeks should be sufficient to prevent the majority of fetal-maternal hemorrhages.
4. Administration of 300 μg of RhIg is also indicated for:
   a. Pregnancy that terminates at 12 weeks of gestation.
   b. Pregnancy that terminates, and the gestational age is unknown.
   c. Amniocentesis, cordocentesis, and CVS.
5. Administration of 50 μg of RhIg is indicated for a pregnancy that terminates before 12 weeks of gestation.
6. More than 300 μg of RhIg is indicated for fetal-maternal hemorrhage that is larger than usual—an attempt to estimate the amount of fetal blood should be made with the Kleihauer-Betke test.

The measurement of fetal-maternal hemorrhage

More than 50% of fetal-maternal hemorrhage at delivery is less than 1 cc. Only 1/300 cases of FMH exceeds the capacity of one vial (300 μg) of RhIg.

Method	Sensitivity (volume [cc] of fetal blood)
Rosette	5
D^u*	25
ELISA	5
Kleihauer-Betke test	5
(the definitive quantitative test)	

*The D^u test specifically looks for weak Rh positivity. In this test it is important to describe specifically the uniformity of reaction. The mixed-field reaction suggests a fetal-maternal hemorrhage of an Rh+ fetus into an Rh− mother. In the uniform-field reaction, the result implies the presence of an incomplete D antigen (D^u).

Minor Antigen Incompatibility

See Table 11-1.
1. Incidence varies with population.
2. Incidence is increased in multiparas and patients with a history of transfusion or intravenous drug abuse and sharing needles.

THE ISOIMMUNIZED PREGNANCY
Effects on the Fetus and Neonate

All complications of erythroblastosis fetalis are due to anemia of varying degrees and the ensuing fetal cardiovascular response.

Fetus

1. Anemia.
2. Hydrops fetalis (accumulation of fluid in the fetal body cavities, hydramnios, placentomegaly).
3. The evaluation of the rate of fetal erythrocyte destruction and the degree of fetal anemia has undergone a tremendous change over the past several years. With the advent of cordocentesis, fetal blood can be directly tested with relatively little risk. This technique also permits the performance of a direct intravascular transfusion if indicated. At this point in time, however, cordocentesis is not being performed at all centers. The student of erythroblastosis fetalis will therefore be frustrated by the current lack of uniformity both in evaluation and treatment.

Neonate

1. Anemia.
2. Kernicterus (a severe form of neonatal jaundice).
3. Neonatal congestive heart failure (always preceded by hydrops fetalis).
4. The treatment of the neonate, if indicated, consists of either a simple transfusion in mild cases or exchange transfusions in more severe cases.

Management of a Sensitized Pregnancy
Serology

1. First sensitized pregnancy.
   a. Titer less than *critical value* (varies depending on the laboratory but is usually 1:16 to 1:32)—repeat serologic tests every 4 weeks.
   b. Titer exceeds the critical value—amniocentesis or cordocentesis at 22 to 24 weeks.

Table 11-1 Hemolytic disease caused by irregular antibodies

Blood Group System	Relative Frequency (%)	Antigens Related to Hemolytic Disease	Hemolytic Disease Severity	Proposed Management
Lewis	16.6	Not a proved cause of hemolytic disease of the newborn	—	—
I	3.2	Not a proved cause of hemolytic disease of the newborn	—	—
Kell	14.1	K	Mild to severe with hydrops fetalis	Amniotic fluid bilirubin studies
		k	Mild	Expectant
		Ko	Mild	Expectant
		Kp^a	Mild	Expectant
		Kp^b	Mild	Expectant
		Js^a	Mild	Expectant
		Js^b	Mild	Expectant
Rh (non-D)	10.1	E	Mild to severe with hydrops fetalis	Amniotic fluid bilirubin studies
	9.7	C	Mild to severe with hydrops fetalis	Amniotic fluid bilirubin studies
	1.9	c	Mild to severe with hydrops fetalis	Amniotic fluid bilirubin studies
Duffy	3.3	Fy^a	Mild to severe with hydrops fetalis	Amniotic fluid bilirubin studies
		Fy^b	Not a cause of hemolytic disease of the newborn	—
		By^3	Mild	Expectant
Kidd	1.6	Jk^a	Mild to severe	Amniotic fluid bilirubin studies
		Jk^b	Mild	Expectant
		Jk^3	Mild	Expectant
MNSs	7.4	M	Mild to severe	Amniotic fluid bilirubin studies
		N	Mild	Expectant
		S	Mild to severe	Amniotic fluid bilirubin studies
		s	Mild to severe	Amniotic fluid bilirubin studies
		U	Mild to severe	Amniotic fluid bilirubin studies
MSSs	—	Mi^a	Moderate	Amniotic fluid bilirubin studies
		Mt^a	Moderate	Amniotic fluid bilirubin studies

Blood group system	Antigen		Severity	Management
Lutheran	Vw		Mild	Expectant
	Mur		Mild	Expectant
	Hil		Mild	Expectant
	Hut		Mild	Expectant
	Lu^a	.4	Mild	Expectant
	Lu^b		Mild	Expectant
Diego	Di^a	—	Mild to severe	Amniotic fluid bilirubin studies
	Di^b		Mild to severe	Amniotic fluid bilirubin studies
Xg	Xg^a	—	Mild	Expectant
P	PP1^pk (Tj^a)	—	Mild to severe	Amniotic fluid bilirubin studies
Public antigens	Yt^a	4.8	Moderate to severe	Amniotic fluid bilirubin studies
	Yt^b		Mild	Expectant
	Lan		Mild	Expectant
	En^a		Moderate	Amniotic fluid bilirubin studies
	Ge		Mild	Expectant
	Jr^a		Mild	Expectant
	Co^a		Severe	Amniotic fluid bilirubin studies
	Co^a-b-		Mild	Expectant
Private antigens	Batty	—	Mild	Expectant
	Becker		Mild	Expectant
	Berrens		Mild	Expectant
	Biles		Moderate	Amniotic fluid bilirubin studies
	Evans		Mild	Expectant
	Gonzales		Mild	Expectant
	Good		Severe	Amniotic fluid bilirubin studies
	Heibel		Moderate	Amniotic fluid bilirubin studies
Private antigens	Hunt	—	Mild	Expectant
	Jobbins		Mild	Expectant
	Radin		Moderate	Amniotic fluid bilirubin studies
	Rm		Mild	Expectant
	Ven		Mild	Expectant
	Wright^a		Severe	Amniotic fluid bilirubin studies
	Wright^b		Mild	Expectant
	Zd		Moderate	Amniotic fluid bilirubin studies

Modified from Weinstein L: Irregular antibodies causing hemolytic disease of the newborn: a continuing problem, Clin Obstet Gynecol 25:321, 1982.

Management of a pregnancy in an Rh- woman

Initial visit:
Maternal blood type — any
Maternal Rh status — negative
Maternal antibody screen — negative

→ Paternal blood type — any
Paternal Rh status

Positive   Negative

28 weeks   Maternal antibody screen   No further
                                                testing
                                                necessary

        Negative   Positive

        Administer 300 g of Rhlg   See next section

40 weeks   Maternal antibody screen
(>12 weeks
after Rhlg)
        Negative   Positive (12% of those
                          who got 28 week Rhlg
        Administer 300 g of Rhlg   will be weakly positive)

                          Deliver if > 1:4
                          See next section
                          for route of delivery

Postpartum   Maternal antibody screen
              Rh status of the neonate

        Positive   Negative

    Administer 300 g   No further testing or therapy
    of Rhlg if no Rhlg
    administered at term

2. Subsequent sensitized pregnancy.
    a. Amniocentesis or cordocentesis at 22 to 24 weeks.
    b. Alternatively, follow the same regimen as for First Sensitized Pregnancy above.

Amniocentesis*

1. Zone I (Fig. 11-1)—unaffected or mildly affected fetus. Repeat amniocentesis every 3 to 4 weeks.
2. Zone II—interpretation requires a trend. Repeat amniocentesis every 1 to 2 weeks.
   a. Decreasing values—mild disease.
   b. Level or increasing values—severe disease (the steepness of the rise reflects to some extent the severity of the disease).
3. Zone III—severe disease. Requires intrauterine transfusion or delivery (treat according to gestational age).

Intrauterine transfusion

In the Figure on p. 158, the intrauterine transfusions that are done by cordocentesis can be done intraperitoneally. The timing of the intraperitoneal transfusions is similar to the timing of the intravascular transfusions. Historically, the intraperitoneal transfu-

*Measurement at OD_{450}—absorbance of bilirubin.

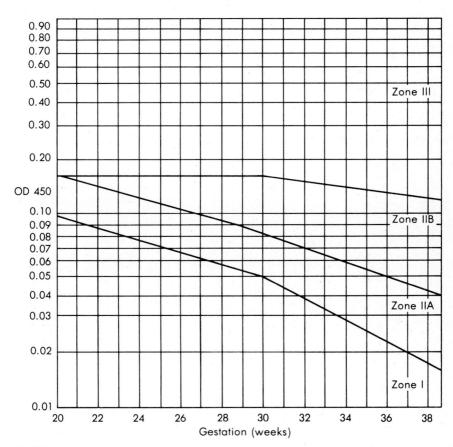

Fig. 11-1

Delta (difference between predicted and expected) optical density of amniotic fluid at 450 nm by weeks gestation (Liley curve), as modified for use at The Ohio State University Hospital. *Zone I*, Consistent with an unaffected or mildly affected infant; *Zone IIA*, consistent with a mildly to moderately affected infant; *Zone IIB*, consistent with a moderately to severely affected infant; *Zone III*, consistent with a severely affected infant.

From The Ohio State University Hospital.

A protocol currently used at The Ohio State University

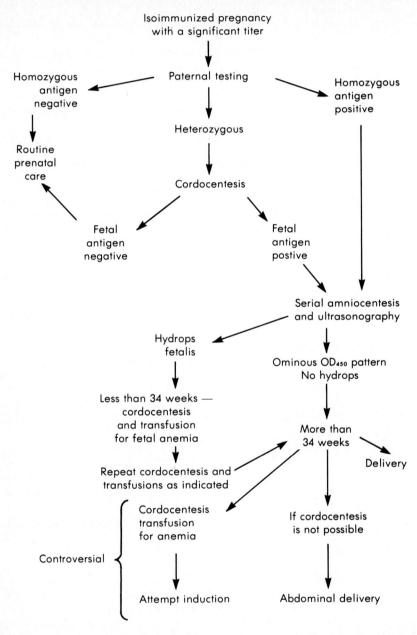

sions have not been done beyond 32 weeks. The success and safety of both techniques depend on the experience of the operator. The blood used for the transfusion is washed type-O Rh− blood. Both intraperitoneal and intravascular transfusions must be performed under ultrasonographic guidance.

There are various formulas for the estimation of the volume of blood to be transfused. For an intraperitoneal transfusion see Table 11-2. For a direct intravascular transfusion see Fig. 11-2.

Table 11-2   Recommended volumes of blood to be injected at intrauterine transfusion

Week of Gestation	Volume (ml)
24	40
25	50
26	60
27	70
28	80
29	90
30	100
31	100
32	100-120

From Queenan JT: Modern management of the Rh problem, Hagerstown, Md, 1977, Harper & Row, Publishers Inc.

The ways of estimating the intervals in between transfusions are also controversial. The accuracy is limited by the variable rate of the destruction of the erythrocytes not only among different patients but also in the same patient at different times. We use 1% hematocrit drop per day.

Other antepartum testing

1. Ultrasonography.
   a. Relatively insensitive—the degree of anemia cannot be ascertained unless hydrops fetalis is present. This, however, does not appear until a very low level of hemoglobin is reached (less than or equal to 4 mg/dl).
2. Fetal heart–rate monitoring (NST, OCT).
   a. Very insensitive—a very significant anemia must be present before appreciable changes in fetal heart rate are present.
3. Doppler fetal blood–flow studies.
   a. There is a correlation between the velocity and volume of the fetal blood flow and the hemoglobin content of the blood. Doppler fetal blood–flow studies are currently under research.

ABO incompatibility

A and B antigens are present in many maternal and fetal tissues. Prior pregnancy, transfusion, or other potential causes of isoimmunization are not necessary for sensitization to occur.

The usual result of ABO incompatibility is a mild neonatal hyperbilirubinemia. Less than 1% of the cases require exchange transfusion. Special antenatal diagnostic procedures are not necessary.

Reasons for the mildness of the hyperbilirubinemia

1. Some of the antibodies directed against the A and B antigens are absorbed in tissues other than erythrocytes where these antigens are present as well. Because of the ubiquitous nature of these antigens, there is an element of maternal immune desensitization.
2. There are fewer A and B antigens than other known antigens on the fetal erythrocytes.
3. In individuals with A and B blood type, the antibody is primarily IgM and as such does not cross the placenta. Individuals with O blood group produce anti-A and -B IgG, which crosses the placenta. Therefore, the ABO incompatibility disease of the neonate occurs primarily in mothers with the O blood type.

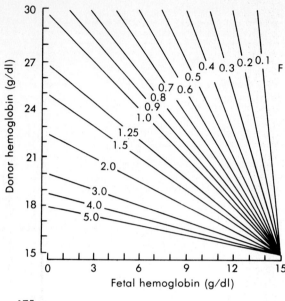

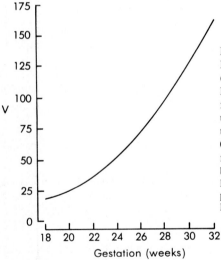

Fig. 11-2
Nomogram for calculating volume of donor blood (ml) necessary to correct fetal anemia. The value F is multiplied by the value V. For example, for a fetus at 24 weeks gestation, the V value is 50. If the pretransfusion fetal hemoglobin is 5 g/dl and the donor blood hemoglobin is 26 g/dl (value F = 0.9), 45 ml of donor blood will need to be transfused to achieve a posttransfusion fetal hemoglobin of 12.5 g/dl (normal mean for gestation).
From Queenan JT: Modern management of the Rh problem, Hagerstown, Md, 1977, Harper & Row, Publishers Inc.

ALLOIMMUNE THROMBOCYTOPENIA

1. Causes
   a. Platelet antigen Pl^{A1}—90% of cases.
   b. Less common platelet antigens—10% of cases.

Platelet Antigen Incompatibility

1. Incidence—1:5000 births.
2. Mechanism—analogous to Rh sensitization.
3. Clinical manifestation—varies from mild petechiae to severe hemorrhage.
4. Immunofluorescence platelet suspension is 90% positive for platelet antibodies.

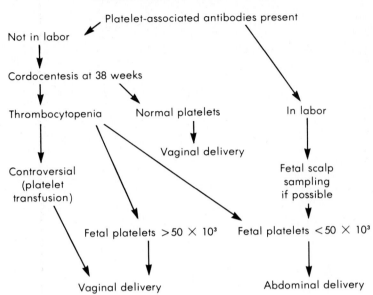

Management of an affected pregnancy

5. Most common antigen involved in platelet isoimmunization—P1[1] (90%).
6. Differentiation from idiopathic thrombocytopenic purpura (ITP)—presence of platelet-associated antibodies in platelet isoimmunization and an absence in ITP. The mother is not affected in platelet isoimmunization. The disease may affect the first pregnancy, and the recurrence rate is 75%.

NONIMMUNE HYDROPS

With the current use of the Rh globulin, the relative incidence of nonimmune hydrops is increasing. Additionally, as ultrasonography becomes more widely used, the antepartum diagnosis of this disease is more commonly made before fetal death.

ETIOLOGY

See box on opposite page.
1. Etiology is unknown—50% of cases.
2. Congenital heart disease or arrhythmias—20% of cases.
3. Chromosomal abnormalities—16% of abnormalities.
4. The diagnosis is made on the basis of the presence of hydrops and the exclusion of isoimmunization. The prognosis is generally poor but depends on the etiology, duration, and severity of the hydrops. See box on opposite page for work-up.

REVIEW QUESTIONS

True or False
1. E,e, C,c, are all part of the rhesus antigen.
True or False
2. E,e, C,c, are considered minor antigens.

Etiology of nonimmune hydrops

A. Fetal

1. Hematologic

Homozygous α-thalassemia
Chronic fetomaternal transfusion
Twin-to-twin transfusion
Multiple gestation with parasitic fetus

2. Cardiovascular

Severe congenital heart disease (atrial septal defect, ventricular septal defect, hypoplastic left heart, pulmonary valve insufficiency, Ebstein's anomaly, sub-aortic stenosis)
Premature closure of foramen ovale
Myocarditis
Large A-V malformation
Tachyarrhythmias: atrial flutter, supraventricular tachycardia
Bradyarrhythmias: heart block
Fibroelastosis

3. Chromosomal

Trisomy 21
Turner's syndrome 45,XO
Other trisomies
Triploidy
Mosaicism

4. Pulmonary

Cystic adenomatoid malformation of lung
Pulmonary lymphangiectasia
Pulmonary hypoplasia
Congenital chylothorax

5. Renal

Congenital nephrosis
Renal vein thrombosis
Posterior urethral valves
Spontaneous bladder perforation

6. Intrauterine infections

Syphillis
Toxoplasmosis
CMV
Leptospirosis
Chagas' disease
Congenital hepatitis
Herpes simplex

7. Congenital anomalies

Achondroplasia
Thanatophoric dwarfism
Sacrococcygeal teratoma

8. Miscellaneous

Meconium peritonitis
Fetal neuroblastomatosis
Tuberous sclerosis
Small-bowel volvulus

B. Placental

Umbilical vein thrombosis
Chorioangioma
True cord knots

C. Maternal disease

Diabetes mellitus
Toxemia
Severe anemia

D. Idiopathic

From Clin Obstet Gynecol 29:1986.

Work-up of nonimmune hydrops

A. Hematologic
1. Complete blood cell count—if anemic, electrophoresis, sickledex, glucose-6-phosphate dehydrogenase
2. VDRL
3. Toxoplasmosis, rubella, cytomegalovirus, and herpes simplex (TORCH) titers
4. Blood type and Rh
5. Antibody screen
6. SMA with computer-23, including liver function tests, bilirubin, BUN, creatinine, electrolytes, albumin, and protein
7. Kleihauer-Betke test
8. MS-AFP
9. Parental HLA type (if recurrent or idiopathic)

B. Urologic
1. Urine analysis
2. CMV culture

C. Ultrasonography
1. Full growth study
2. Amniotic-fluid volume, placental thickness
3. Morphologic survey for anomalies
4. Cardiac evaluation: rhythm and chamber size
5. Major vessel sizes
6. Skin thickness
7. Internal free fluid

D. Amniotic fluid or fetal blood sample
1. Karyotype
2. TORCH titers
3. Specific infection IgM's if suspicious
4. Viral cultures
5. ΔOD 450
6. AFP
7. Fetal blood film and indices
8. Fetal plasma albumin and total protein

E. At delivery
1. Karyotype if not done
2. Autopsy
3. Viral studies
4. Photographs
5. X-ray examination

From Clin Obstet Gynecol 29: 1986.

Select the best answer.
3. The rate of sensitization in a rhesus-incompatible pregnancy after delivery without RhIg administration is:
   a. 15%-20%
   b. 10%
   c. 1%-2%
4. The rate of sensitization in a rhesus-incompatible pregnancy with RhIg administration after delivery only is:
   a. 15%-20%
   b. 10%
   c. 1%-2%
   d. 0.2%
5. The rate of sensitization in a rhesus-incompatible pregnancy with both antepartum and post-partum RhIg administration is:
   a. 15%-20%
   b. 10%
   c. 1%-2%
   d. 0.2%

6. Half-life of RhIg is:
    a. 100 days
    b. 50 days
    c. 25 days
    d. 10 days
7. The definitive quantitative test for estimating the volume of fetal maternal hemorrhage is:
    a. Rosette method
    b. Du method
    c. ELISA method
    d. Kleihauer-Betke method
8. ABO incompatibility is a common cause of:
    a. Hydrops fetalis
    b. Neonatal hyperbilirubinemia
    c. Platelet antigen incompatibility
9. In most cases of non-immune hydrops
    a. Congenital heart disease can be identified on ultrasound
    b. Cardiac arrhythmia can be identified on ultrasound
    c. Chromosomal abnormalities are present
    d. The etiology of hydrops cannot be identified by ultrasound

ANSWERS

1. True
2. True
3. a
4. c
5. d
6. c
7. d
8. b
9. d

BIBLIOGRAPHY

Frigoletto FD, Jr, Jewett JF, and Konugres AA, editors: Rh hemolytic disease: new strategy for eradication, Boston, 1982, GK Hall & Co.

Frigoletto FD et al: Ultrasonographic fetal surveillance in the management of the isoimmunized pregnancy, N Engl J Med 315:430, 1986.

Gabbe SG, Niebyl JR, and Simpson JL: Obstetrics: normal and problem pregnancies, New York, 1986 Churchill Livingstone Inc.

Grannum PA et al: In utero exchange transfusion by direct intravascular injection in severe erythroblastosis fetalis, N Engl J Med 314:1431, 1986.

Hobbins JC et al: Percutaneous umbilical blood sampling, Am J Obstet Gynecol 152:1, 1985.

Kennedy MS et al: Problems with antenatal use of Rh immune globulin: results of a nationwide survey, Transfusion 23:434, 1983.

Nicolaides KH et al: Lancet 1988.

Nusbacher J, and Bove JR: Sounding boards—Rh immunoprophylaxis: is antepartum therapy desirable? N Engl J Med 303:935, 1980.

Pollack W: Rh hemolytic disease of the newborn: its cause and prevention, Reprod Immuno, Prog Clin Biol Res 70:185, 1981.

Queenan JT: Modern management of the Rh problem, Hagerstown, Md, 1977, Harper & Row, Publishers Inc.

Proceedings of the McMaster Conference on Prevention of Rh Immunization, Vox Sang 36:50, 1979.

The selective use of Rho(D) immune globulin (RhIg), Tech Bull no 61, March 1981 (update—November 1983), ACOG.

Intrauterine Growth Retardation

12

Steven G. Gabbe
Jay D. Iams

Poor fetal growth, or *intrauterine growth retardation (IUGR),* is arbitrarily defined statistically to include those infants whose weight is at or below the 10th percentile for the gestational age at birth. Although 70% of these infants will be normally or constitutionally small, this group will also include infants with markedly increased perinatal morbidity and mortality, up to 6 to 10 times greater than a normal population (the mortality rates for infants with IUGR are 120/1000 births, including infants with anomalies, and 100/1000 births in nonanomalous infants). The detection and management of IUGR depends on two principal data points that are the focus of much prenatal care: (1) the gestational age of the fetus and (2) the estimated weight and growth pattern of the fetus throughout pregnancy. Although weight can be reliably measured ($\pm$10%) throughout pregnancy by ultrasonography, accurate assessment of the duration of pregnancy within $\pm$10 days can really only be made in the first half of gestation. Thereafter, the range of normal is too broad and the key historical events are too remote to be confident of gestational age beyond $\pm$21 days.

CLASSIFICATION OF IUGR (TABLE 12-1)

IUGR may be classified as *symmetric,* in which the fetal head and body are equally small, or *asymmetric,* in which the head is less affected than the torso. Patterns of growth for asymmetric and symmetric IUGR are shown in Figs. 12-1 and 12-2, respectively.

Table 12-1 Classification of IUGR

	Asymmetric	Symmetric
Estimated fetal weight <10%	Yes	Yes
Head circumference/abdominal circumference	↑	Nl
Femur length/abdominal circumference	↑	Nl
Abdominal circumference <10%	Yes	Yes
Amniotic fluid	Nl or ↓	Nl or ↓
Anomalies	—	May be present

Nl, Normal.

65

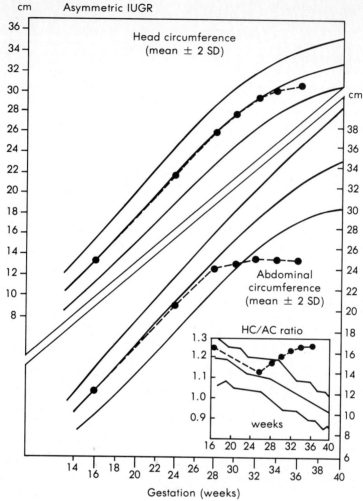

Fig. 12-1
Asymmetric growth retardation, demonstrating maintenance of head circumference (HC) growth but slowed abdominal circumference (AC) growth. The HC/AC ratio is increased.
From Chudleigh P, and Pearce JM: Obstetric ultrasound: how, why and when, New York, 1986, Churchill Livingstone.

Symmetric

Symmetric IUGR is a condition caused by factors that are inherent to the fetus or that affect the fetus from early in pregnancy (e.g., chromosomal, genetic, or infectious teratogens). Overall, cell number is decreased. Symmetric IUGR cannot be distinguished from wrong dates in late pregnancy.

Asymmetric

Cell size, rather than number, is decreased in asymmetric IUGR. Brain growth is relatively normal except in advanced cases. The abdominal circumference (AC) is re-

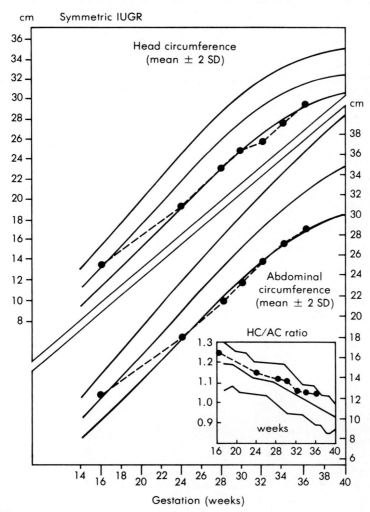

Fig. 12-2
Symmetric growth retardation with growth of both head circumference (HC) and abdominal
circumference (AC) at or below the 5th percentile. The HC/AC ratio is normal.
From Chudleigh P, and Pearce JM: Obstetric ultrasound: how, why and when, New York, 1986, Churchill
Livingstone.

duced because of smaller cell size and decreased glycogen stores in the fetal liver.
Asymmetric IUGR is defined by abnormal elevated head circumference/abdominal circumference (HC/AC) or femur length/abdominal circumference (FL/AC) ratios.

ETIOLOGY
Normally Small (70%)

1. Constitutionally small stature
2. No increase in fetal/perinatal morbidity
3. A *retrospective* diagnosis

Antepartum Factors Associated with Poor Fetal Growth

Medical complications

Hypertension, pregnancy-induced hypertension (PIH)
Renal disease
Severe cardiopulmonary disease
Hemoglobinopathies
Lupus anticoagulant

Obstetrical complications

Multiple gestation
Antepartum hemorrhage
Postmaturity

Previous gestational complications

Recurrent fetal wastage (abortion, congenital anomaly, prematurity)
Perinatal death
Previous IUGR (Table 12-2)

Socioeconomic factors

Low socioeconomic status and poor nutrition
Low weight, short stature, poor weight gain
Social drug abuse (alcohol, tobacco)

Intrinsic Growth Failure (10% to 15%)

1. Genetic
2. Infections
   a. Toxoplasmosis
   b. Cytomegalovirus
   c. Rubella
   d. Syphilis
3. Drugs: alcohol, aminopterin, coumadin, phenytoin, heroin, methadone, and trimethadione

Extrinsic Growth Failure (10% to 20%)

1. Placental disease: infarction, hemangiomas, premature placental separation, and single umbilical artery
2. Disorders leading to reduction in uteroplacental blood flow (see box above)

ESTABLISHING FETAL AGE USING ULTRASONOGRAPHY
Accuracy

The accuracy of an ultrasonographic estimate of fetal age is inversely related to fetal age. Ultrasonography estimates age by measuring size, much as we all do when first meeting an infant or child. Just as we overestimate the age of large children and underestimate the age of smaller children, estimates of fetal age based on ultrasonography do the same, especially after 20 to 24 weeks gestation. Before that time, the range in normal growth of ultrasonographically measured fetal body parts is narrow enough that ultrasonography may be reliably used to estimate fetal age; individual variations in

Table 12-2 The tendency to repeat gestational age and birthweight in successive births

Weight of First Birth	No. of Subjects Studied	Second Birth	
		Small for Gestational Age (%)	Relative Risk of IUGR (%)
>90th percentile	8470	1.6	0.2
10th-90th percentile	57,602	6.7	1.0
<10th percentile	10,457	23.0	3.4

From Bakketieg LS et al: Am J Obstet Gynecol 135:1086, 1979.

Table 12-3 Ultrasonographic assessment of fetal age

Measurement	Gestational Age (menstrual weeks)	Range (days)
Crown-rump length	5 to 12	± 3
Biparietal diameter	12 to 20	± 8
	20 to 24	± 12
	24 to 32	± 15
	> 32	± 21
Femur length	12 to 20	± 7
	20 to 36	± 11
	36+	± 16

growth have not yet been expressed. The optimal method for ultrasonographic assessment of fetal age varies with gestational age, as shown in Table 12-3.

Other fetal measurements show a similar range. Long bones, including the humerus, tibia, radius, and ulna, can all be measured accurately, as can outer and inner orbital diameters. Recently, transcerebellar diameter has been touted as a fetal measurement that is relatively spared by IUGR and is therefore useful in dating in cases where IUGR is suspected.

The accuracy of gestational-age estimates by ultrasonography increases as more variables are measured. A composite of biparietal diameter (BPD), abdominal circumference, head circumference, and femur length improves predictive accuracy by 8% at 12 to 18 weeks and up to 28% at 36 to 42 weeks.

In later gestation, the accuracy of fetal-age determination is enhanced by serial measurements. Sabbagha, Hughey, and Depp (see bibliography) have reported growth-adjusted sonographic age (GASA) using BPD and AC before 26 weeks and then 10 to 12 weeks later with an error of ±7 days. Two to three parameters studied at least 2 weeks apart at 24 to 32 weeks have an error of ±10 days. With suspected IUGR, sustained growth of all variables indicates a "normal" small fetus or error in dates.

Estimation of Fetal Weight

Composite tables estimating fetal weight have been constructed by several authors and are usually based on a combination of (1) head size, as measured by BPD or head circumference, (2) femur length, and (3) abdominal circumference. Tables by Hadlock et al and Shepard et al (see bibliography) are currently in most common use.

DETECTION OF IUGR

All pregnancies should be screened for IUGR by serial measurement of fundal height, but the accuracy of this clinical measure is less than ideal (see Table 12-4). When poor

Table 12-4   Prediction of size of infants at birth by measurement of symphysis fundus height

	Below 10th Percentile (%)	Above 90th Percentile (%)
Sensitivity	70/263 (27)	104/277 (38)
Specificity	2337/2656 (88)	2321/2642 (88)
Predictive value positive	70/389 (18)	104/425 (25)
Predictive value negative	2337/2530 (92)	2321/2494 (93)

From Persson B et al: Br J Obstet Gynaecol 93:206, 1986.

IUGR: Most Predictive Ultrasonographic Criteria for Antenatal Diagnosis

Oligohydramnios
EFW below 10th percentile
Elevated HC/AC

From Benson CB et al: Radiology 160:415, 1986.

growth is suspected by fundal height measurement or when risk factors are present, ultrasonography should be used to detect or exclude IUGR.

Ultrasonographic Detection of IUGR

Ultrasonographic findings associated with IUGR include:
1. Elevated HC/AC that is greater than 2 SD above mean: 85% will have IUGR
2. FL/AC ratio is greater than 23.5
3. Estimated fetal weight (EFW) is less than 10th percentile for age
4. Diminished or absent amniotic fluid
5. Advanced placental grade
   A single parameter is not a good predictor of IUGR, but as shown in the box above, the combination of several is helpful.

MANAGEMENT OF IUGR
Antepartum Management

1. Review and reestablish dates to confirm diagnosis.
2. Rule out abnormal karyotype with amniocentesis or cordocentesis.
3. Look for fetal anomaly on ultrasonogram.
4. Remove risk factors for poor growth.
   a. Smoking.
   b. Poor nutrition.
   c. Toxins, medications.
   d. Excessive physical activity.
5. Increase rest to improve fetal blood flow.
6. Antepartum fetal assessment (see Chapter 6) of fetal well-being and pulmonary status.

Timing of Delivery

Deliver as soon as pulmonary maturity is achieved to remove fetus from the hostile environment.

Intrapartum Management

Continuous fetal heart-rate monitoring should be used, supplemented by scalp-blood pH measurement.

NEONATAL OUTCOME
Immediate Morbidity of Asymmetric IUGR

1. Asphyxia
2. Meconium aspiration
3. Polycythemia
4. Hypoglycemia
5. Hypocalcemia
6. Hypothermia
7. Pulmonary alveolar hemorrhage

Long-Term Follow-up

Impaired physical and neurologic development are most common in the symmetrically growth-retarded infants and those infants with arrested head growth before 26 weeks' gestation. Asymmetrically growth-retarded infants usually display some catch-up growth.

REVIEW
QUESTIONS

1. Which of the following are important parameters in predicting long-term neurologic sequelae in infants with asymmetric growth retardation?
   a. Head circumference at birth
   b. Time of onset of growth retardation
   c. Presence of intrapartum asphyxia
   d. Gestational age at delivery
   e. All of the above
2. Which of the following ultrasonographic parameters can be used independently of gestational age to detect IUGR?
   a. Abdominal circumference
   b. Head circumference/abdominal circumference ratio
   c. Femur length/abdominal circumference ratio
   d. Transcerebellar diameter
   e. Head circumference
3. If serial fundal height measurements are carefully performed, the clinical diagnosis of IUGR can be expected to be accurate in approximately:
   a. 10% of cases
   b. 25% of cases
   c. 50% of cases
   d. 80% of cases
4. Which of the following has been associated with asymmetric growth retardation?
   a. Fetal rubella infection
   b. Maternal smoking
   c. Pregnancy-induced hypertension
   d. Fetal trisomies
   e. Maternal heroin addiction

5. Oligohydramnios may be diagnosed by ultrasonography when the largest vertical pocket of amniotic fluid is less than:
    a. 7 cm
    b. 1 cm
    c. 5 cm
    d. 4 cm
    e. 3 cm
6. Neonatal morbidity commonly associated with IUGR includes all of the following *except:*
    a. Asphyxia
    b. Meconium aspiration
    c. Polycythemia
    d. Respiratory distress syndrome
    e. Hypoglycemia

ANSWERS

1. e
2. c
3. b
4. c
5. b
6. d

BIBLIOGRAPHY

Benson CB, Doubilet PM, and Saltzman DH: Intrauterine growth retardation: predictive value of U/S criteria for antenatal diagnosis, Radiology 160:415, 1986.
Campbell S: Ultrasound measurement of the fetal head to abdomen circumference ratio in assessment of growth retardation, Br J Obstet Gynaecol 84:165, 1977.
Hadlock FP et al: A date-independent predictor of intrauterine growth retardation: femur length/abdominal circumference ratio, AJR 141:979, 1983.
Mintz MC, and Landon MB: Sonographic diagnosis of fetal growth disorders, Clin Obstet Gynecol 31:44-52, 1988.
Persson B et al: Prediction of size of infants at birth by measurement of symphysis fundus height, Br J Obstet Gynaecol 93:206, 1986.
Sabbagha RE, Hughey M, and Depp R: The assignment of growth-adjusted sonographic age (GASA): a simplified method, Obstet Gynecol 51:383, 1978.
Seeds J: Impaired fetal growth: definition and clinical diagnosis, Obstet Gynecol 64:303, 1984.
Seeds J: Impaired fetal growth: ultrasonic evaluation and clinical management, Obstet Gynecol 64:577, 1984.
Shepard MJ et al: An evaluation of two equations for predicting fetal weight by ultrasound, Am J Obstet Gynecol 142:48, 1982.

Preeclampsia-Eclampsia

13

Frederick P. Zuspan

Preeclampsia is a syndrome of unknown etiology that is characterized by the sequential development of facial and hand edema, hypertension, and proteinuria after the twentieth week of gestation. If only hypertension is present, the diagnosis is gestational hypertension. When both hypertension and proteinuria are present, the diagnosis of preeclampsia can then be made. Once the disease progresses and a patient with preeclampsia develops a seizure, the patient has eclampsia. Eclampsia portends the possibility of death for the mother (0.5% to 17% of cases) and for the fetus (10% to 37% of cases). The higher figures are observed in developing countries. Eclampsia can occur during the antepartum or intrapartum periods or during the first five postpartum days.

The demography of preeclampsia includes the following:
1. Occurs in 6% to 8% of pregnancies.
2. Principally a disease of the first-term pregnancy (85% of cases).
3. Occurs in 14% to 20% of multiple gestations.
4. Occurs in 30% of patients with major uterine anomalies.
5. Occurs in 25% of patients with chronic hypertension and 25% with chronic renal disease.
6. Some women may have repetitive severe disease, and it is most likely that this is because of a genetic tendency (e.g., a recessive gene).

The major goal of prenatal care is detection of early preeclampsia and aggressive therapy to prevent severe complications. All severe complications of preeclampsia-eclampsia should be preventable with prompt diagnosis.

DIAGNOSIS
Blood-Pressure Recordings

The object is to compare blood-pressure values of early gestation to late gestation and eliminate the cardiovascular alterations of the enlarging uterus on the great vessels. All blood-pressure recordings in pregnancy should be taken in the lateral recumbent position or with a 15- to 30-degree tilt to the left side.
1. Record the systolic blood pressure—I Korotkoff sound (opening sound).
2. Record IV Korotkoff sound (muffled).
3. Record V Korotkoff sound (disappears).

Findings are significant if the blood pressure is greater than 140/90 mm Hg or there is a rise of systolic pressure that is greater than 30 mm Hg or a rise of diastolic pressure that is greater than 15 mm Hg. The IV Korotkoff sound should be used because pregnancy is a condition with high cardiac output. A specific level of diastolic pressure should be used rather than a simple rise in blood pressure. The figure that has been chosen to make a diagnosis of gestational hypertension is the diastolic pressure level of 90 mm Hg, and if proteinuria is present, the diagnosis is termed *preeclampsia*. A rise certainly should be taken as a warning sign, but the specific diagnosis and classification of preeclampsia cannot be made without a diastolic blood pressure level of at least 90 mm Hg along with proteinuria.

PATHOGENESIS

The etiology is unknown, but the pathogenesis is understood.
1. Associated with:
    a. Increased placental mass, as seen in multiple gestation and diabetes.
    b. Cardiovascular/renal disease.
    c. First-term pregnancy.
    d. Uterine anomalies.
2. Systems involved include:
    a. The *uterus,* with its uteroplacental lesion where there is failure of trophoblasts to invade the spiral arteries. This results in less dilation, causing a relative decrease in blood flow. Additionally, the total adrenergic denervation that occurs in normal pregnancy in the uterus is less complete, resulting in more adrenergic nerves that can constrict the spiral arteries at their base.
    b. The *renal lesion* that causes proteinuria is glomeruloendotheliosis, which is a reversible lesion, but once established, it is present until delivery.
    c. The major *cardiovascular* lesion is generalized *vasospasm,* resulting in hypertension. As the disease progresses, sequestration of fluid leaves the vascular compartment for the third space, resulting in a decreased blood volume and increased hematocrit.
    d. The alteration in the cardiovascular system of increased sensitivity to pressor hormones and agents is associated with a decrease in prostacyclins and an increase in constricting thromboxanes.
3. Shock organs: the major systems.
    a. The uteroplacental bed.
    b. The kidney.
    c. The cardiovascular system.
4. Shock organs: the minor systems.
    a. The reticuloendothelial system, with a decrease in platelets and an increase in fibrin split products.
    b. The brain, with edema and hemorrhage.
    c. The liver, with necrosis and hemorrhage.
    d. The minor-system involvement indicates the seriousness of the disease and may cause death in the mother.

The cardiovascular changes in preeclamptic pregnancies include those listed in Table 13-1.

THE INFANT OF THE PREECLAMPTIC MOTHER

The problems for the baby are related principally to the degree of prematurity but may also include IUGR if maternal vasoconstriction has been present for a protracted period of time. Most offspring do well if they are more than 32 weeks of gestation. Interruption of pregnancy is usually because of maternal indication. Problems of the offspring relate to prematurity and not the preeclampsia-eclampsia.

CLASSIFICATION OF THE DISEASE

There are different degrees of seriousness of this disease. As a general rule, the earlier the onset, the more serious for the patient and her fetus because the pregnancy may need interruption for maternal indications.

Table 13-1   Cardiovascular changes in preeclamptic pregnancies

States	Normal Pregnancy (Compared to Prepregnant State)	Preeclampsia (Compared to Normal Pregnancy)
Cardiac output	Increased	Same/increased/decreased
Blood volume	Increased	Decreased
Peripheral resistance	Decreased in first and second trimester	Increased
Arterial blood pressure	Same in first and second trimester	Increased
Uteroplacental blood flow	Increased	Decreased
Cerebral blood flow	Increased	No change
Hepatic blood flow	Increased	No change
Renal blood flow	Increased until third to fourth week	Decreased

Gestational hypertension. In gestational hypertension, the blood pressure exceeds 140/90 or the systolic pressure increase is greater than 30 or the diastolic pressure increase is greater than 15 after the twentieth week of gestation. No proteinuria is present. (This is sometimes referred to as *pregnancy-induced hypertension [PIH].*)

Preeclampsia (mild). Mild preeclampsia is the presence of gestation hypertension and persistent proteinuria, with a protein concentration greater than 300 mg per liter. (Please note that edema no longer enters into the diagnosis of preeclampsia.)

Preeclampsia (severe). In severe preeclampsia, preeclampsia has progressed and one or more of the following signs or symptoms are present:

1. Systolic blood pressure greater than 160 mm Hg
2. Diastolic blood pressure greater than 110 mm Hg
3. Increased liver enzymes and/or jaundice
4. Platelets less than 100,000 per mm^3
5. Oliguria (less than 400 ml of urine in 24 hours)
6. Proteinuria (protein concentration greater than 3 g per liter or 4+ on random sample)
7. Retinal hemorrhages
8. Pulmonary edema
9. Coma
10. Hypogastric or epigastric pain

Assume severe disease is a medical emergency.

MANAGEMENT PROTOCOLS
Gestational Hypertension: Expectant Outpatient Management

1. See patient twice per week.
2. Monitor fetal well-being by confirming fetal kick count of greater than six per hour on two 1-hour evaluations each day. The patient rests on her side during the evaluations.
3. Educate patient to recognize increase in severity of disease.
4. Weigh twice a week.
5. Monitor blood pressure at home or office twice a week.
6. Test for proteinuria twice a week by dipstick.
7. Limit physical activity: complete bed rest with bathroom privileges.
8. Maintain normal diet without salt restriction.

Management of Preeclampsia (Gestational Hypertension with Proteinuria)

Patient should be hospitalized and the seriousness of the disease should be evaluated. Laboratory data include 24-hour urine protein, serum creatinine and uric acid, electrolytes, complete blood cell count (CBC), liver profile, and coagulation profile. Repeat results as indicated.

Clinical condition	Hospitalization
	Management
Patients who need hospitalization, i.e., have the diagnosis of preeclampsia	Measure urine output
	High-protein diet
	Fetal surveillance: monitor kick counts every day for two 1-hour periods— fetal well-being indicated by at least six kicks per hour
	Bed rest with bathroom privileges
	Weigh daily
	Measure blood pressure four times per day
	Consider induction if cervix is favorable and gestation is greater than 36 weeks
	Definitive treatment
Preeclampsia (severe) with immature fetus and/or fetal growth retardation	Prevent convulsions: use IV magnesium sulfate (4-6 gm load dose over 5 minutes, then 1-2 gm/hour)
	Control blood pressure: use IV hydralazine if diastolic pressure is persistently greater than 100
	Deliver by inducing labor and/or cesarean section after adequate observation and laboratory workup
Severe preeclampsia-eclampsia	Stop convulsions with magnesium sulfate program
	Control blood pressure with hydralazine program
	Deliver by inducing labor and/or cesarean section after baseline laboratory work of 2- to 4-hour observation

Anesthesia

Anesthesia for delivery could be any modality except spinal anesthesia. A spinal anesthetic is contraindicated because of the deranged maternal physiology. Epidural anesthesia under good conditions is quite satisfactory after adequate hydration, as is general anesthesia. If delivery is vaginal, local anesthesia or pudendal block is satisfactory. Pediatric standby is necessary in case the baby needs resuscitation.

Magnesium sulfate therapy

The standard of care in the United States is the use of magnesium sulfate to control convulsions. It is not a hypotensive drug, and benefits include an increase in uterine blood flow to protect the fetus and an increase in prostacyclins to prevent uterine vasoconstriction.

1. Administer parenterally. Excreted principally in the urine, and only 1% to 2% recovered in the feces. If oliguria, decrease dose because overdose may result.

2. Magnesium and calcium have a complex interdependent influence on the excitability of the components of the neuromuscular junction. If an overdose of magnesium is given, calcium chloride (1 g intravenously) can reverse the process.
3. If administered intravenously (the method of choice), take 5 minutes to give magnesium sulfate. The initial dose should be 4 to 6 g intravenously to saturate body tissues. Then give by controlled infusion pump at 1 to 2 g per hour.
4. Patient monitoring includes:
    a. Each hour, check deep tendon reflexes, which should be hypoactive but present.
        (1) Reflexes are absent if the serum magnesium concentration is greater than 5 mmol/l.
    b. Count respirations hourly (respiratory paralysis observed when concentration exceeds 6.5 mmol/l; cardiac arrest occurs above 12 mmol/l.
    c. Monitor hourly urine output by Foley catheter (should be at least 25 cc per hour or 100 cc per 4-hour period).
    d. Serum magnesium may be obtained as a guidepost to therapy but is usually not needed. Cord-blood magnesium helps guide the pediatrician.

Excretion of magnesium sulfate in the newborn is usually complete by 36 to 48 hours after birth, and adverse effects on the fetus are rare. Magnesium sulfate does not sedate either the mother or the fetus.

Control of blood pressure

The diastolic blood pressure should not be permitted to consistently exceed 100 mmHg. If this occurs, IV hydralazine in 2.5 to 5 mg IV-bolus doses is given. If additional hydralazine is needed after two doses, it is administered by a constant infusion pump in which 100 mg of hydralazine is instilled into a plastic bag containing 200 ml of saline. Infusion rate is dictated by the blood-pressure level and should be monitored by a pulse Doppler blood-pressure cuff.

The *standard of care in the United States* is the use of magnesium sulfate to control convulsions and the use of hydralazine to control blood pressure.

The drugs listed in Table 13-2 can also be used in pregnancy hypertension.

Vasodilators, such as sodium nitroprusside and diazoxide, produce significant side effects and are not used.

Diuretic agents are not used because they may adversely effect the fetus. No evidence exists that either diuretics or antihypertensive agents prevent the development of preeclampsia.

Decision for delivery in severe preeclampsia or eclampsia

Once the patient's seizure tendency and blood pressure are controlled, a decision should be made as to whether or not delivery should take place. The more serious the condition of the patient, the greater the need to proceed to delivery. (Delivery is the definitive cure for the disease, and all medications and therapy are identified as temporizing measures.)

1. Establish gestational age by history, lung maturity, or ultrasonography.
2. Try to achieve delivery as soon as possible—there is no magic waiting period for stabilization. All laboratory tests should be returned within 2 to 4 hours. A decision for delivery can then be made.
3. Laboratory tests: electrolytes, liver function battery, and complete hemogram and clotting profile, including platelets and fibrin split products.
4. Evaluate condition of cervix, and if it is favorable and has a good Bishop score, proceed with oxytocin induction if the presentation of the fetus is vertex and the

Table 13-2 Antihypertensive drugs used to treat hypertension in pregnancy

Drug	Action	Oral Dose (mg)	Parenteral Dose (mg)
Methyldopa	Inhibition of vasoconstricting impulses from vasoregulatory center in medulla oblongata, inhibition of impulses from hypothalamus	500 (3 to 4 times daily) (tablet size 250)	250-500
Propranolol	β-adrenergic blockade, usually associated with decreased cardiac output	20-40 (4 times daily)	—
Hydralazine	Direct relaxation of arterioles, action on muscle, increased cardiac output	20-40 (4 times daily) when prolonged tachyphylaxis may occur	2.5-5
Labetalol	α- and β-blockade	100 (2-3 times daily)	100
Prazosin	α-adrenergic blockade	0.5-5 (2-3 times daily)	—

fetus is greater than 1500 g. If the cervix is unfavorable and urgency for delivery is not apparent, consider prostaglandin gel (2 mg) ripening, which may also promote uterine contractions.

5. If fetus is less than 1500 g, consider cesarean section.
6. If fetus is greater than 1500 g, begin trial of labor using diluted intravenous oxytocin (10 units/1000 cc lactated Ringer's solution) and begin at 1 mU per minute with a controlled infusion device. Use fetal monitoring, and when membranes rupture, apply internal scalp clip. If patient does not deliver in 8 to 12 hours, consider cesarean section.
7. If time permits a 48-hour waiting period, it is permissible if lung maturity is poor, to consider maternal adrenal steroids.
   a. Betamethasone (2 doses of 12 mg 12 hours apart)
   b. Dexamethasone (8 mg qid for 1 day)
   c. Either betamethasone or dexamethasone should accelerate pulmonary maturity if the fetus is less than 35 weeks gestation. Steroids do not worsen the hypertension.

Management of central venous pressure and pulmonary capillary wedge pressure (Swan-Ganz catheter)

If an arterial or venous catheter is chosen for use in the patient, it is necessary to first establish that the patient has a good blood-clotting mechanism. (A catheter is seldom necessary.)

1. Swan-Ganz monitoring helps avoid fluid overloads and prevents iatrogenic pulmonary edema.
2. Swan-Ganz monitoring is used to show that the patient is unable to cope with circulating volume that is necessary to maintain the cardiac index and ventricular filling pressure. Patients with preeclampsia do not have the capacity for vasodilation.
3. Volume expanders are potentially dangerous and should be monitored by Swan-Ganz data.

Postnatal Care

1. Continue therapeutic doses of magnesium sulfate for at least 24 hours, then gradually reduce.
2. Control blood pressure with antihypertensive drugs. Patient may need a prescription for oral medications if diastolic blood pressure exceeds 100 mmHg when she goes home.
3. Diuresis should occur by 72 hours after birth.
4. Oral contraceptives may be given at the 6-weeks' examination if the blood pressure is normal.

PREVENTION

1. Identify the potentially high-risk patient, i.e., one with first-term pregnancy, diabetes, chronic renal or cardiovascular disease, major uterine anomalies, multiple gestation, or genetic predisposition. If any of these factors are present, see patient at frequent-interval rate (i.e., every 2 to 3 weeks) after 20 weeks gestation.
2. Encourage bed rest—half an hour at noon and one hour before evening dinner. If gestational hypertension develops, patient must restrict her activities to home bed rest and be seen at least twice a week.
3. Encourage a diet of at least 1 g of protein per kilogram of body weight per day to prevent a negative nitrogen balance. (Neither diet nor salt restriction have been shown to prevent preeclampsia.)
4. No restriction on salt intake.

Baby Aspirin and Calcium Studies

Studies have now shown that baby aspirin (i.e., 40 to 80 mg of aspirin per day) may be enough to increase prostacyclins, decrease the thromboxanes, and prevent the occurrence of severe preeclampsia. Studies have yet to show whether or not the administration of baby aspirin on a daily basis from the twentieth week of gestation is preventive. There have been suggestions in studies in developing countries that a high calcium intake (i.e., greater than 2 g per day) may be beneficial in the prevention of severe complications of pregnancy. Further studies are needed to establish these as realistic therapy programs.

REVIEW
QUESTIONS

1. The basic etiology of preeclampsia-eclampsia is:
   a. Disruption of aldosterone-angiotensin system
   b. Excessive salt intake and retention
   c. Decreased protein intake
   d. Dissimulated intravascular coagulopathy
   e. Unknown
2. Treatment of severe preeclampsia-eclampsia includes:
   a. Therapeutic levels of parenteral magnesium sulfate
   b. Diuretic therapy
   c. Morphine sulfate as needed
   d. Dilantin and phenobarbital therapy
   e. Diazepam therapy

3. The decision for delivery in preeclampsia should be based on:
   a. Condition of the cervix
   b. Condition of the mother
   c. Condition of the fetus
   d. Response to therapy
   e. All of the above
4. The treatment of hypermagnesemia is:
   a. Stop magnesium sulfate
   b. Calcium chloride intravenously
   c. Assisted ventilation if needed
   d. All of the above
5. The blood pressure during pregnancy:
   a. Should be taken by recording IV Korotkoff sound for diastolic reading.
   b. Is increased by activity.
   c. Should be taken in the lateral recumbent position.
   d. All of the above.
6. The severity of the bood pressure in pregnancy is:
   a. Directly related to fetal outcome.
   b. Inversely related to fetal outcome.
   c. Not related to fetal outcome.
   d. None of the above.

ANSWERS

1. e
2. a
3. e
4. d
5. d
6. a

BIBLIOGRAPHY

Pritchard JA, and Stone SR: Clinical and laboratory observations of eclampsia, Am J Obstet Gynecol 99:754, 1967.

Robertson WP et al: The placental bed biopsy: review from three European centers, Am J Obstet Gynecol 155:401, 1986.

Sibai BM, Graham JM, and McCubbin JH: A comparison of intravenous and intermuscular magnesium sulfate regimens in preeclampsia, Am J Obstet Gynecol 150:728, 1984.

Wallenberg H et al: Low-dose aspirin prevents pregnancy-induced hypertension and preeclampsia in angiotensin sensitive primigravida, Lancet 1(8471):1, 1986.

World Health Organization Study Group (Zuspan, FP, chairman): The hypertensive disorders of pregnancy, Tech Rep Series 758, Geneva, 1987, World Health Organization.

Zuspan FP, and Talledo OE: Factors affecting delivery in eclampsia condition of the cervix and uterine activity, Am J Obstet Gynecol 100:672, 1968.

Chronic Hypertension in Pregnancy

14

Frederick P. Zuspan

Acute and chronic hypertension in pregnancy constitute the most common medical problem (8% to 11% of pregnancies) seen in pregnancy. Between one third to one half the cases of hypertension in pregnancy are chronic hypertensive disease. The most common diagnosis is essential vascular hypertension, for which there is no known cause. Chronic hypertension in pregnancy is diagnosed if the patient has a sustained elevation of arterial blood pressure that is greater than 140/90 mmHg before the twentieth week of gestation. A persistent diastolic blood pressure of greater than 80 mmHg before the twentieth week of gestation should warrant suspicion. Hypertension is classified as mild, moderate, or severe, depending on the absolute level of the blood pressure (BP) reading, with or without evidence of end-organ damage. The clinical syndrome of acute hypertension (i.e., preeclampsia) superimposed on existing chronic hypertensive disease is the most serious for both mother and fetus. A simplified classification of chronic hypertensive disease is shown in the box on p. 182.

PATHOPHYSIOLOGY AND BLOOD-PRESSURE REGULATION

The brachial artery blood pressure is highest when a patient is sitting, lower when she is lying on her back, and lowest when she is lying on her side. Uterine size and compression of the inferior vena cava and aorta are factors that alter blood-pressure recordings after the twentieth week of gestation.

1. Use two-headed stethoscope to teach patient how to take her own blood pressure.
2. Take blood pressure with patient in left lateral recumbent position, using upper arm. May use only 15- to 30-degree tilt of body.
3. Use upper arm, and lower to near heart level to record blood pressure. Aneroid gauge manometer preferred.
4. Record systolic, IV, and V Korotkoff sounds. The IV Korotkoff sound is preferable because pregnancy is a condition with high cardiac output.
5. If mean arterial blood pressure is greater than 100, prognosis for fetus worsens.

$$\text{Mean BP} = \frac{S + 2D}{3}$$

   where S is systolic and D is diastolic. Fetal loss is directly proportional to elevation of blood pressure.
6. Use home blood-pressure recordings if you suspect chronic hypertension or if office blood pressure is persistently greater than 140/90. Preferred recording time is in morning (lowest) and before rest in the afternoon (highest). Ask pa-

---

Chronic Hypertensive Disease
Hypertension before the Twentieth Week of Gestation

Primary

Essential or idiopathic—most common type observed

Secondary (to a known cause)
Renal

Parenchymal (glomerular nephritis, chronic pyelonephritis, interstitial nephritis, polycystic kidney), renal vascular

Adrenal gland

Cortical: Cushing's syndrome, hyperaldosteronism
  Medullary: pheochromocytoma
  Other: coarctation of aorta, thyrotoxicosis

From Zuspan FP, and O'Shaughnessy RW: Chronic hypertension in pregnancy. In Pitkin RM, and Zlatnik FJ, editors: Yearbook of obstetrics and gynecology, Chicago, 1979, Year Book Medical Publishers Inc.

tient to record I, IV, and V Korotkoff sounds. Take blood pressure at least two to three times per week. Home blood-pressure reading is most accurate.

THE SUSPICION AND DIAGNOSIS OF THE DISEASE

Consider a patient at potential risk for the hypertensive diseases of pregnancy if one or more of the following are present:
1. Diastolic blood pressure in nonpregnant state or before 20 weeks gestation exceeds 80 mmHg.
2. History of antecedent hypertension.
3. History of secondary causes of hypertension (such as renal disease).
4. Positive family history of hypertension.
5. Hypertension in previous pregnancy.

EARLY EVALUATION OF THE PREGNANT HYPERTENSIVE PATIENT

1. Include a funduscopic examination in the physical examination.
2. Evaluate heart size by palpation, and if necessary, do a chest x-ray examination.
3. Auscultate over the renal arteries and abdomen to rule out a bruit consistent with renovascular hypertension.
4. Palpate the femoral and radial arteries simultaneously to rule out coarctation of the aorta.
5. Teach the patient how to take her own blood pressure, using a two-headed stethoscope, in the lateral recumbent position. Ask her to take blood pressure readings three times a week—during a morning, an evening before she rests, and a weekend when she does not work.

Screening laboratory data should include the following:
1. Complete urinalysis—to test for proteinuria or abnormal microscopic sediment that suggests renal disease.
2. A 24-hour urine sample—for protein and creatinine clearance to rule out renal disease.
3. Serum electrolytes—to rule out primary hyperaldosteronism.

4. If the blood pressure is episodic, urinary catecholamines—to rule out pheochromo-cytoma.
5. Ultrasonography of kidneys—to rule out a unilateral contracted kidney.
6. EKG and chest x-ray examination are optional, depending upon the severity of the hypertension.

Renal disease is more prevalent than appreciated; studies at the University of Chicago have shown that, clinically, only 1% of chronic renal disease is diagnosed. When renal biopsy by electron microscopy was done, 17% of patients had chronic renal disease that was unsuspected. Renal biopsy is not currently recommended in pregnancy except under very special circumstances.

HOME BLOOD-PRESSURE DATA

The findings comparing home and office blood-pressure recordings indicate that only 31% of office and home blood-pressure recordings agree. In other words, 69% of the blood-pressure recordings are different, and in more than 50% of these cases, the office blood-pressure recording is higher than the home blood-pressure recording. This may lead to unnecessary use of medications. Rayburn et al (see bibliography) have also shown that home blood-pressure recordings decrease the need for antihypertensive medications (48% versus 76% of pregnant hypertensive patients) as well as hospitalization (11% versus 76% of pregnant hypertensive patients).

The benefits of home blood-pressure recording are:
1. Alters perception of physician and nurse toward blood pressure recorded in the office. Antihypertensive therapy should not be started because of one or two office readings of mild hypertension.
2. Underscores the role of emotions, anxiety, and environment in blood-pressure recordings.
3. Makes the patient her own advocate, and further reinforces the role of bed rest.
4. Diminishes the use of antihypertensive drugs during pregnancy.
5. Decreases the need for hospitalization.

MANAGEMENT

If at all possible, preconceptional counseling is important for the woman who has chronic hypertension. She may well have had a tragic experience with a previous pregnancy and may or may not have developed preeclampsia. It is important to establish baseline data on this patient and to teach her how to monitor her own blood pressure before conception. If the patient is on diuretic medication, she should be advised to gradually discontinue taking it before conception. If she has not discontinued taking the medication before conception, this must be taken into consideration when the patient is first seen after conception. It may take 3 to 4 weeks to gradually eliminate the medication in order to prevent rebound fluid retention. An appropriate diet that curtails heavy salt use is recommended. This can be achieved by eating fresh and frozen food and avoiding food in cans and bottles.

Diagnosis and Initial Assessment During Pregnancy

1. In-depth history (look for history of renal disease or repeated UTI and at family history) and physical examination.
2. Basic baseline laboratory tests (usual prenatal determinations plus tests for electrolytes, serum creatinine and blood urea nitrogen (BUN), urea clearance, and 24-hour urinary protein).
3. Patient records her own blood pressure.

4. Observation by patient of the effect of bed rest on blood pressure.
5. Frequent prenatal visits (at least every 2 weeks).
6. If home diastolic blood-pressure recording consistently exceeds 84 mmHg in early pregnancy, consider pharmacotherapy for control of blood pressure. (There is no proof to date that pharmacotherapy will alter fetal salvage, but it will control major alterations in maternal blood pressure. Also, it does not prevent preeclampsia.)
7. Major emphasis should be on half an hour of bed rest at noontime and an hour and a half of bed rest before preparing the evening meal—this may be the most important therapy for fetal health. Start no later than 16 weeks gestation. (See Fig. 14-1.)
8. A well-balanced diet, with at least 70 g of protein per day, is fundamental to maintain zero nitrogen balance. If overt hypertension is present, salt intake should be restricted by eating fresh or frozen food and nothing out of a bottle or a can (this is a 4 g sodium chloride diet). The kidney can regulate sodium metabolism over a wide range of daily salt intake, and in most instances, severe salt restriction in the diet is not needed.
9. Therapeutic abortion is rarely necessary.
10. Establish firm date for estimated date of delivery. Ultrasonography is advisable.

Pharmacotherapy

1. Start antihypertensive medication when home diastolic blood pressure consistently exceeds 84 mmHg or consistent office blood pressure is greater than 90 mmHg.
2. Current drug of choice is methyldopa (Aldomet) in divided doses of 750 to 2000 mg per day.

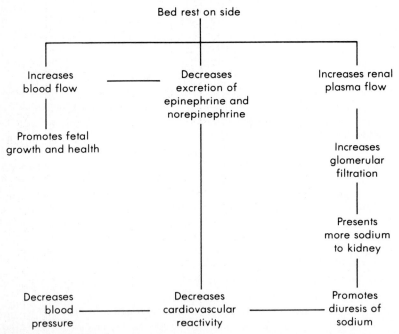

Fig. 14-1
Role of bed rest in fetal/maternal health.

3. Continue additional bed rest to minimize drug therapy. Examine work habits of patient carefully.
4. Consider using β-blocker such as propranolol or atenolol. Labetalol (α- and β-blocker) has also been used. (See Table 14-1.) All drugs cross placenta/fetus, and newborns make good adjustments unless prematurity is a major factor. These drugs do not cause birth defects. Current recommendations suggest avoiding lactation if patient will be on β-blocker after birth. Parlodel should *not* be used for lactation suppression.
5. Hydralazine may be used but should not be a first-choice drug. Can be used in conjunction with methyldopa. Oral use associated with tachyphylaxis.

MANAGEMENT GENERALIZATIONS

1. Intrapartum fetal evaluation (NST) should begin at 30 weeks gestation and occur on each subsequent visit.
2. Biochemical testing is of no value; biophysical testing is more reliable.
3. Careful dating of gestation and serial ultrasonography to rule out IUGR is necessary. IUGR is usually not seen until after 30 to 32 weeks of gestation. Need a minimum of three ultrasonograms.
4. Chronic hypertension is associated with a four- to eight-fold increase in abruptio placentae—care should be taken when the patient complains of abdominal discomfort.
5. Do not permit patient to go beyond term because placenta may have dysmaturity. Often an earlier delivery may be necessary.
6. Observe for preeclampsia, which is indicated by an increase in blood pressure and development of proteinuria. The patient can help you diagnose these.
7. Hospitalize patient if preeclampsia or IUGR intervenes.

Antepartum Fetal Evaluation (Biophysical Testing)

1. Serial ultrasonography to date gestation should be done at around 10 to 12 weeks, at 20 to 24 weeks, and at 30 to 32 weeks. During the third ultrasonogram, observe for IUGR.
2. NST on each visit from 30 weeks on, and nipple stimulation or oxytocin challenge test (OCT) as needed. Vibratory stimulation of fetus will abbreviate the NST.
3. Fetal movement activity count—instruct patient to lie on her side for two 1-hour periods and do fetal-kick count. If greater than six per hour, this indicates fetal health.
4. If preterm delivery is anticipated, glucocorticoids with betamethasone or dexamethasone may be given to enhance fetal lung maturity if mother's condition is stable and there is no fetal distress. These drugs do not worsen hypertension.
5. Convert an unfavorable cervix to a favorable cervix with vaginal prostaglandin (2

Table 14-1   Commonly used drugs in treating hypertension in pregnancy

Drug Name	Type	Usual Dose
Propranolol	β-blocker	20 to 40 mg bid to qid
Atenolol	β-blocker	25 to 50 mg bid to tid
Labetalol	β-blocker with α component	100 mg bid or tid
Hydralazine	Direct action—not α- or β-blocker	20 to 30 mg bid to qid

mg in a diaphragm or intracervical insertion of 0.5 mg). This may alter the cervical condition and permit vaginal delivery using oxytocin. Method to make up prostaglandin gel: 20 mg prostaglandin E_2 (Prostin E2) suppository mixed with 40 cc of KY Jelly, then dispensed in 4-cc plastic syringe (2 mg) for use with vaginal diaphragm.

Labor and Delivery

1. Deliver no later than term, and deliver before term if superimposed preeclampsia intercedes or fetal distress or IUGR are observed.
2. Continuously monitor patient during labor.
3. Perform early rupture of membranes for scalp-clip application and judicious use of scalp pH as needed.
4. Regional anesthesia with epidural is satisfactory and ideal. Guard against hypotension with fluid load before anesthesia.
5. Pediatrician should be available for evaluation of baby. Assume all antihypertensive agents cross placenta. Newborn usually does well.

The majority of women with mild chronic hypertension will do well during pregnancy, and the need for sterilization is not apparent, except as an option. If severe hypertension is present, surgical sterilization (if not after delivery then as an interim procedure by laparoscopy) should be seriously discussed. As a general rule, the woman with chronic hypertension most likely should *not* be given oral contraceptives. It is usually necessary to send the patient home with an antihypertensive medication that she has been on during pregnancy, but often at a reduced dose. Have her readjust dose by home blood-pressure recordings and verbal consultations with the obstetrician. Her postpartum blood pressure at 6 weeks will probably continue to be elevated unless she is on antihypertensive medication.

LONG-TERM CONTRACEPTION

Women who have chronic hypertension should not be placed on oral contraceptives. Some form of barrier contraception is preferable. Those women who have completed their childbearing can be offered a permanent form of contraception.

REVIEW
QUESTIONS

1. The severity of the blood pressure in pregnancy is:
   a. Directly related to fetal outcome
   b. Inversely related to fetal outcome
   c. Not related to fetal outcome
   d. None of the above
2. Chronic hypertension can usually be diagnosed:
   a. Before pregnancy
   b. Most easily in multipara
   c. Because parents often have genetic component
   d. All of the above
3. The differential diagnosis between acute and chronic hypertension:
   a. Is very difficult in primipara
   b. Is aided by renal biopsy
   c. Has deleterious effect on fetus
   d. All of the above

4. The blood pressure during pregnancy:
   a. Should use IV Korotkoff sound for diastolic reading
   b. Is increased by activity
   c. Should be taken in the lateral recumbent position
   d. All of the above

ANSWERS

1. a
2. d
3. d
4. d

BIBLIOGRAPHY

Rayburn WF, Zuspan FP, and Biehl EJ: Self–blood pressure monitoring during pregnancy, Am J Obstet Gynecol 148:159, 1984.
Redman CWG et al: Fetal outcome in trial of antihypertensive treatment in pregnancy, Lancet 2:753, 1976.
Reiss RE et al: Retrospective analysis of blood pressure course during preeclamptic and matched controls, Am J Obstet Gynecol 156:894, 1987.
Rubin PC et al: Obstetric aspects of the use of pregnancy-associated hypertension of the β-adrenoceptor antagonist, atenolol, Am J Obstet Gynecol 150:389, 1984.
Sibai BM, Abdella TN, and Anderson GD: Pregnancy outcome in 211 patients with mild chronic hypertension, Obstet Gynecol 61:571, 1983.
Sibai BM, Grossman RA and Grossman H: Effects of diuretics on plasma volume in pregnancies with long-term hypertension, Am J Obstet Gynecol 150:831, 1984.
Zuspan FP: Chronic hypertension in pregnancy, Clin Obstet Gynecol 27:854, 1984.
Zuspan FP, and O'Shaughnessy RW: Maternal physiology and diseases: chronic hypertension in pregnancy. In Pitkin RM, and Zlatnik FJ, editors: Yearbook of obstetrics and gynecology, Chicago, 1979, Year Book Medical Publishers Inc.

Postterm Pregnancy

Frederick P. Zuspan

Postterm pregnancy is defined as the continuation of pregnancy beyond 295 days (*term gestation* is between 38 to 42 weeks duration). Approximately 5% to 7% of pregnancies go beyond 42 weeks gestation, but the true incidence of postterm pregnancy is unknown because of multiple factors.

1. Several related and unrelated factors are associated with pregnancies beyond 41 weeks gestation. The lowest perinatal morbidity and mortality is seen between 39 to 41 weeks gestation.
2. The majority of "diagnosed" postterm pregnancies are the result of factors such as inappropriate dating of the pregnancy or a prolonged follicular phase. Hence the patient who has been taking her basal body temperature may be the only patient for whom the true estimated date of confinement (EDC) and actual postdate gestation can be accurately diagnosed.
3. Prolonged gestation is seen with congenital anomalies, absent pituitary as seen in anencephaly, hypoplastic fetal adrenals, placental sulphatase deficiency, and fetal osteogenesis imperfecta.
4. Recurrence rate may be as high as 50%.
5. Postterm pregnancy is seen more frequently in primigravida, and a positive correlation exists with ethnicity (Australians, Greeks, and Italians).

Some confusion about the pathophysiology of postterm pregnancy exists. It is important to remember that there are two types of postterm gestation. In the first type (95% of cases), the placenta is normal, and the fetus continues to grow and does not have any of the stigmata characteristically described as being seen in a fetus in a postterm pregnancy. The patient who has a normal placenta and goes beyond 295 days ends up with a macrosomic fetus with associated cephalopelvic disproportion (CPD); shoulder dystocia is not uncommon in these fetuses, and the incidence of cesarean section is higher because of CPD. In the second type of postterm pregnancy (5% of cases), the placenta is dysmature, and the fetal prognosis is poor.

The feto-placental unit dictates whether a potential problem may exist in any given pregnancy that goes beyond 41 weeks. Some consideration should be given to an understanding of its growth and development, which includes the following:

1. Placental function declines after 36 weeks, and placental growth no longer continues after 34 to 36 weeks of gestation. Placental aging may then begin.
2. The dysmature placenta has altered placental function, a decrease in thickness, and an increase in infarction, fibrin, and calcium deposition, resulting in diminished placental reserve.
3. Uterine sensitivity to oxytocin is often decreased; hence uterine inertia is seen more frequently.

4. The cervix does not know when the fetus is to be delivered and frequently is unfavorable, with a low Bishop score.
5. Amniotic-fluid volume diminishes as gestation progresses: estimated volume — 1000 ml at 38 weeks, 300 to 400 ml at 42 weeks, and less than 300 ml after 42 weeks gestation. Ultrasonography shows whether or not the amniotic-fluid volume is diminished. If it is, this may be an ominous sign for the fetus and probably indicates a dysmature placenta. It may be associated with cord compression problems during labor.

DIAGNOSIS

Pregnancy dating is the single most important issue when trying to diagnosis postterm gestation — it is the actual key to making the diagnosis.
1. Establish a known and recorded last menstrual period — believe what patient tells you and calculate EDC.
2. If the patient has been using the basal body temperatures method, it is the most reliable method of dating the EDC.
3. Conducting an early pelvic examination before 12 weeks of gestation in a nonobese patient is helpful (because uterine size equals gestational age).
4. An ultrasonographic examination performed at the tenth to twelfth week of gestation is accurate within a range of plus-or-minus 7 days — a good case can be made for an early ultrasonographic examination of all patients because of this one issue. If an ultrasonographic examination is not done at 10 to 12 weeks gestation, one should be done at 16 to 20 weeks of gestation to confirm the EDC.
5. Quickening in a primigravida at 18 to 20 weeks gestation or a multigravida at 16 to 18 weeks gestation is also helpful in dating the pregnancy.
6. Uterine measurement from symphysis to uterine fundus by tape measure is most accurate when 28 cm equals 28 weeks of gestation.

If a discrepancy exists in history, clinical examination, and uterine size, an ultrasonographic examination should be done to firm up the EDC.

PATHOPHYSIOLOGY

Meconium staining of amniotic fluid — present in 20% to 30% of cases in normal-term gestation, but in postdate pregnancies the percentage of patients that have meconium staining is increased to as high as 50%. This may or may not be a sign of chronic placental aging.

FETAL AND NEONATAL FINDINGS

The diagnosis of postterm gestation usually affects only the fetus and not the mother and is often made as an after-the-fact diagnosis in the nursery or delivery room. The newborn may exhibit the classic findings associated with a dysmature placenta, which are:
1. First stage: long nails, skin with parchmentlike wrinkling and peeling, a long thin infant who appears malnourished and lacks subcutaneous fat.
2. Second stage: identical to the first stage with the addition of meconium in amniotic fluid with staining of membranes, placenta, and fetal skin.
3. Third stage: amniotic fluid, fetal skin, and membranes are markedly stained yellow; a wrinkled, shriveled, "old-man" appearance of the fetus, who often may appear to be apprehensive.

Problems for the newborn range from no problems to a stillbirth, with multiple problems between the two extremes. During the intrapartum period, the diminished amniotic fluid may result in variable cord sign decelerations of the fetal heart. If the placenta is too dysmature, late decelerations may also be seen. Once the baby is delivered, polycythemia and hypoglycemia may be present. However, if thick meconium is present, immediate meconium aspiration for the newborn may be a possibility. A pediatrician should evaluate the newborn as soon as is practical. If a pediatrician is not present, the obstetrician may be obligated to put the baby in an incubator after using a DeLee suction trap when the baby's head first emerges from the perineum. Actual intubation may be necessary if a meconium plug is present in the trachea. This is usually not seen unless thick, tenacious meconium exists.

PREGNANCY MANAGEMENT

It is obvious that before a course of action can be determined, the diagnosis of postterm pregnancy must be made with some degree of certainty. Problems exist principally for the fetus in regard to the presence or absence of chronic intrauterine hypoxia and growth.

Three schools of thought concerning pregnancy management currently exist:
1. No induction. The risk of postdate pregnancy is not well known, but the risk of an induction may be greater. Data are available from randomized prospective studies to substantiate this position.
2. Routine induction. A routine of inducing all patients who have reached 42 weeks of gestation does eliminate the problem of postterm gestation. Because the cervix is often unfavorable, the cesarean-section rate will be higher than the current incidence of 20% to 25% for all pregnancies. The case for routine induction has gained momentum in recent times because of the litigious medical-legal milieu that exists.
3. Selective induction. Selective induction may be carried out when the cervix is favorable with confirmed pregnancy dates or when there is evidence of a failing fetoplacental functioning unit.

Once a patient reaches 42 weeks gestation, one of the preceding management methods can be instituted; the the following fetal assessment programs are often helpful when the method of management is being chosen (see also Chapter 6):
1. Sonography—growth curves, fetal size, and, most importantly, the amount of amniotic fluid, which is the single most important factor in decision making in induction of labor.
2. Cardiotachometry—biophysical testing using NST, breast/nipple stimulation or formal CST with oxytocin if the results of the NST and breast/nipple stimulation are not satisfactory. Testing should begin at the end of the forty-first week of gestation and be done on a biweekly basis.
3. Fetal activity score—the patient is instructed to rest on her side for two 1-hour periods each day and record the number of kick counts. If six or more counts per hour take place, this is considered normal fetal activity.
4. Biophysical profile—done under ultrasonography with the use of a scoring system.
5. Umbilical artery and uterine artery Doppler velocimetry— role is uncertain at present in these patients.
6. Estrogen/creatinine ratios—originally thought to be helpful but are no longer done. Hence biophysical testing is the procedure of choice.

LABOR MONITORING

1. If the patient has a postterm pregnancy, labor monitoring using direct fetal scalp monitoring is important.
2. Scalp pH should be available and done if persistent abnormalities of the fetal heart are noted, including multiple variable decelerations as well as late decelerations.
3. Cervical ripening has been attempted with some degree of success using agents such as a Foley catheter, locally applied estrogens, vaginal prostaglandins, intracervical laminaria, and intracervical vaginal prostaglandin gel. These agents are all used to convert an unfavorable cervix to a favorable cervix in an attempt to decrease the incidence of cesarean section.

THE DELIVERY

1. If a dysmature placenta did not exist, be aware of CPD with an increased incidence of shoulder dystocia caused by macrosomia.
2. Cesarean-section rate with postterm gestations will be greater than the current average of 20% to 25%.
3. Have adequate anesthesia available for unknown complications that may exist.
4. If available, a pediatrician should be present in the delivery room.

REVIEW
QUESTIONS

More than one correct answer is possible.
1. Fetal outcome in postterm pregnancy is determined by:
   a. Length of gestation
   b. Fetal lung maturity
   c. Congenital anomalies
   d. Placental grading on ultrasonogram
   e. Functional type of placenta
2. Fetal/newborn problems encountered in postterm pregnancy include:
   a. Macrosomia
   b. Increased blood viscosity
   c. Meconium-stained amniotic fluid
   d. Dysmature placenta
   e. All of the above
3. Problems associated in managing postterm pregnancy include:
   a. Accuracy in dating conception
   b. Determining type of placenta (i.e., normal versus dysmature)
   c. Low Bishop score on cervix
   d. Lack of sensitivity to infused oxytocin
   e. All of the above
4. Which of the following are correct statements in regard to prolonged gestation?
   a. It may be associated with fetal congenital anomalies.
   b. There may be decreased amniotic fluid.
   c. There may be cord compression patterns during labor on fetal heart tracing.
   d. It is seen more frequently in older, multiparous patients.

ANSWERS

1. e
2. e
3. e
4. a, b, c

BIBLIOGRAPHY

Ballantyne JW: The problem of postmature infant, J Obstet Gynaecol Br Emp 2:36, 1902.

Beicher NA, Vans JH, and Townsend L: Studies in prolonged pregnancy, Am J Obstet Gynecol 103:476, 1969.

Clifford SH: Postmaturity with placental dysfunction, J Pediatr 44:1, 1954.

Cole RA, Howie PW, and MacNaughten MC: Elective induction of labor: a randomized prospective trial, Lancet 1:767, 1975.

Freeman RK et al: Postdate utilization of the contraction stress test for primary fetal surveillance, Am J Obstet Gynecol 140:128, 1981.

Gibb DMF et al: Prolonged pregnancy: is induction of labor indicated? A prospective study, Br J Obstet Gynaecol 84:292, 1982.

Naeye RL: Causes of perinatal mortality: excess and prolonged gestations, Am J Epidemiol 108:429, 1978.

Resnik R: Postterm gestation: a symposium, J Reprod Med 33:249, 1988.

Vorheer RH: Placental insufficiency in relation to postterm pregnancy and fetal postmaturity, Am J Obstet Gynecol 124:67, 1975.

Labor and Delivery

16

Edward J. Quilligan

Proper management of labor, delivery, and the puerperium is one of the most important tasks of the obstetrician-gynecologist. As in antenatal care, the goal of intrapartum care is maximal safety for mother and infant in a style that facilitates a positive beginning to the parent-child relationship. Most women will do relatively well during pregnancy, labor, and delivery, and a minimum of medical intervention is necessary to meet these goals. Some, however, will require substantial intervention to achieve a safe and comfortable delivery. Deciding who needs and who does not need the various interventions available to the obstetrician is a continuing challenge, faced anew with each laboring patient. It requires a thorough understanding of the normal labor process and its myriad variations.

THE PROCESS OF LABOR

1. *Labor* is uterine activity that results in progressive dilation and/or effacement of the uterine cervix over a brief period of time (less than 24 to 36 hours).
2. *Effacement* is the thinning of the cervix (see Fig. 16-1). The normal length of the cervix in a nonpregnant woman is approximately 5 cm—the degree of effacement is expressed as the percentage remaining of this length (e.g., a woman in early labor may have a cervical length of 3 cm—her cervix would therefore be 40% effaced).
3. *Dilation* is the diameter of the cervical os, which is expressed in centimeters. In women who are pregnant for the first time, both the internal os and the external os are closed. In *parous* women (those who have given birth before), the external os may be as much as 3-cm dilated, but the internal os is normally 1 cm.

Before labor, the cervix of most women will efface and even dilate to some degree. The extent to which this occurs before labor is termed *cervical ripening* and is a significant determinant of the length of actual labor that will be required to reach complete cervical dilation (10 cm) and effacement (100%). Labor may be compared to a journey—the final destination—delivery—is the same for all, but the distance from the starting point differs from one woman to another, resulting in the well-known wide variations in the length of labor (from less than 3 hours to more than 24 hours [see Table 16-1]). Cervical dilation and effacement occur as the result of both biochemical and physical factors. The physical process of each labor contraction pulling the cervix against the presenting fetal part occurs once labor has begun. The biochemical process shown in the box on p. 197 occurs both before labor, independent of uterine contractile activity, and during labor, along with contractions (see Fig. 16-2).

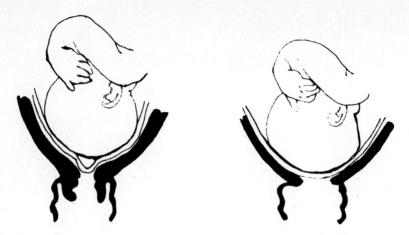

Fig. 16-1
The fetal vertex applied to the cervix. The cervix is dilated and pulled upward over the presenting part.

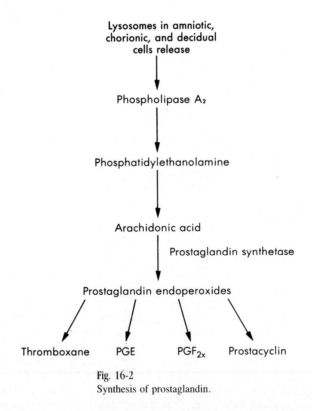

Lysosomes in amniotic,
chorionic, and decidual
cells release

Phospholipase A₂

Phosphatidylethanolamine

Arachidonic acid

Prostaglandin synthetase

Prostaglandin endoperoxides

Thromboxane   PGE   PGF₂ₓ   Prostacyclin

Fig. 16-2
Synthesis of prostaglandin.

Biochemical Alterations in the Cervix as Labor Approaches

Collagen and protein concentrations decrease
Hyaluronic acid increases
Prostaglandin E_2 released
Water content increases

Table 16-1   Average durations of various phases of labor

Phase	Duration for Nulliparas (hr)	Duration for Multiparas (hr)
Latent phase	6-11	4-8
Active phase	4-6	2-3
Second stage	1-2	0.5-1

STAGES OF LABOR

Labor is described in three stages (see Table 16-1):

1. The first stage starts with the onset of progressive uterine contractions and concludes with complete cervical dilation and effacement. It is further subdivided into two phases:

   a. The latent phase, beginning with the first regular contractions and continuing until the cervix reaches 3- to 4-cm dilation. The rate of cervical dilation in this phase is slow—less than 0.5 cm per hour.

   b. The active phase, which follows the latent phase, is when the rate of cervical dilation increases to 1 cm/hr or more. This rate continues through complete cervical dilation.

2. The second stage begins with complete cervical dilation and ends with the delivery of the infant.

3. The third stage begins with the delivery of the infant and ends with the delivery of the placenta and fetal membranes.

THE PROGRESS OF LABOR

In addition to the state of the cervix at the time labor begins, the course of labor is determined by the following three factors: the *power* (contractions), the *passenger* (fetal size), and the *passageway* (pelvic size). These three factors are traditionally known in obstetrics as the *three p's*.

Power: Uterine Contractions

The muscles of the uterus are in three layers: anteroposterior, circular, and figure eight. These muscles communicate with each other by gap junctions. Gap junctions increase in the uterine musculature in late pregnancy because of the effects of both estrogen and prostaglandins E_2 and $F_{2\alpha}$. Uterine contractions occur throughout pregnancy at relatively infrequent intervals (less than 3 to 4 an hour) and are called *Braxton Hicks contractions*. Both the strength and frequency of contractions increase as labor begins at term. (Preterm labor may have a more subtle onset.) This increase in strength and frequency is caused by an increase in prostaglandin E_2 and $F_{2\alpha}$ within the uterus; these locally active hormones act by increasing cytosolic calcium, leading to activation of myosin light chain kinase. This enzyme in turn produces phosphorylation of myosin and interaction of myosin and actin filaments. The increase in the number of gap junctions leads to an increase in sensitivity to circulating oxytocin, further increasing uterine-contraction frequency and strength.

Uterine contractions in labor normally occur every 2 to 5 minutes in the active phase and last 30 to 90 seconds. The uterine muscle should relax completely for at least 60 seconds between contractions. Assessment of uterine activity may be accomplished in the following three ways:

1. Palpation
2. External tocodynamometry
3. Internal tocodynamometry

Palpation of the uterus by an experienced labor observer is suitable for any labor that is progressing normally. When the progress of labor seems slow and whenever drugs affecting uterine activity are given, uterine-contraction frequency and strength should be assessed with a contraction monitor, or *tocodynamometer*.

A *tocodynamometer* is a device used to record uterine activity, continuously which is usually done simultaneously with a continuous recording of the fetal heart rate. Uterine contractions may be recorded indirectly with an *external tocodynamometer*, a pressure-sensitive disc that is held on the maternal abdomen by a belt. This device will reliably measure the frequency and duration of contractions in most women but cannot assess the intensity of contractions. Direct measurement of intrauterine pressure is accomplished via a saline-filled catheter that is inserted through the cervix alongside the presenting part, which is then connected to a strain gauge. This *internal tocodynamometer* can record not only frequency and duration but also intensity of contractions (Fig. 16-3). Baseline resting-uterine tonus between contractions is also measured with this technique. Table 16-2 displays the normal values for frequency, intensity, and resting tone.

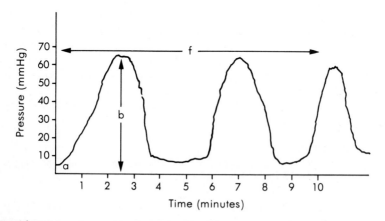

Fig. 16-3
Typical uterine contractions recorded with an intrauterine catheter. *a,* Tonus; *b,* intensity; *f,* frequency.

Table 16-2   Intrauterine pressure measurement

Measurement	Normal Values
Frequency	2-4/10 min
Intensity	30-100 mmHg
Tonus	10-15 mmHg

The Passenger: Fetal Size, Presentation, and Position

The size of the fetus obviously has an effect on the character of labor. Infants who are greater than 3800 g, and especially those greater than 4500 g, may be expected to have difficulty with descent and delivery.

The *presentation* of the fetus is that part of the fetal anatomy that is "presenting" for delivery through the cervix, as follows:

1. *Vertex*—head presenting normally
2. *Face*—face presenting
3. *Brow*—forehead presenting
4. *Breech*—buttocks or feet presenting
5. *Frank breech*—buttocks with hips flexed and legs extended
6. *Complete breech*—buttocks with hips flexed and legs flexed
7. *Footling breech*—one (single footling) or both (double footling) feet presenting
8. *Shoulder*
9. *Compound*—two fetal parts presenting (e.g., head and hand)

The *position* of the fetus describes the relationship of the fetal presenting part to the maternal pelvis; the maternal pelvis is described as right or left and as anterior or posterior (Fig. 16-4). The fetal presenting part is referenced from a specific point, depending on the presentation. The vertex is referenced from the occiput, the breech from the fetal sacrum, and the face from the fetal chin. For example, a fetus whose occiput was on the maternal right anterior side of the pelvis (who was therefore looking toward the maternal left posterior) would be described as being in the right occiput anterior (ROA) position. Other common positions in vertex presentation include left occiput anterior (LOA), left occiput transverse (LOT), left occiput posterior (LOP), right occiput transverse (ROT), and right occiput posterior (ROP). To name these positions, start each time with the maternal pelvic side, then the fetal reference point, and finally the anterior, transverse, or posterior aspect of the maternal pelvis. The same system applies for other presentations (e.g., a fetus is said to be in the left sacrum anterior [LSA] position when the fetal sacrum in a breech presentation is located at about the 10 o'clock position in the left anterior region of the maternal pelvis).

Mechanisms of labor

The cardinal mechanisms of labor in the vertex presentation are described in Figs. 16-4 to 16-7, and are listed as follows:

1. Flexion of the fetal head.
2. Descent of the head—head usually enters the pelvis with the sagittal suture oblique or transverse.
3. Internal rotation—sagittal suture rotates to occiput anterior or to occiput posterior (less common).

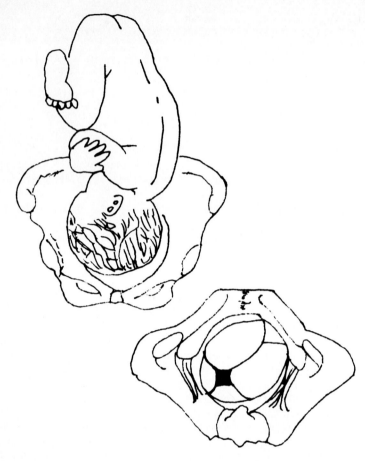

Fig. 16-4
Fetal head entering pelvis. NOTE: Posterior fetal skull (occiput) is in left anterior quadrant of maternal pelvis *(LOA)*.

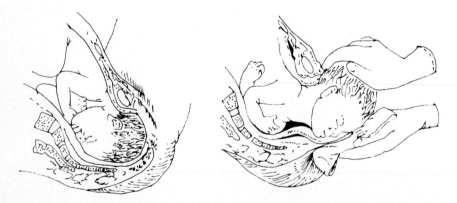

Fig. 16-5
The fetal head being born by a process of deflection. NOTE: Position of the operator's hands protecting the maternal perineum and guiding the fetal head.

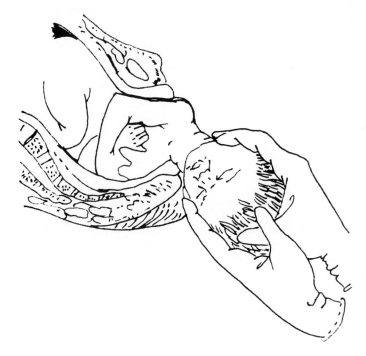

Fig. 16-6
Delivery of the anterior shoulder by slight downward traction on the fetal head.

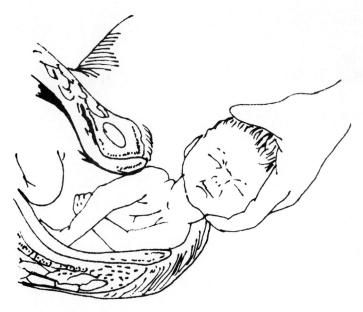

Fig. 16-7
Delivery of posterior shoulder by gently lifting the fetal head upward.

4. Extension of the fetal head (if occiput anterior) beneath the maternal pubic symphysis to deliver the head.
5. Restitution—the head rotates 45 degrees to line up with the shoulders, which are oblique in the maternal pelvis.
6. External rotation—head rotates another 15 degrees to line up with the shoulders, which are now aligned in the anteroposterior diameter of the pelvis.
7. Delivery of the shoulders—with gentle downward traction on the head, the anterior shoulder slides beneath the symphysis. The posterior shoulder then delivers over the perineum, followed by the infant's body.

The Passageway: Pelvic Size
Parts of the maternal bony pelvis

1. *Inlet*—bounded anteriorly by the top of the symphysis, posteriorly by the sacral promontory, and laterally by the pectinate lines.
2. *Midpelvis*—bounded anteriorly by the midpoint on the symphysis, posteriorly by the midpoint on the curve of the sacrum, and laterally by the ischial spines.
3. *Outlet*—bounded anteriorly by the inferior border of the symphysis, posteriorly by the tip of the sacrum, and laterally by the ischial tuberosities.

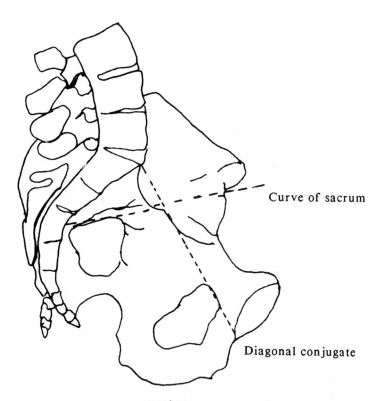

Curve of sacrum

Diagonal conjugate

Fig. 16-8
Lateral view of pelvis.

Clinical evaluation of the pelvis

The inlet is estimated by assessing the diagnonal conjugate from the inferior border of the symphysis to the sacral promontory; greater than 12 cm is normal (Fig. 16-8). The midpelvis is evaluated by examining the curve of the sacrum (it should not be flat) and by noting the prominence of the ischial spines. The outlet may be judged by finding the angle of the pubic rami to be 90 degrees or more and the distance between the ischial tuberosities to be 9 cm or more.

Types of pelvis (Fig. 16-9)

1. *Gynecoid*—anteroposterior and lateral dimensions are proportional throughout.
2. *Android*—transverse diameters and pubic arch narrower than the gynecoid pelvis.
3. *Anthropoid*—narrow lateral diameters with large anteroposterior dimensions.
4. *Platypelloid*—narrow anteroposterior diameters with wide lateral dimensions.

MEASUREMENT OF THE PROGRESS OF LABOR

Fig. 16-10 describes the course of cervical dilation and descent of the fetal head in graphic fashion. During the latent phase of labor in the primigravida, complete efface-ment customarily occurs before appreciable dilation. In the multigravida, effacement and dilation more often proceed simultaneously. Descent of the presenting part may occur during both the first and second stages of labor, especially in the primigravida; most descent occurs in the second stage. The *station* of the presenting part is the term

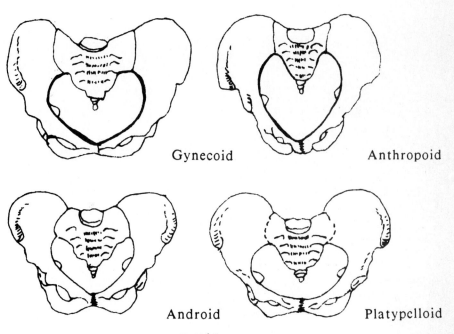

Fig. 16-9
Various pelvic types.

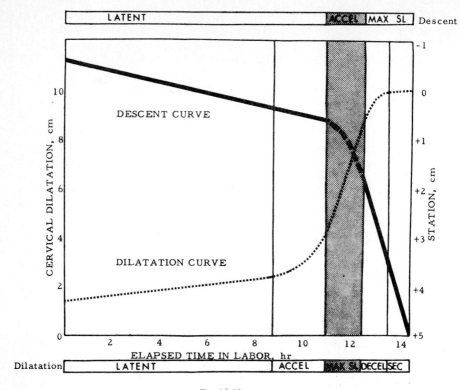

Fig. 16-10
Friedman curve.

used to describe descent, as measured in centimeters above or below the ischial spines. Station is said to be *minus* when above the spines and *plus* when below the spines.

ABNORMAL LABOR

Abnormalities may occur in any stage of labor. The diagnosis of labor disorders is greatly facilitated by creating a graphic display of cervical dilation and descent of the presenting part over time (see Figs. 16-10 and 16-11), which is called a *Friedman curve*. It is helpful to remember the three *p's* as possible causes of dysfunctional labor; abnormalities of contraction strength or frequency, fetal size or presentation, or pelvic dimension may alone or in combination lead to abnormal labor.

Oxytocin Administration

Labor problems caused by weak, inefficient, or infrequent uterine contractions may be treated safely and effectively with intravenous oxytocin. When administered in an intravenous fashion with an infusion pump with continuous monitoring of contraction frequency, intensity, and fetal heart rate, oxytocin has an excellent safety record; failure to follow these simple precautions may lead to disastrous consequences should uterine overstimulation occur.

The infusion is customarily begun with a mixture of 10 U in 1000 ml of D5W/ normal saline, infusing 0.5 mU/min. The rate is doubled every 30 minutes until 3 contractions occur within 10 minutes or until a dose of 10 mU/min is reached; the dose is

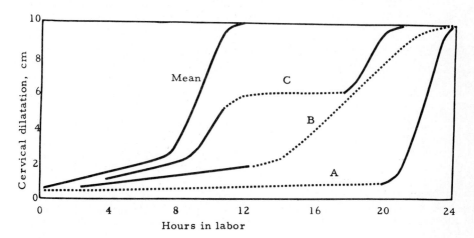

Fig. 16-11
Aberrant labor patterns. *A*, prolonged latent phase. *B*, protracted active phase. *C*, Arrested active phase.

then increased more slowly if necessary by 2 mU/min every 30 minutes until the desired contraction frequency is achieved. If the pregnancy is less than 37 weeks, higher doses may be required. A contraction intensity of 50 mm Hg, as measured by an intrauterine pressure catheter, is the desired contraction strength. Complications of oxytocin include:

1. *Uterine overstimulation,* or *polysystole*—more than 5 contractions/10 min.
2. *Fetal distress*—late decelerations of the fetal heart rate.
3. *Water intoxication*—caused by antidiuretic properties of oxytocin; occurs only at very high doses.

Treatment of all complications is the same—turn off the infusion immediately. The half-life is short, so this will be effective in most cases. If excessive uterine activity persists after the infusion is stopped, it may be necessary to arrest contractions with a bolus of β-mimetic (e.g., terbutaline 0.25 mg subcutaneously).

Prolonged Latent Phase

Poorly coordinated or ineffective contractions during the latent phase (see Fig. 16-11, *A*) may lead to maternal exhaustion. Treatment with a dilute solution of intravenous oxytocin is usually effective in producing more effective, coordinated contractions, which in turn result in progressive cervical dilation. For some patients, sedation with narcotics and/or hypnotics may be helpful.

Protracted Active Phase

Progress of less than 1.5 cm/hr in a multigravida or less than 1.2 cm/hr in a primigravida is abnormally slow in the active phase (see Fig. 16-11, *B*). The etiology is usually uncoordinated uterine activity but may be fetal-pelvic disproportion. Therapy with intravenous oxytocin is continued as long as there is progress.

Arrested Active Phase

An *arrested active phase* is defined as lack of progress in dilation for 2 hours or more in the active phase (Fig. 16-11, *C*). The etiology may be inadequate uterine activity but is more commonly Cephalopelvic disproportion (CPD). This diagnosis requires that there be no progress in cervical dilation or descent for 2 hours or more despite contractions of 50 mm Hg with a frequency of 3 in 10 minutes.

The etiology may be small pelvic capacity or large fetal size or a combination of the two. Positional disproportion occurs when the vertex is in a persistent occiput posterior position or when the head is deflexed as it comes through the birth canal (e.g., brow or face).

Treatment of arrest in the active phase requires documentation of adequate uterine activity without cervical change for 2 hours. If the cause is a persistent occiput posterior position, placing the mother on the side where the occiput lies may be of help. All cases of arrested active phase caused by CPD will require delivery by cesarean section.

Arrest of Descent in Second Stage

Arrest of descent in second stage is defined by failure of the presenting part to descend for 1 hour or more after complete cervical dilation. It may be caused by the following:
1. CPD
2. Inadequate contractions
3. Poor expulsive effort

Treatment includes trying various methods and positions to facilitate pushing. If an epidural anesthetic has been placed, it may be allowed to wear off to allow the patient to experience the "urge" to push. Placing the patient in the upright position may be helpful in some cases. If contractions are inadequate in strength or frequency, oxytocin augmentation may be employed.

If the patient is exhausted and not pushing well as a result, assisting delivery with vacuum extraction or low forceps may be helpful. Station must be at +2 or below, and anesthesia must be adequate to use this option safely. In addition, the fetus must be estimated to weigh less than 3700 g. When fetal size or pelvic capacity is in doubt, delivery by cesarean section is the wisest choice.

THE PROCESS OF DELIVERY—VAGINAL

1. When the presentation of the fetus is vertex:
   a. Spontaneous delivery—see Mechanisms of Labor.
   b. Forceps or vacuum extractor—used primarily to assist descent and lift head over the perineum. May be used to rotate vertex to occiput anterior. Forceps should never be applied if station of vertex is above +2.
2. When the presentation of the fetus is breech:
   a. Frequency—3.5% of pregnancies after 38 weeks.
   b. In labor:
      (1) Vaginal delivery only when presentation of fetus is frank breech, fetus weighs 2500 to 3700 g, and there is an adequate maternal pelvis.
      (2) All others should be delivered by cesarean section.
   c. Before labor—may consider external cephalic version under tocolysis after 36 weeks.
      (1) External version—to perform, need uterine relaxation and expertise.
         (a) Patient should be 37 weeks pregnant.
         (b) Do ultrasonographic examination to see position of fetus.
         (c) Do fetal NST to assure that fetus is reactive.
         (d) Start infusion of ritodrine hydrochloride at 100 µg/min and run for 30 minutes.

(e) Grasp fetal head and buttocks through the mother's abdomen and turn fetus either backwards or frontwards.

(f) Check fetal heart rate frequently when turning fetus—if bradycardia occurs, stop.

(g) When fetus is in vertex position, stop ritodrine and do fetal NST.

Surgical Treatment of Perineum during Vaginal Delivery—Episiotomy

During delivery of the vertex, the perineum distends and the physician must judge whether it is going to tear. If the physician judges that it will tear, a prophylactic incision *(episiotomy)* is preferred.

Types of episiotomy

1. *Median* (Fig. 16-12) incision straight back towards the rectum.
   a. May extend through the sphincter of the rectum (3-degree laceration).
   b. May extend through rectal mucosa (4-degree laceration).
   c. Repair (Fig. 16-13) each specific layer: vaginal mucosa, deep perineal structures, and subcutaneous tissue and skin should be closed in layers, using absorbable suture.
2. *Median lateral*—incision from midpoint on fourchette to 45 degrees lateral to midline. Seldom used except for short perineum.
   a. Repaired as above—in layers

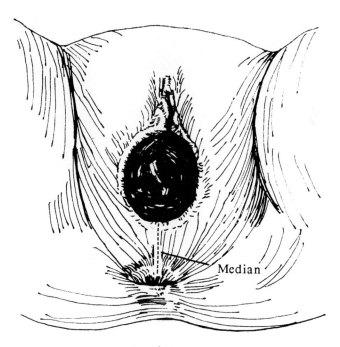

Fig. 16-12
Median episiotomy.

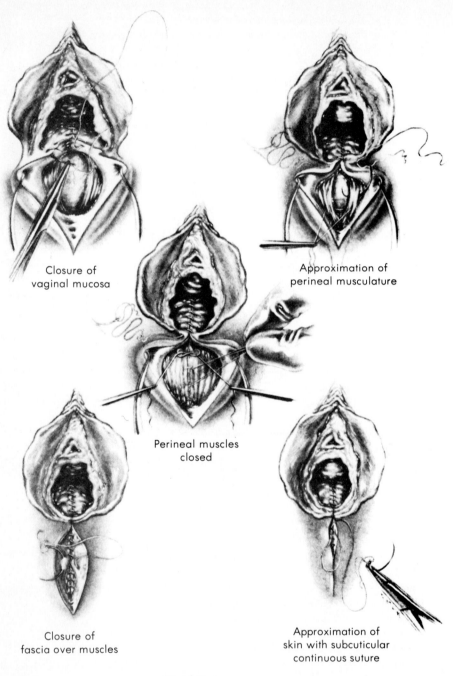

Closure of
vaginal mucosa

Approximation of
perineal musculature

Perineal muscles
closed

Closure of
fascia over muscles

Approximation of
skin with subcuticular
continuous suture

Fig. 16-13
Repair of median episiotomy.

Types of tears

1. Vaginal and perineal tears
    a. Vaginal—sulcus—lateral vaginal wall. Secure all bleeders and suture.
    b. Perineal:
        (1) 1 degree—involves only skin and vagina; may require a suture.
        (2) 2 degrees—skin, vagina, and deeper perineal tissues; repair as episiotomy.
        (3) 3 degrees—involves sphincter or rectum; repair as episiotomy after sphincter has been reapproximated.
        (4) 4 degrees—involves rectal mucosa; repair rectal mucosa, sphincter, and other tissues, layer by layer.
2. Cervical lacerations—usually at 9 o'clock position on the cervix; repair if deep or bleeding with figure eight stitches.
3. Hematomas—may occur in episiotomy site, in labia, or in vaginal vault.
    a. Treatment if small and not enlarging—simply observe; if enlarging—open, try to identify bleeders, and tie them and pack if necessary.

ABDOMINAL DELIVERY—CESAREAN SECTION

1. Types include:
    a. *Low uterine segment transverse*—a transverse incision in the lower uterine segment under the bladder peritoneum.
    b. *Low vertical*—a vertical incision in the lower uterine segment and lower part of body of uterus. Used primarily for premature breech delivery.
    c. *Classic*—incision through upper body of uterus or fundus. Seldom used unless there are significant adhesions and scarring in lower uterine segment.

Indications for Cesarean Section

1. Failure to progress in labor and CPD. This is the indication for about 30% of cesarean sections.
2. Repeat cesarean section—a patient who has previously delivered children by cesarean section may elect a repeat cesarean birth. This is the reason for 30% of cesarean sections. There is now excellent evidence that 60% to 80% of patients who had low transverse cesarean sections may safely undergo vaginal birth after cesarean (VBAC). (This approach is recommended by the American College of Obstetricians and Gynecologists.) May use oxytocin and/or epidural anesthesia with patients who are VBAC.
3. Breech presentation.
4. Fetal distress.
5. Placenta previa or premature separation of the placenta.

POSTDELIVERY COMPLICATIONS

1. Vaginal bleeding—need to rule out vaginal or cervical lacerations. Usually the bleeding is from the uterus, as with the following:
    a. Uterine relaxation—treatment is to give oxytocin first (up to 100 mU/min) and massage uterus; if that doesn't work, give 15-methyl prostaglandin 15 to 25 mg IM.
    b. Uterine rupture—diagnosis by intrauterine palpation; repair rent or do hysterectomy.
    c. Retained placenta or placental tissue—diagnosed by manual palpation; treatment—remove tissue manually or with a large curet.

2. Uterine inversion—diagnosed by seeing inside of uterine fundus at introitus or in vagina—need to replace uterus immediately; may also cause shock in patient.

MONITORING THE FETUS DURING LABOR
Use of Heart Rate

1. Intermittent auscultation
   a. Standard intrapartum care of the normal patient in the first stage of labor includes auscultation of the fetal heart rate for at least 30 seconds, beginning at the peak of a contraction. Frequency of listening is increased to every 5 minutes during the second stage of labor.
   b. The normal fetal heart rate is between 110 and 160 beats per minute. Rates outside these limits may indicate fetal compromise and should be investigated.
2. Continuous electronic fetal heart–rate monitoring methods
   a. External—ultrasonographic transducer on the maternal abdomen.
   b. Internal—fetal scalp electrode.
3. Baseline rate (Fig. 16-14, A)
   a. 120 to 160 is normal.
   b. The *baseline rate* is the rate over time. Changes in fetal heart rate that last less than 2 minutes are referred to as *periodic changes* (see below). Abnormalities in baseline rate may be either of the following:
      (1) Tachycardia—160 to 180—moderate; greater than 180—severe.
          (a) Causes of tachycardia:
              • Maternal fever
              • Maternal medication (e.g., atropine or β-mimetics)
              • Fetal anemia
              • Mild fetal hypoxia
              • Fetal tachyarrhythmia—look for maternal stimulants and fetal cardiac anomalies
      (2) Bradycardia—100 to 200—moderate; less than 100—severe.
          (a) Causes of bradycardia:
              • Fetal heart block—may occur with maternal lupus and anti-SSA/SSB antibodies or with cardiac anomaly
              • Maternal medication (e.g., β-blockers)
              • Severe fetal hypoxia

Periodic Changes

1. Acceleration—an increase in fetal heart rate of 15 beats per minute that last 15 to 120 seconds (Fig. 16-14, B).
2. Decelerations—may be variable, early, or late.
   a. Variable decelerations (Fig. 16-14, C and box):
      (1) Variable in timing relative to contractions.
      (2) Variable in shape and severity.
      (3) Most common type of deceleration; 70% of labors usually have rapid deceleration, with rapid return to baseline.
      (4) Patterns of variable deceleration:
          (a) Acceleration at start of pattern—good sign.
          (b) Smooth acceleration at the end of the deceleration and slow return to baseline are signs of fetal distress.
      (5) Caused by compression of the umbilical cord.

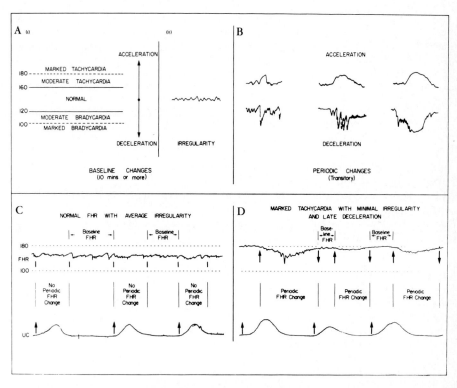

Fig. 16-14
Classification of fetal heart-rate patterns.

Fetal Heart Rate Deceleration Patterns

Variable
Mild

Duration less than 30 seconds or heart rate that doesn't go below 80 beats/min

Moderate

Level of heart rate less than 80 beats/min regardless of duration

Severe

Less than 70 beats/min for more than 60 seconds

Late
Mild duration

15 to 60 seconds

Moderate duration

30 to 90 seconds

Severe duration and depth

30 to 90 seconds: rate of less than 100, or decrease of 45 beats/min or more

Early
Non-pathologic

(see text)

   (6) Treatment
      (a) Change mother's position to relieve pressure on cord.
      (b) Administer 100% oxygen if prolonged or severe.
      (c) May try to replace amniotic fluid via intrauterine pressure catheter infusion of saline if prolonged or severe.
      (d) Delivery required if severe variable deceleration is unresponsive to above measures.

  b. Early decelerations (Fig. 16-15, *A*):
    (1) Caused by head compression with vagal stimulation.
    (2) Start coincident with onset of contraction and mirrors shape of contraction—seldom less than 100 beats per minute.
    (3) No treatment required—a benign condition.

  c. Late decelerations (Fig. 16-15, *B* and box on p. 211):
    (1) Caused by fetal hypoxia, poor maternal oxygenation, interference with intervillous blood flow, excessive uterine activity, maternal hypotension, premature separation of the placenta, and placental infarction.
    (2) Treatment includes:
      (a) 100% O_2 to the mother.
      (b) Improve/protect maternal uterine blood flow, correct hypotension, stop oxytocin, turn mother to left side.
      (c) Immediate delivery required if associated with a flat baseline fetal heart rate.
      (d) If fetal heart rate accelerates in response to scalp or acoustic stimulation, patient may be observed and fetus assessed with scalp blood pH if possible.

3. Prolonged decelerations
  a. Drop in heart rate that is usually rapid and lasts longer than 2 minutes; recovery usually rapid.
  b. Etiology uncertain.
  c. Treatment as for late decelerations, with immediate delivery required if prolonged more than 10 minutes.

4. Heart-rate variability
  a. *Variability* is a term used to describe both short-term (beat to beat) changes in fetal heart rate and long-term cyclic changes in fetal heart rate that occur at 4 to 6 cycles per minute.
  b. Short-term normal variability is 5 to 10 beats per minute; absent is 0 to 2 beats per minute (Fig. 16-15, *C*).
  c. Long-term normal variability is 5 to 10 beats per minute and absent is 0 to 2 beats per minute (see Fig. 16-15, *C*).
  d. Etiology of decreased variability:
    (1) Fetal sleep changes—decrease in quiet sleep versus REM sleep; usually will produce decreased, but not absent, variability; lasts less than 90 minutes.
    (2) Drugs (e.g., atropine, diazepam, narcotics).
    (3) Congenital CNS malformations (e.g., anencephaly).
    (4) Hypoxia—usually associated with later or severe variable decelerations; when this combination is seen, delivery is required.

5. Fetal heart–rate irregularities
  a. Must differentiate true fetal arrhythmia from technical recording artifact—look at raw fetal ECG.

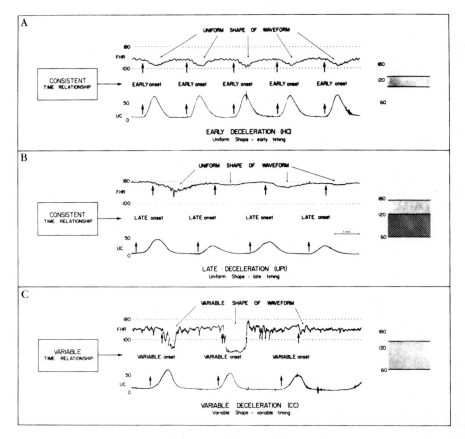

Fig. 16-15
Classification of fetal heart-rate patterns.

b. Arrhythmias may include premature atrial contractions, paroxysmal atrial tachycardia, various degrees of heart block, and vagal cardiac arrest.

6. Auxiliary tests of fetal well-being in labor
   a. Scalp stimulation: if pinching or rubbing the fetal scalp causes an acceleration of the fetal heart rate of more than 15 beats per minute for more than 15 seconds, the fetal scalp pH will be greater than 7.20.
   b. Sound stimulation test: if a mixed-frequency sound (e.g., artificial larynx) placed on the mother's abdomen elicits an acceleration of more than 15 beats per minute for more than 15 seconds, the fetal scalp pH will be greater than 7.20.
   c. Fetal scalp blood sampling for pH: can only be used when the cervix is more than 3 to 4 cm dilated and membranes are, or can be, ruptured.
      (1) Normal—greater than 7.25.
      (2) Intermediate—7.20 to 7.25—repeat if fetal heart rate pattern is not improved or delivery not accomplished in less than 30 minutes.
      (3) Abnormal—less than 7.20.
      (4) Use when fetal heart–rate tracing is suspicious and stimulation tests are not reassuring.

REVIEW QUESTIONS

1. A 24-year-old woman enters labor at 41 weeks in her first pregnancy. She is found to be 3 cm dilated and completely effaced with the vertex at zero station. Contractions are occurring every 5 minutes, lasting 45-60 seconds. The fetal heart rate is 120 beats/minute. What is your plan of management?
   a. Send her home to await the active phase of labor. She should return when the contractions are every 3 minutes or when the bag of water breaks.
   b. Admit her to the hospital, and observe her labor which is normally progressive at this point.
   c. Administer oxytocin to augment contractions. The frequency and duration are insufficient to expect a normally progressive labor.
   d. Rupture the amniotic sac and place an internal scalp electrode to confirm fetal heart rate. If the rate of 120/minute is confirmed, plan an immediate scalp pH to rule out fetal distress.
   e. Stimulate the fetal scalp with your finger to look for an acceleration of 15 beats per minute to exclude fetal distress.
2. Some time later, she is found to be 5 cm dilated, completely effaced, with the vertex at zero station. The amniotic fluid is stained with meconium and the fetal heart rate is 156, with sudden drops during contractions to 100-110. The rate returns to 150-160 shortly after the contraction is complete. Your plan of management is:
   a. Continue to observe her normally progressive labor. Intervention is not necessary at this time.
   b. Place an internal scalp electrode to record the fetal heart rate more accurately, and an internal pressure catheter to measure the strength of contractions. Administer oxygen to the mother, and change her position to relieve cord compression. These measures are necessary because the fetal heart rate changes and meconium suggest the possibility of fetal compromise.
   c. The fetal heart rate changes and meconium stained fluid indicate fetal distress is present. Because she is only 5 cm dilated, labor may be expected to last an additional number of hours. The fetus will clearly not tolerate additional labor of that duration, and prompt cesarean section is therefore the best choice.
   d. Administer oxytocin to augment labor. The fetus is beginning to show evidence of compromise; labor should therefore be hastened to avoid fetal distress later.
   e. Lavage the intrauterine cavity with warmed saline to remove the meconium before delivery.
3. The woman eventually dilates her cervix completely, and the baby's head is now found to be at +1 station. The anterior fontanelle is immediately beneath and slightly to the left of the maternal symphysis pubis. This position of the fetal head is said to be:
   a. LOA
   b. LOP
   c. ROA
   d. ROP
   e. None of the above
4. This position of the fetal head requires:
   a. Cesarean section—it is not a safe practice to attempt delivery from this position through the vagina.
   b. Forceps rotation to a more favorable position to allow vaginal delivery.
   c. Oxytocin augmentation to achieve contractions of sufficient strength to force the head to rotate to a more favorable position.

    d. Additional maternal pushing to rotate the head, compared to the other more favorable positions, is all that is necessary.

    e. This is the ideal position to begin the second stage of labor, which should proceed normally in this case.

5. Following delivery of an apparently healthy infant, the patient begins to bleed heavily. The most likely cause and treatment are:

    a. Laceration of the cervix and/or vagina, which will require surgical repair.

    b. Coagulopathy induced by consumption of clotting factors during labor and delivery. Treat with cryoprecipitate or fresh frozen plasma.

    c. Uterine atony, which is treated with massage and intravenous oxytocin.

    d. Heavy bleeding is normal after delivery. No special treatment is necessary unless the hemoglobin falls by more than 2 gm/dl from pre-delivery levels.

    e. Immediate embolization of both uterine arteries is the only way to avoid hysterectomy for this patient.

ANSWERS

1. b
2. b
3. d
4. d
5. c

BIBLIOGRAPHY

Edusheim TG et al: Fetal heart rate response to vibratory acoustic stimulation predicts fetal pH in labor, Am J Obstet Gynecol 157:1557, 1987.

Freeman RK, and Garite TD: Fetal heart rate monitoring, Baltimore, 1981, Williams & Wilkins.

Friedman EH: Labor: clinical evaluation and management, East Norwalk, Conn, 1967, Appleton-Century-Crofts.

Partiarco MS et al: A study on intrauterine fetal resuscitation with terbutaline, Am J Obstet Gynecol 157:384, 1987.

Seitchik J, and Castillo M: Oxytocin augmentation and dysfunctional labor, Am J Obstet Gynecol 145:526, 1983.

Seitchik J, Holden AEC, and Castillo M: Amniotomy and oxytocin treatment of functional dystocia and route of delivery, Am J Obstet Gynecol 155:585, 1986.

Anesthesia in Obstetrics

17

Kathryn J. Zuspan

A thorough understanding of obstetrical anesthesia and analgesia is critical to providing good obstetrical care. Communication between the obstetrician, anesthesiologist, and obstetrical nurse is vital. Anyone administering obstetrical anesthetics must be able to recognize and manage the wide variety of complications that are unique to the obstetrical patient. Skill in intubation and resuscitation is mandatory.

MATERNAL PHYSIOLOGY AND OBSTETRICAL ANESTHESIA

A thorough appreciation of the changes in maternal physiology during pregnancy is fundamental to good obstetrical anesthetic care. These changes both alter the pregnant patient's response to anesthetic agents and increase her risks, as shown in Table 17-1.

FETAL CONSEQUENCES OF ANESTHESIA IN PREGNANCY
During Pregnancy

Anesthetics given during gestation (e.g., for cervical cerclage, appendectomy, or other unavoidable procedures) have the potential to produce teratogenic effects, spontaneous abortion, or premature labor. No evidence at present links anesthetic agents with preterm labor or spontaneous abortion. The only human studies linking anesthetic agents with fetal anomalies suggested a possible association with librium, valium and meprobamate given in the first 6 weeks of gestation. Recommendations for anesthetic choices in pregnancy are given in Table 17-2.

Intrapartum Analgesia/Anesthesia

Anesthetics given during labor and delivery may be needed for pain relief during labor, operative vaginal delivery, or cesarean section. Neonatal respiratory depression is a possible side effect associated with drugs given for pain relief and sedation in labor and with general anesthetic agents as well. Neurobehavioral effects, ranging from mild to severe, have been reported with many anesthetic agents.

Postpartum Anesthesia

Anesthesia may be required after delivery (e.g. for tubal ligation). If the mother is breast-feeding, there is potential for passage of the drugs given for anesthesia into the milk and then to the infant. Although most drugs do cross into breast milk in detectable amounts, it is usually the case that the amount is pharmacologically insignificant (see Chapter 20). Neonatal effects can be minimized when necessary by temporary cessation of nursing while continuing to pump the breast to maintain milk production and by limiting the quantity of drug received by the postpartum breast feeding patient.

Table 17-1   Changes in physiology and their effect on anesthetic management

System and Change	Anesthetic Significance
Respiratory	
Respiratory mucosa more vascular and edematous	Because of increased risk of difficult intubation, use smaller endotracheal tube (e.g., 6.0 or 7.0); avoid nasal intubation
Lowered functional residual capacity; increased oxygen consumption; hyperventilation present	Because of increased risk of fetal and maternal hypoxia, give supplemental O_2 by face mask (vs. nasal cannula) for regional anesthesia; for general anesthesia—preoxygenation for 3 min or 4 deep breaths by face mask before induction
Cardiovascular	
40% increase in cardiac output	More rapid induction and emergence from general anesthesia
Engorgement of venous plexus (e.g., veins in epidural space)	Increased risk of intravascular placement of epidural catheter; also decreases the size of epidural space so less drug is needed to acquire epidural block
Gastrointestinal	
Increased intragastric pressure; delay in gastric emptying; relaxation of gastroesophageal sphincter; decreased gastric and intestinal motility	Because of increased risk of aspiration, give prophylaxis before any major anesthetic with a nonparticulate antacid (e.g., sodium citrate 30 cc PO); for general anesthesia, use rapid-sequence induction technique—this requires use of cricoid pressure and a cuffed endotracheal tube with stylet; avoid positive pressure ventilation before intubation; extubation is done when patient is awake
Reproductive	
Increased size and weight of uterus	Because of increased risk of aortocaval compression in supine position leading to maternal hypotension and decreased uteroplacental blood flow, use wedge under patient's right hip to give left lateral uterine displacement

MANAGEMENT OF PAIN DURING LABOR

Relief of pain during labor does more than make the experience more pleasant for the mother. In some cases, as shown in Fig. 17-1, the autonomic changes caused by unrelieved labor pain can result in fetal acidosis. Pain in the first stage of labor is the result of uterine contractions and cervical changes and is transmitted via the spinal

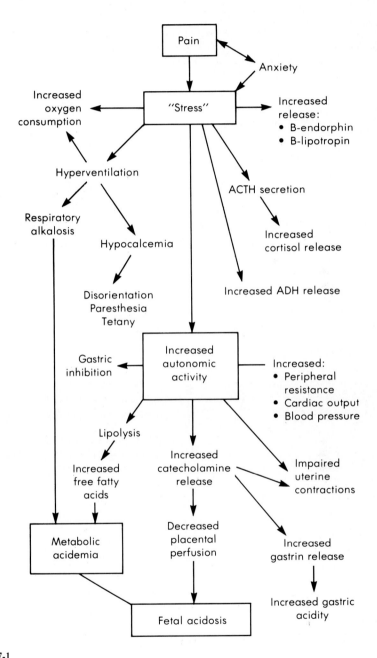

Fig 17-1
Physiologic changes related to labor pain.
From Cousins MJ, and Bridenbough PO: Neural blockade in clinical anesthesia and management of pain, ed 2, Philadelphia, 1986, JB Lippincott Co.

nerves from T10 to L1 (Fig. 17-2). Pain in the second stage of labor additionally involves stretching of the vagina, vulva, and perineum. These impulses travel through spinal nerves entering S2 to S4. The agents used for spinal and epidural analgesia/anesthesia are shown in Table 17-3. An overview of available techniques for pain relief in labor is shown in Table 17-4. The various needle placements for spinal, epidural, and caudal blocks are shown in Fig. 17-4.

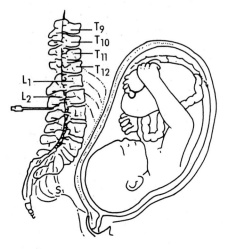

Fig. 17-2
Pain pathways involved in labor, extending from T-10 to L-1 for the pain of uterine contractions and cervical dilation, and involving S-2 to S-4 for the pain of vaginal and perineal distention. Also indicated is the appropriate placement for a lumbar epidural catheter.
From Ostheimer GW: Regional anesthesia techniques in obstetrics, 1980, Breon Laboratories, Inc.

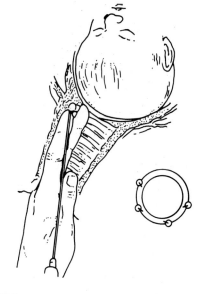

Fig. 17-3
Technique of paracervical block for anesthesia during labor; injections of local anesthetic are placed at 3, 5, 7, and 9 o'clock. This technique has a high rate of associated fetal bradycardia.
From Zuspan FP, and Quilligan EJ: Operative obstetrics, East Norwalk, Conn, 1988, Appleton-Century-Crofts.

Table 17-2   Recommendations for anesthesia in the pregnant surgical patient

Type of Case	Recommendation
Elective	Defer to 6 weeks after delivery when maternal physiology has returned to normal
Urgent	Defer to second or third trimester to avoid fetal exposure in vulnerable first trimester
Emergency (in first trimester)	No technique is better than the other; key is to avoid hypoxia, hypotension, and hypovolemia; consider regional anesthesia because no animal or human studies have demonstrated teratogenicity

Table 17-3   Local anesthetics in obstetrics

Name	Use	Associated Problems
Lidocaine	Spinal/ epidural	"Floppy but alert babies"—the once popular hypothesis that epidural lidocaine led to hypotonic neonates has been proven *wrong*
Chloroprocaine	Epidural	If given into the subarachnoid space, there is the potential for neurotoxicity, which is described as an *adhesive arachnoiditis*— thus it cannot be used for spinal anesthesia
Bupivacaine	Spinal/ epidural	If given intravascularly (i.e., via an epidural vessel), there is the potential for cardiotoxicity (described as *seizures* followed by cardiac arrest, which is difficult to reverse)
Tetracaine	Spinal	Given epidurally there is excellent motor block but inadequate sensory block—thus it is used for spinal, not epidural, anesthesia

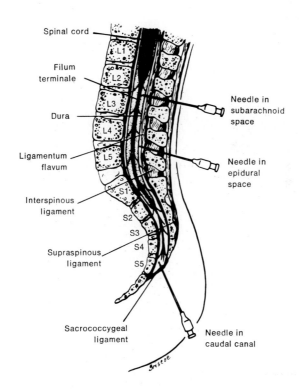

Fig. 17-4
Schematic diagram of lumbosacral anatomy; showing needle placement for subarachnoid, lumbar epidural, and caudal bolck.
From Shnider, SM: Anesthesia for obstetrics, Baltimore, 1979, The Williams & Wilkins Co, p. 98.

Table 17-4 Labor pain relief techniques

Technique	Comments
Relaxation Technique	
Psychoprophylaxis (Lamaze method)	This is not "natural childbirth"; the patient is taught to concentrate on breathing techniques during the various stages of labor, which will distract the patient and thus relieve discomfort. The husband or support person is taught to assist and encourage the patient through labor; this technique may be used alone or in combination with other forms of analgesics
Systemic Drugs	
Sedatives, tranquilizers	Group includes phenothiazine derivatives, hydroxyzine, and benzodiazepines; used to allay anxiety, promote sleep, and potentiate narcotics; examples include promethazine (Phenergan), propiomazine (Largon), and diazepam (Valium); an antagonist for diazepam is physostigmine (Antilirium)
Narcotics	Used to relieve labor pain; maternal side effects include postural hypotension, nausea and vomiting, obtunded reflexes, and respiratory depression; neonatal side effects include neurobehavioral changes and respiratory depression; examples include meperidine (Demerol), alphaprodine (Nisentil), butorphanol (Stadol), nalbuphine (Nubain), pentazocine (Talwin), fentanyl (Sublimaze), and morphine; an antagonist is naloxone (Narcan)
Dissociative drugs	Used to provide intense maternal analgesia and sleep without loss of consciousness; an example is ketamine (Ketalar); diazepam is usually also given in an effort to eliminate ketamine's possible psychomimetic side effect; an antagonist is physostigmine (Antilirium)
Paracervical Block (Fig. 17-3)	Used to provide analgesia in the first stage of labor; involves injecting local anesthetic into the vaginal mucosa at various sites on the cervix; maternal side effects—rare; neonatal side effects—high incidence of fetal bradycardia

Table 17-4 cont'd
• Epidural Analgesia
(Fig. 17-4)

Used to provide excellent analgesia and anesthesia for labor and delivery; this technique decreases maternal and fetal metabolic acidosis; no negative effects are found on uterine blood flow, uterine contractions, or the progress of labor; the epidural analgesic does not prolong the first stage of labor. Though the second stage may be prolonged because of the epidural analgesic, the patient should be allowed to push for up to 4 hours without intervention if good fetal monitoring is used and the fetus is stable—using this technique, the forcep and cesarean-section rates are not increased. The epidural analgesic should be initiated as soon as the patient notes discomfort and the obstetrician is committed to delivery; there is no need to wait for a particular cervical dilatation. The epidural analgesic is placed after the patient receives a 500-1000 ml lactated Ringer's solution bolus; aspiration of the catheter followed by a test dose of local anesthetic is used to further test catheter placement before injection of the full dose of the appropriate concentration and volume of local anesthetic—this helps rule out possible intravascular or subarachnoid placement of the catheter. Following the dose, the patient's blood pressure is monitored every few minutes for 20 minutes. With the sympathectomy that occurs as the epidural block sets up, hypotension is possible and can be avoided by increasing the intravenous fluid rate or by repositioning the patient—when this fails, ephedrine is used; the epidural analgesic can be redosed at intervals or given as a constant infusion; narcotics may be added to the local anesthetic—this improves analgesia and decreases the concentration of local anesthetic needed, thereby diminishing the amount of motor block

Local Anesthetics used with Epidural Analgesia/Anesthesia (Table 17-4)

Lidocaine (Xylocaine), bupivacaine (Marcaine, Sensorcaine), and chloroprocaine (Nesacaine)

Contraindications to Epidural Analgesia/Anesthesia
Absolute

Coagulation disorders, some neurologic disorders, maternal hypotension, generalized sepsis, and localized infection at insertion site

Relative

Aortic stenosis, pulmonary hypertension, placenta previa without bleeding, and abruptio placentae without bleeding

ANESTHESIA FOR VAGINAL DELIVERY

The epidural anesthetic is one method of pain relief applicable to both labor as well as all manners of delivery, including spontaneous and instrumental vaginal births and cesarean section. This makes it a popular choice among laboring women, obstetricians, and anesthesiologists. The need for anesthesia will vary greatly among parturients. Some women will require very little or no medication, whereas others will need a great deal. Working within the framework of maximal safety for both mother and neonate, the goal of obstetric anesthesia is to allow each woman to experience childbirth as she wishes. A wide variety of choices are available for vaginal delivery anesthesia.

Local infiltration

1. Local infiltration is useful for spontaneous delivery before cutting and repairing an episiotomy.
2. The usual drug of choice is 1% lidocaine. Other local anesthetics may be substituted.

Pudendal block

1. A pudendal block (Fig. 17-5) is useful for spontaneous or instrumental vaginal deliveries.
2. The most commonly used agent is 1% lidocaine.
3. The pudendal block is designed to anesthetize the internal pudendal and perineal nerves bilaterally in an effort to relax the perineal muscles and anesthetize the perineal skin.
4. Local infiltration, described above, may be used additionally to improve the perineal pain relief.

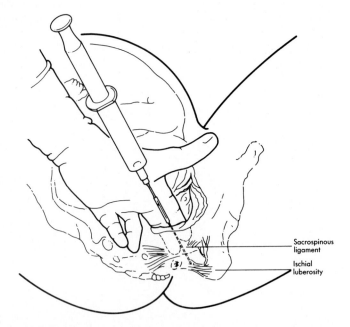

Sacrospinous
ligament

Ischial
tuberosity

Fig. 17-5
Pudendal block—transvaginal approach.
From Ostheimer GW: Regional anesthesia techniques in obstetrics, 1980, Breon Laboratories, Inc.

Epidural anesthesia

1. Epidural anesthesia is useful for spontaneous or instrumental vaginal deliveries.
2. The most commonly used local anesthetic drugs are listed in Table 17-3.
3. A *perineal, sit-up,* or *top-up* dose of local anesthetic is given through the epidural catheter. This is used to attain motor block, perineal relaxation, and anesthesia. It is given late in the second stage of labor, with the patient in the sitting position. The epidural anesthetic is dosed with a larger volume and stronger concentration of local anesthetic than that used earlier in labor.

Caudal anesthesia

1. Caudal anesthesia (Figs. 17-4 and 17-6) is useful for spontaneous or instrumental vaginal delivery.
2. The same local anesthetics as those used for epidural anesthesia are used for caudal anesthesia.
3. Once popular, caudal anesthesia has largely been replaced by epidural anesthesia.
4. The caudal canal is the most caudal extension of the epidural space. Local anesthetic given through a needle or catheter placed at this point provides rapid onset of muscle relaxation and perineal anesthesia; however, there are some disadvantages. Unlike epidural anesthesia, larger volumes of local anesthetic are needed, and the technique is more difficult to perform and more painful to the patient. Also, there is the danger of an accidental injection of local anesthetic directly into the fetal presenting part, which is in close proximity.
5. Precautions and contraindications are similar to those for epidural anesthesia.

Spinal or saddle block anesthesia

1. Spinal or saddle block anesthesia is useful for instrumental vaginal delivery.
2. Local anesthetics commonly used for spinal or saddle block anesthesia are listed in Table 17-3.

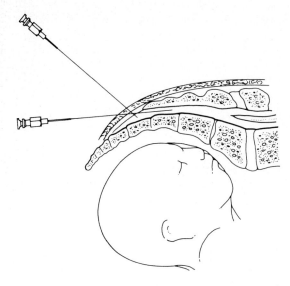

Fig. 17-6
Insertion of needle into caudal canal. Note proximity of fetal head.
From Ostheimer GW: Regional anesthesia techniques in obstetrics, 1980, Breon Laboratories, Inc.

3. In *saddle block anesthesia,* which is a form of spinal anesthesia, anesthesia is maximized in the anatomic areas that would touch a saddle if the patient were riding a horse. The traditional spinal technique is used, but a smaller dose of hyperbaric local anesthetic is given, and the patient is in the sitting position. The result is sacral anesthesia.
4. Precautions and contraindications are similar to those for epidural anesthesia. There is also a greater risk of spinal headache.
5. Spinal headaches can be treated in a variety of ways, including bedrest, analgesics, fluids, intravenous caffeine, and the epidural blood patch—the latter has the greatest success rate. The blood patch involves performing an epidural procedure on the patient. At the level of the previous dural puncture, blood from the patient is drawn and immediately injected through the needle into the epidural space. This creates a clot "patch" over the dural puncture site until the dura seals over the puncture hole. Relief is typically immediate.

Inhalational analgesics

1. Inhalational analgesics are useful for spontaneous or instrumental deliveries.
2. Oxygen and nitrous oxide with enflurane (Ethrane) or methoxyflurane are commonly used. They are inhaled continuously in low concentrations or intermittently in higher concentrations.
3. Inhalational analgesics provide maternal pain relief; however, there is also a risk of maternal aspiration, respiratory depression, or loss of consciousness.

ANESTHESIA FOR CESAREAN SECTION

The choice of anesthetic for cesarean delivery depends on several variables. The medical status of the pregnant woman and her fetus, as well as the skills of the obstetrician and anesthesiologist, should be considered. In some cases, the emergent nature of the procedure is the dominant variable. In cases of fetal distress, a general anesthetic is often the best choice unless an epidural catheter is already in place.

The estimated surgical time factor is another consideration. The interval from uterine incision to delivery (UD interval) should be less than 3 minutes, regardless of the anesthetic method chosen. UD intervals of less than 3 minutes are associated with higher Apgar scores and a decreased risk of acidosis. For general anesthesia, the interval between abdominal incision and delivery of the infant (A–D interval) is also important because intervals of more than 8 minutes have been associated with low Apgar scores and acidosis.

Regardless of the method chosen, the following general caveats apply to all patients undergoing cesarean delivery:

1. A prophylactic oral dose of a nonparticulate antacid should be given to help prevent aspiration pneumonitis. Aspiration remains the leading cause of anesthesia related deaths in the obstetrical population. A dose of 30 cc of sodium citrate is commonly used.
2. A wedge is placed under the patient's right hip to produce left lateral uterine displacement, thus avoiding maternal hypotension secondary to aortocaval compression when the patient is supine on the operating room table.
3. Patients are well oxygenated. For cases involving local, spinal or epidural anesthesia, the patient receives supplemental oxygen by face mask versus nasal cannula. For cases involving general anesthesia, the patient receives 100% oxygen by face mask for 3 minutes or four deep breaths before induction and intubation and is maintained on at least a 50% oxygen concentration during the case.
4. The pediatrician or other personnel who will resuscitate the infant should be

made aware of any anticipated neonatal effects of agents used during delivery. The anesthetic choices for cesarean section follow.

Epidural anesthesia

The technique, precautions, and contraindications of epidural anesthesia for cesarean section are the same as those for labor. Unlike with labor, the epidural for cesarean section requires a greater preload of intravenous lactated Ringer's solution; 1500 to 2000 ml is appropriate. A stronger concentration and larger volume of local anesthetic is used, and the level of the block is extended to T4 to T6. The epidural catheter may be redosed at appropriate intervals during the cesarean section to maintain the surgical level of anesthesia.

Spinal anesthesia

The technique, precautions, and contraindications to spinal anesthesia are similar for labor and cesarean section. A 1500 to 2000 ml preload of lactated Ringer's solution is needed. A larger dose of hyperbaric local anesthetic produces a level of anesthesia to T4 to T6.

General anesthesia

All pregnant patients undergoing general anesthesia require intubation using a rapid-sequence induction. This involves using cricoid pressure and avoiding positive pressure ventilation before muscle paralysis for intubation. The patient is extubated when she is awake and in control of her gag reflexes. These measures are used to avoid maternal aspiration.

A variety of drugs and techniques are used. Some of the typical agents are discussed below.

Before induction, the patient receives oxygen and glycopyrrolate (Robinul), a synthetic anticholinergic used to reduce airway secretions, decrease the volume and acidity of stomach contents, and block cardiac vagal inhibitory reflexes.

Induction of anesthesia and intubation are done using thiopental (Pentothal) and succinylcholine (Anectine). Thiopental, a barbiturate, has a short-acting depressant effect on the CNS. Succinylcholine, an ultrashort-acting skeletal muscle relaxant, facilitates endotracheal intubation.

Following intubation, anesthesia is maintained using oxygen, nitrous oxide, an inhalational agent, a muscle relaxant, narcotics, and tranquilizers. Oxygen is given in a 50% to 100% concentration. Nitrous oxide, often withheld until after delivery, is added to reduce the chance of maternal recall and lower the inhalational anesthetic requirements. Low concentrations of enflurane, the most commonly used inhalational agent, serve to increase uterine blood flow and decrease the risk of maternal recall. In low concentrations, enflurane does not cause neonatal depression nor uterine bleeding. Different muscle relaxants are used, depending on the surgeon's speed.

Succinylcholine is short-acting, atracurium (Tracrium) and vecuronium (Norcuron) have intermediate duration, and pancuronium (Pavulon) has a long duration of action. Incidentally, these muscle relaxants cross the placenta but have no effect on neonatal respiration or Apgar scores. Following delivery, narcotics and tranquilizers are used to deepen the level of anesthesia. The shorter-acting drugs, such as fentanyl, are often chosen so that the mother will be alert after delivery for bonding with the neonate. At the end of the cesarean section, the muscle relaxants (with the exception of succinylcholine) are reversed. This is done with one of the cholinesterase inhibitors. These anticholinergic drugs include pyridostigmine (Regonol), neostigmine (Prostigmin) or edrophonium (Tensilon). Gylcopyrrolate or atropine are also given to block the bradycardia and excessive secretions that are often seen with the anticholinergic drugs.

Local infiltration of the anterior abdominal wall

1. Rarely used, this technique is appropriate for an emergency cesarean section when no one trained in anesthesia is available.
2. No preoperative sedation is used. Gentle handling of the patient and the instruments is critical.
3. The most common agent is 5% procaine (novocain) with epinephrine added.

ANESTHESIA/ANALGESIA FOR THE POSTPARTUM PERIOD

Most women will require only minimal amounts of oral analgesics, such as acetaminophen or ibuprofen, after delivery. For some, however, these drugs will not be sufficient. Those who deliver abdominally are naturally going to have a greater need for analgesia; others who might need additional pain relief include women with perineal lacerations involving the rectal sphincter, or with perineal or pelvic hematomas, or women who have undergone elective tubal ligation. Traditionally, such patients have been offered parenteral doses of narcotics, such as meperidine or morphine, or oral agents, such as acetaminophen with codeine. Although reasonably effective as analgesics, these narcotics all have unfortunate side effects, including somnolence, nausea, or vomiting. Lactating women are often reluctant to use them, although neonatal effects from short-term use are essentially nil. Two new techniques, patient-controlled analgesia (PCA) and epidural narcotics, have addressed these problems and have increasingly involved the anesthesiologist in postpartum pain management.

PCA

PCA allows the patient to have more direct control over her own analgesia. The patient's intravenous line is connected to a PCA pump that dispenses systemic drug, usually a narcotic, when the patient pushes a button. The pump is programmed to dispense the analgesic up to a predetermined maximal dose per unit of time, after which no drug is given until a preset period of time elapses. This reduces the risk of overdose. Various narcotics have been used, and patient satisfaction is excellent with this method. Surprisingly, the total amount of narcotic dispensed with PCA pumps is less than that given when the nurse gives intramuscular narcotic injections on patient request.

Epidural Narcotics

With epidural narcotics, an increasingly popular technique, women who have delivered with an epidural anesthetic receive narcotics through the epidural catheter. Pain relief is excellent using minimal doses of drug without the motor block seen with local anesthetics. The duration of analgesia depends on the narcotic used. Fentanyl, for example, gives 2 hours of analgesia, meperidine 4 to 5 hours, and morphine 12 to 20 hours. Possible side effects range from common complaints of pruritis and nausea and vomiting to the rare chance of respiratory depression. Additional monitoring of these patients is required because of the latter possibility.

SUMMARY

Providing anesthesia and analgesia for the parturient is a complex and exciting task. It involves choosing and tailoring the techniques to meet the needs, desires, and skills of the patient, neonate, obstetrician, and anesthesiologist. Communication, teamwork, respect, and an understanding of obstetrical anesthesia are essential.

REVIEW
QUESTIONS

More than one answer is possible.

1. Anesthesia given to the mother may have some effect on the fetus/neonate during the following times:
   a. During gestation.
   b. During labor and delivery.
   c. During postpartum period in breast-feeding mothers.
   d. During childhood (excluding teratogenic effects).

2. In order to optimize the safety of the mother and neonate before the incision is made for a cesarean section, all mothers should receive which of the following:
   a. Oxygen by nasal cannula.
   b. Left lateral uterine displacement.
   c. A preoperative medication to relax the patient.
   d. A nonparticulate antacid.

3. In order to reduce the chance of low Apgar scores and neonatal acidosis, the following time frames should be observed:
   a. The uterine incision-to-delivery time should be less than 3 minutes for general anesthesia.
   b. The uterine incision-to-delivery time should be less than 5 minutes for epidural anesthesia.
   c. The abdominal incision-to-delivery time should be less than 8 minutes for general anesthesia.
   d. The abdominal incision-to-delivery time should be less than 8 minutes for epidural anesthesia.

4. The anesthesiologist attempts to limit fetal drug exposure before cesarean delivery under general anesthesia. Therefore which of the following are true?
   a. The anesthesiologist gives no drugs that cross the placenta before delivery.
   b. The anesthesiologist avoids giving the mother muscle relaxants before delivery because these can paralyze the fetal lungs and affect neonatal respirations.
   c. Statements a. and b. are true.
   d. Statements a. and b. are false.

True or False

Epidural anesthesia for relief of labor pain:

5. Decreases the flow of blood to the fetus.
6. Increases the likelihood of a forceps delivery or cesarean section.
7. Is provided by local anesthetics that cross the placenta and are detected in the fetus and newborn.
8. Can cause "floppy but alert" hypotonic neonates at delivery if lidocaine is used.
9. Can decrease maternal anxiety and thus reduce the associated neonatal metabolic acidosis.

ANSWERS

1. a, b, c
2. b, d
3. a, c
4. d
5. F
6. F

7. T
8. F
9. T

BIBLIOGRAPHY

Bonica JJ: Principles and practice of obstetric analgesia and anesthesia, Philadelphia, 1967, FA Davis Co.

Covino BG, and Vassallo HG: Local anesthetics: mechanisms of action and clinical use, New York, 1976, Grune & Statton Inc.

Datta S et al: Neonatal effect of prolonged anesthetic induction for cesarean section, Obstet Gynecol 58:331, 1981.

Kuhnert BR, Linn PL, and Kuhnert PM: Obstetric medication and neonatal behavior: current controversies, Clin Perinatol 12:423, 1985.

Ostheimer GW: Manual of obstetric anesthesia, New York, 1984, Churchill Livingstone Inc.

Ramanathan S et al: Oxygen transfer from mother to fetus during cesarean section under epidural anesthesia, Anesth Analg 61:576, 1982.

Shnider SM, and Levinson G: Anesthesia for obstetrics, ed 2, Baltimore, 1987, Williams & Wilkins.

Zuspan FP, and Quilligan EJ: Douglas-Stromme Operative obstetrics, ed 5, East Norwalk, Conn, 1988 Appleton-Century-Crofts.

Neonatal Resuscitation

18

Susan W. Aucott
John J. Moore

Resuscitation of the newborn, like that of older children and adults, follows the basic principles of *a*irway, *b*reathing, and *c*irculation (ABC). In addition, the infant must make the transition from intrauterine to extrauterine life. An organized, team approach to newborn resuscitation allows prompt and adequate support of this physiologic process, especially when complicated by distress at birth.

MECHANISMS OF FETAL DISTRESS

Any interruption in the chain linking the maternal and fetal cardiorespiratory system can result in fetal distress (see Table 18-1).

PHYSIOLOGIC TRANSITION

For the fetus to survive in the extrauterine environment, several transitions must be made successfully.

1. The onset of respirations after birth allows the infant to oxygenate independently. Significant intrathoracic pressures must be generated in order to overcome the intraalveolar surface tension in the fluid-filled lungs. Without adequate respiration, the pH drops rapidly because of the combined respiratory and metabolic acidosis. Other transitions rely on the onset of respirations, making it the primary focus of neonatal resuscitation.
2. Fetal circulation obtains oxygenated blood from the placenta via the umbilical vein. Vascular resistance across the pulmonary bed is very high during fetal life. Therefore blood bypasses the lungs by shunting from the right to left atrium through the foramen ovale and from the pulmonary artery to the aorta through the ductus arteriosus. At birth, clamping of the umbilical cord causes a sudden drop in venous return and right atrial pressure, allowing closure of the foramen ovale. The simultaneous onset of respiration and expansion of the lungs decreases the pulmonary vascular resistance. Increased pulmonary blood flow improves the pH and oxygenation, causing constriction of the ductus, thus establishing the adult circulation pattern. Accomplishment of adequate respirations thus greatly affects this transition as well.
3. It is difficult to establish temperature homeostasis for the wet infant brought into the relatively cold, dry environment of the delivery room. Cold stress results in increased oxygen consumption, making the fetal transition more difficult.

PRINCIPLES OF RESUSCITATION
Team Concept

In the distressed or premature infant, the normal physiologic transition may not take place. A team of individuals who are skilled in neonatal resuscitation should be on

Table 18-1   Mechanisms of fetal distress

Condition	Result	Etiologies
Mother		
Hypoxia	Inadequate O_2 delivery to fetus	Maternal heart, lung, or muscle disease; anesthesia accident
Shock	Inadequate uterine placental perfusion	Infection, hemorrhage
Drugs/toxins	Maternal vasodilation, hypotension, and decreased cardiac output	Demerol, phenobarbital, general anesthesia, $MgSO_4$
Uterine Circulation		
Anesthesia	Local vasodilation with decreased uterine perfusion	Spinal anesthesia, epidural anesthesia
Maternal vascular disease	Poor local blood flow	Diabetes, SLE, hypertension
Acute blood loss	Fetal hypovolemia, anemia	Placenta previa, acute fetal-maternal bleed, twin-to-twin transfusion
	Maternal and/or fetal blood loss; compression of placenta by clot, causing sudden increase in fetal venous pressure	Abruption

hand for any delivery that is suspected to involve fetal distress.

Team members (at least three) may consist of physicians, nurses, or respiratory therapists, provided they are trained in neonatal resuscitation and available within 3 minutes, 24 hours a day. Individual roles (see Table 18-2) should be assigned before the onset of resuscitation to ensure an effective resuscitation. Such teams are most effective if they work together on a regular basis and routinely participate in "mock code" drills using mannequins. In order to maintain the skills of the personnel, regular simulation drills become particularly important in perinatal services with a low volume of complicated resuscitations.

Protocol

Use of a protocol in the form of a flow sheet (Fig. 18-1) greatly facilitates resuscitation. This form of protocol can be held by one of the team members and serve simultaneously as orders, instant "crib" sheet, and documentation of the events of the resuscitation. The latter may be accomplished by tracing the paths taken directly on the protocol sheet.

Equipment

Necessary equipment should be assembled and checked in advance (see Table 18-3).

Assessment

After the infant is delivered, the initial step is a quick assessment of the infant as he or she is dried off (see Fig. 18-1). The Apgar score provides a numerical assignment of

Table 18-1   Mechanisms of fetal distress—cont'd

Condition	Result	Etiologies
Placenta/Cord		
Obstruction	Interruption of oxygenated blood returning from placenta	Knot, prolapse
Acute blood loss	Fetal hypovolemic anemia	Marginal insertion, cord rupture
Baby		
Meconium	Aspiration and pneumonitis	Reflection of earlier asphyxial event
Infection	Shock, hypotension, respiratory distress	Bacterial, viral, other
Congenital anomalies	Impedes onset of respiration and oxygenation	Hypoplastic lungs, airway obstruction, diaphragmatic hernia
	Inadequate cardiac output or severe shunting	Congenital heart disease
	Abdominal catastrophe	Gastroschisis, omphalocele, bowel obstruction and/or perforation
Hemolytic disease	Hydrops: severe anemia, congestive failure, edema	Rh incompatibility, nonimmune hydrops
Drugs/toxins	Depressed respiratory drive, hypotension	General anesthesia or systemic drugs via mother; local injections directly into fetus

the assessment. Examine the heart rate, color, respiratory effort, tone, and reflex irritability to establish the extent of resuscitation required (see Table 18-4).

A brief physical examination also allows identification of major anomalies pertinent to resuscitation.

Anomaly	Comment
Bowel	
Omphalocele, gastroschisis, scaphoid abdomen (diaphragmatic hernia)	No bagging with bag and mask —in order to avoid bowel distension. With exposed bowel, wet saline towels are necessary to prevent rapid water and heat loss.
Spinal	
Myelomeningocele, encephalocele	Care must be taken to avoid injury to neural tissue.

Resuscitation
  Airway

Drying and rubbing the infant's back usually provides sufficient stimulation for respiration. Stimulation should be brief, lasting 10 to 15 seconds. If little or no response in

Arrive in L & D

Review history, Set up equipment

Delivery

Receive Infant – Start resuscitation clock

Place in infant warmer

Meconium protocol if appropriate

MINIMAL P.E./STIMULATE & DRY (15 Sec max)

(_____) _____) Apgar 1 minute/5 minutes

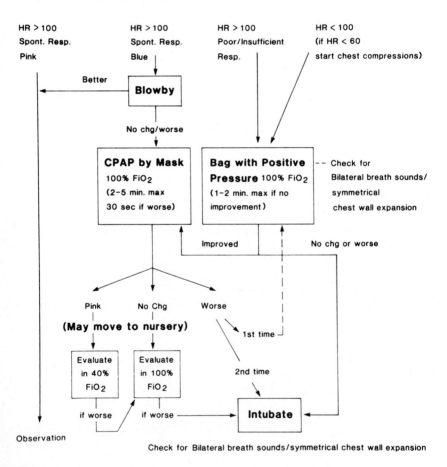

HR > 100	HR > 100	HR > 100	HR < 100
Spont. Resp.	Spont. Resp.	Poor/Insufficient	(if HR < 60
Pink	Blue	Resp.	start chest compressions)

Observation

Check for Bilateral breath sounds/symmetrical chest wall expansion

Fig. 18-1
Protocol for neonatal resuscitation.

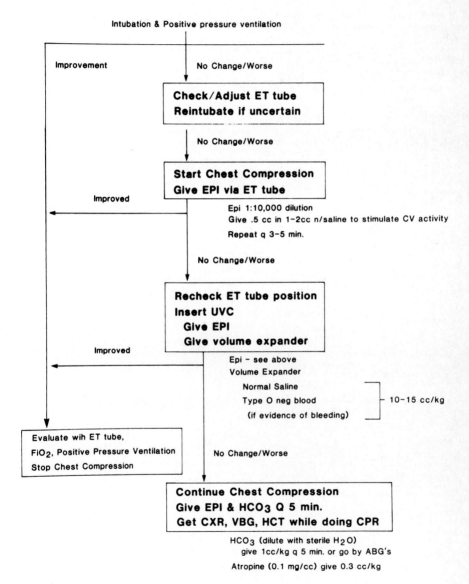

Intubation & Positive pressure ventilation

Improvement

No Change/Worse

**Check/Adjust ET tube
Reintubate if uncertain**

No Change/Worse

**Start Chest Compression
Give EPI via ET tube**

Improved

Epi 1:10,000 dilution
Give .5 cc in 1–2cc n/saline to stimulate CV activity
Repeat q 3–5 min.

No Change/Worse

**Recheck ET tube position
Insert UVC
  Give EPI
  Give volume expander**

Improved

Epi – see above
Volume Expander
  Normal Saline
  Type O neg blood   ⎤ 10–15 cc/kg
  (if evidence of bleeding) ⎦

Evaluate wih ET tube,
FiO$_2$, Positive Pressure Ventilation
Stop Chest Compression

No Change/Worse

**Continue Chest Compression
Give EPI & HCO$_3$ Q 5 min.
Get CXR, VBG, HCT while doing CPR**

HCO$_3$ (dilute with sterile H$_2$O)
  give 1cc/kg q 5 min. or go by ABG's
Atropine (0.1 mg/cc) give 0.3 cc/kg

Fig. 18-1 cont'd.

Table 18-2 Team roles for neonatal resuscitation

Team Member	Position	Role
1	Head	Airway management, O_2 administration, intubation
2	Side	Dry, stimulate, assess heart rate, chest compressions
3	Side	Recorder, medications, IV, umbilical line

Table 18-3 Equipment for neonatal resuscitation

Equipment*	Sizes	Comments
Radiant warmer	—	Heat source
Warm blankets	—	—
Oxygen	—	Warmed and humidified
Infant mask	0, 1	—
Inflation bag with manometer	—	Provide positive pressure ventilation
Laryngoscope/blades	0, 1	For intubation
Suction	—	Both bulb syringe (routine) and wall suction (for meconium removal)
Endotracheal tubes	2.5, 3.0, 3.5	—
Umbilical catheter tray	—	—
Drugs	—	Appropriate dilutions

*Includes major equipment only. Exhaustive lists are available in references cited in bibliography.

heart rate or respiratory effort is elicited, more aggressive resuscitative efforts are needed (see Fig. 18-1). For infants without meconium staining, deep suctioning should be avoided because the vagal stimulation causes reflex bradycardia. If the oropharynx needs to be cleared, a bulb syringe is adequate. Hyperextension is not indicated because a neutral position provides an appropriate airway in the newborn.

If meconium-stained fluid is present, no stimulation should be given until the airway is cleared. The most effective means of clearing the airway of meconium lies in the hands of the obstetrician. Thorough suctioning of the mouth and pharynx after delivery of the head allows removal of meconium before onset of respirations. When the fluid contains thick or particulate matter, further suctioning must be done after birth. Deep tracheal suctioning via intubation clears the trachea to avoid aspiration of meconium.

Direct mouth suctioning, or even use of a DeLee suction apparatus, is not appropriate. In order to comply with the Centers for Disease Control guidelines for potential exposure to AIDS, wall suction should be used.

Breathing

Infants who are not pink centrally or who show signs of respiratory distress, such as grunting, retracting, or unequal expansion of the chest, need supplemental oxygen.

Table 18-4 How to assign the Apgar score

Sign	Action to Assign Score	Observations		
		Assign score of 0	Assign score of 1	Assign score of 2
Heart rate	Count cord pulse or auscultate heart	Absent	<100	>100
Color	Visual assessment	Blue, pale	Body pink, extremities blue	Completely pink
Respiratory effort	Visual assessment	Absent	Slow, irregular	Strong cry
Tone	Manipulate extremity	Limp	Some flexion of extremities	Active motion
Reflex irritability	Flick sole of foot	No response	Some motion	Cry

Table 18-5 Indications for various methods of assisted oxygenation in neonatal resuscitation

Oxygen Delivery Method	Indication	Comments	Troubleshooting (if infant remains cyanotic)
Blowby	Spontaneous respirations and good heart rate but cyanotic	Place bag and mask near face to increase inspired O_2	1. Inadequate respirations 2. Congenital heart disease
Continuous positive airway pressure (CPAP) with mask	Remains blue with spontaneous respirations and good heart rate despite blowby	Augmented form of blowby; place mask on infant's face to form seal; maximum pressure is 8 cm of water	1. See above 2. Iatrogenic airway obstruction (nose occluded) 3. Inadequate seal of mask to face
Positive pressure with bag and mask	Cyanosis not improved with CPAP; absent or irregular respiratory effort; heart rate less than 100	If giving first breath, use 35 cm of water for term, 30 cm of water for preterm—then use 20-25 cm of water at 50-80 breaths per minute; assess effectiveness by chest rise and breath sounds	1. See above 2. Inadequate inspiratory pressure 3. Pneumothorax 4. Inadequate cardiac activity
Positive pressure via endotracheal tube (ET)	Unable to obtain adequate air exchange with bag and mask; no improvement or deterioration despite adequate air exchange with bag and mask for 1-2 min; need intubation for ventilation with bowel anomalies	Pressures and rate as above; assess effectiveness by chest rise and breath sounds	1. See above 2. ET mispositioned 3. Hypoplastic lungs (e.g., Potter's syndrome)

Oxygen should be delivered by one of the methods shown in Table 18-5, in accordance with the indication. (See also Fig. 18-1)

Appropriate sizes for the endotracheal tube (ET) and laryngoscope blade are determined by the size of the infant (Table 18-6). The correct position of the ET is shown in Fig. 18-2.

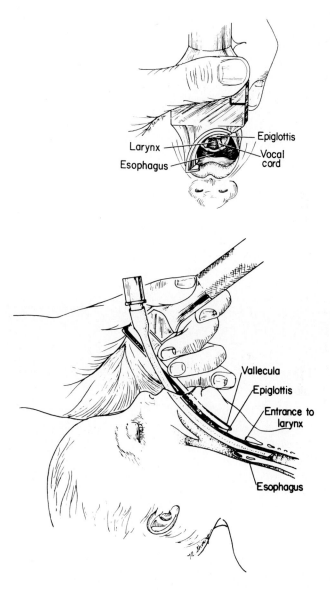

Fig. 18-2
Placement of an endotracheal tube; top shows view seen when intubating a neonate, with clearly visible vocal cords marking entry to the larynx; bottom shows lateral view indicating proper depth of insertion.

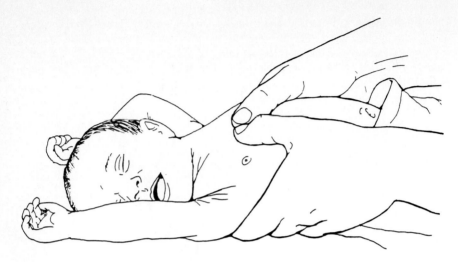

Fig. 18-3
Most effective method of cardiac massage in neonates, stabilizing the chest with both hands by encircling the thorax and using both thumbs to compress the heart.

Table 18-6   Equipment for intubation of the neonate

Size of Neonate	Tube Size	Blade Size	Length of Tube Inserted (mouth to tip)
< 1 kg (2 lb)	2.5	0	7 cm
1-2.5 kg (2-5 lbs)	3.0	0	9 cm
> 2.5 kg (5 lb)	3.5	0 or 1	10-11 cm

Circulation

Cardiac massage should be started if the heart rate remains below 80 beats per minute despite adequate ventilation (see Fig. 18-1). Chest compressions are done in the mid-sternal position, either with two fingers or by using both thumbs while encircling the infant's chest with your hands. The second method (Fig. 18-3) provides better stability and delivery of more effective compressions. The depth of the compression is ½ to ¾ inch at a rate of 120 times per minute. Assess effectiveness by umbilical or femoral pulse.

Drugs

Drugs are rarely necessary in neonatal resuscitation. Most infants respond to ventilatory management alone. When the heart rate remains less than 80 beats per minute despite adequate ventilation, drugs can be administered via an umbilical venous catheter or via the ET for epinephrine. Appropriate doses, indications, and timing are shown in Table 18-7 and Fig. 18-1.

Table 18-7 Drugs for neonatal resuscitation

Drug	Indications	Dose	Dilution	Side Effects or Precautions
Epinephrine (Adrenalin)	To restore myocardial contractility in cardiac arrest—given for flat-line ECG and persistent bradycardia; will increase BP	0.5 cc	1:10,000	Rise in BP with cerebrovascular hemorrhage from overdose
Normal saline	Shock for volume expansion	10-15 cc/kg		
Blood (0−)	Shock for volume expansion	10-15 cc/kg		Transfusion reaction; transmission of infection
Sodium bicarbonate	Metabolic acidosis, which occurs in cardiac arrest	1 mEq/kg	0.5 mEq/cc	High sodium levels; hyperosmolarity; intracranial hemorrhage
Neonatal Narcan	Narcotic depression	0.005-0.010 mg/kg	0.02 mg/cc— repeat every 10-15 min	Contraindicated if mother is suspected narcotic user (will put infant into withdrawal); observe infant for recurrent respiratory depression, as Narcan's effect may be shorter than the narcotic's effect
Dextrose	Hypoglycemia, blood sugar below 30 mg percent	2 cc/kg bolus, then 3-4 cc/kg/hr	10%	Hyperglycemia; retake Dextrostix in 10 min and at least every 30 min thereafter; use infusion pump to regulate

Table 18-8   Postresuscitation neonatal stabilization

System	Response	Comment
Cardiac	Stop CPR when heart rate is greater than 100 with adequate pulse pressure	Continue to monitor heart rate; determine blood pressure; assure adequate urine output
Respiratory		
No or inadequate respirations	After heart rate and pulse are normal, decrease ventilation rate to 40-60 breaths per minute	Evaluate with ABG
Spontaneous respirations	Gradually slow rate until remains only on CPAP; if remains pink, try blowby oxygen	Evaluate with ABG
Metabolic		
Hypoglycemia	Obtain blood glucose level	May need IV fluids of D10W at 80-100 ml/kg/d
Thermal	Maintain body temperature	Radiant warmer, dry, warm blankets

ABG, Arterial blood gas.

Postresuscitation stabilization (Table 18-8)

Postresuscitation stabilization of the neonate is outlined in Table 18-8.

ACKNOWLEDGMENT

This work is supported by the March of Dimes Foundation.

REVIEW
QUESTIONS

1. When meconium-stained fluid is present, all of the following are true except:
   a. The obstetrician has a major role in preventing meconium aspiration by suctioning the infant's pharynx on the perineum.
   b. Meconium staining is the one exception to the deep suctioning rule.
   c. The current recommendation is to use a DeLee suction trap to clear the airway of meconium.
   d. When meconium is not thick or particulate, deep tracheal suctioning is not necessary.
2. Deep tracheal suctioning:
   a. Causes vagally induced bradycardia.
   b. Should be done only for removal of meconium.
   c. Both of the above.
   d. Neither of the above.

3. For adequate resuscitation, the resuscitation team:
   a. Should assign roles after the baby is delivered and the need for resuscitation is assessed.
   b. Should have at least three members.
   c. Must consist of physicians.
   d. All of the above.
4. After delivery of the infant:
   1. The initial step is to provide an airway.
   2. Cold stress increases oxygen consumption.
   3. The primary mechanism for heat production is shivering.
   4. A radiant warmer and warm blankets provide a heat source.
      a. 1 and 3 are true.
      b. 2 and 4 are true.
      c. All are true.
      d. None are true.
5. If an infant is blue with poor respiratory effort:
   a. Oxygen must be delivered by positive pressure ventilation via bag and mask.
   b. Oxygen must be delivered by positive pressure ventilation via bag and mask if no bowel anomalies are present.
   c. Oxygen must be delivered by positive pressure ventilation via endotracheal tube.
6. Weight is a factor in infant resuscitation for all of the following except:
   a. Endotracheal tube size.
   b. Ventilation rate.
   c. Ventilation inspiratory pressures.
   d. Drug doses.
   e. Endotracheal tube insertion depth.

ANSWERS

1. c
2. c
3. b
4. b
5. b
6. b

BIBLIOGRAPHY

Cardon BS et al: Combined obstetric and pediatric approaches to preventing meconium aspiration syndrome, Am J Obstet Gynecol 126:712, 1976.
McIntyre KM, and Lewis AJ, editors: Textbook of advanced cardiac life support, 1987, American Heart Association.
Recommendations for presentation of HIV transmission in health-care settings, Morbid Mortal Week Rep 36:2S, 1987.
Standards for CPR and ECC. VI. Neonatal advanced life support, JAMA 225:2959, 1986.

Postpartum Care

19

Michael Foley

Many physiologic, anatomic, and psychologic changes occur following childbirth. Some changes are well-known and eagerly anticipated by all involved with the birth process, but others are less welcome and/or less well known. The process of postpartum resolution may take many weeks or months, depending on diverse factors such as the mode of delivery, blood loss, the method of infant feeding, the health and temperament of the infant, and most especially the infant's sleep habits.

ANATOMIC RESOLUTION

1. The uterus:
   The uterus undergoes a tenfold involution during the first 6 weeks after delivery, from a weight of approximately 1000 g to 50-100 g.
2. The cervix:
   The marked vascularity, glandular hypertrophy, and hyperplasia characteristic of pregnancy persist for the first week after delivery but regress completely by 6 weeks postpartum.
3. Ovarian function:
   In lactating women, elevated prolactin levels suppress ovulation, usually for 4 to 6 months or more. Prolactin levels fall to normal nonpregnant levels by the third week in nonlactating women but remain elevated for 6 weeks or more in lactating women. Thereafter, prolactin increases with each nursing episode, returning to normal between feedings. After delivery, estrogen levels fall quickly in both lactating and nonlactating women. Serum levels of FSH are similar in both lactating and nonlactating women, suggesting that the ovary is unresponsive to FSH in the presence of elevated prolactin; this is similar to the situation in women with nonpuerperal hyperprolactinemia.
4. Vagina:
   During the puerperium, the vaginal vault decreases in size, returning to normal by the third postpartum week. Lactating women display a thin, pale vaginal epithelium with minimal elasticity and rugation for the duration of nursing or until ovulation returns.

	Relationship of lactation to return of menses	
	Nonlactating women	*Lactating women*
Average days to first	70-75	190
PP ovulatory cycle	(10-12 weeks)	(27 weeks)
Average days to menses	70% by 84 days	70% by 252 days
	mean = 7-9 weeks	mean is dependent on duration of lactation

MANAGEMENT OF THE PUERPERIUM
General Concerns

1. Hospitalization:
   The new mother should be hospitalized for 1 to 3 days for uncomplicated vaginal delivery and 3 to 5 days for uncomplicated cesarean birth. During this period, the new mother should be educated about infant care and feeding, family planning, and "danger signs" of illness for herself and her baby.
2. Physical activity:
   After uncomplicated vaginal birth, physical activity, including stair-climbing, walking, driving, and muscle toning exercises, may begin without delay and progress to normal levels as common sense dictates: women whose infants are awake much of the night may need to progress more slowly than those mothers who get a full night's sleep soon after birth. Recovery after cesarean delivery is also somewhat slower.
3. Sexual activity:
   Sexual activity may be resumed safely when bleeding has subsided (10 to 21 days for vaginal birth; 17 to 30 days for cesarean delivery) and when any perineal tears or incisions have healed. Couples should be cautioned to expect that a variety of changes may affect the sexual relationship, including fatigue, a crying baby, the maternal/paternal roles dominating the wife/husband roles, fear of perineal pain, and lactation-induced libidinal suppression.
4. Work:
   A 6 to 8 week period of "disability" is customary after delivery. However, delivery is not analagous to other medically disabling conditions. Although the duration of labor, mode of delivery, and blood loss may predictably affect the rate of recovery, it is the infant's sleep patterns that most affect the mother's (and father's) ability to function in most jobs. Determination of postpartum "disability" is more an economic benefit to be won at the bargaining table than a medical decision.
5. Postpartum examination:
   An examination scheduled at 6 weeks postpartum confirms uterine resolution and perineal or incisional healing and affords an opportunity to discuss family planning and contraception. A routine Pap smear and a breast examination should also be performed.

Perineal Care

1. Median episiotomy
   Local cleansing, sitz baths, and oral analgesics such as ibuprofen or codeine with acetaminophen are usually sufficient.
2. Mediolateral episiotomy, third or fourth degree extensions, or large periurethral tears
   These may require use of additional measures such as stool softeners, urethral catheters, and strong analgesia. The perineum should be inspected for hematoma formation and cellulitis whenever the patient has had significant lacerations or is unable to void postpartum.
3. Lochia
   Mild vaginal bleeding, called lochia, is normally present for 2 to 3 weeks following vaginal birth and for 3 to 4 weeks after cesarean delivery. Initially the color is bright red, but it later becomes maroon before fading to pink or tan. The patient should be discouraged from using tampons during this time because of the risk of toxic shock syndrome, but they may be used later if they are changed frequently.

Maternal-Infant Bonding

The early postpartum period is a sensitive time during which close mother-infant interaction facilitates subsequent attachment and beneficial parenting behavior. The postpartum unit should be a place that enhances this process, both by its policies and physical layout. Signs of aberrant parental attachment to the infant should be noted and referral to the appropriate social service agency made if necessary.

Coping with Unexpected Outcomes

All families expect an ideal outcome to pregnancy. Anything less than the "perfect" child they had fantasized is likely to lead to some degree of a normal grief reaction. If the child has a minor birth defect or if the birth process itself was less than ideal, this grieving may be short-lived, as the joy accompanying the arrival of the child predominates. If, however, the mother or child has a serious unanticipated problem, then grief may be the dominant emotion. Fetal or perinatal death, a major (either life-threatening or disfiguring) birth defect, and unexpected hysterectomy are all naturally associated with significant grieving.

Symptoms of normal grief include fatigue, insomnia, GI upset, guilt, anger and hostility, and affective changes. It is not commonly appreciated that grieving may normally last as long as 18 months. It is not uncommon to find the family and friends of the couple whose baby has died expressing the erroneous idea that another pregnancy will fill the void of the lost child; this decision should be postponed until the grieving process has been completed.

Guidelines for Managing Perinatal Loss

1. Keep the parent informed; be forthright and honest.
2. Anticipate the various steps in the grieving process.
3. Encourage continuous presence of mother's support person(s).
4. Encourage the couple to see, hold, and touch the infant; if they decline, be thorough in describing the baby's appearance both in the chart and verbally; take pictures of the baby so they may later see if they choose.
5. Teach the family about the grieving process.
6. Prepare the couple for hospital paperwork, e.g., death certificates, autopsy permits, etc.
7. Encourage funeral or memorial services.
8. Help the couple decide how to tell siblings, family, and friends.
9. Encourage the couple to maintain control of as many choices as possible.
10. Discuss subsequent pregnancy and contraception.
11. Expect that much of what is said during this time will need to be repeated; provide both written and verbal counseling.
12. Schedule follow-up visits for counseling.

COMPLICATIONS OF THE PUERPERIUM
Infections
Endometritis

a. Caused by cervicovaginal flora, e.g., anaerobes and gram-negative organisms most commonly
b. More common with cesarean delivery (10% to 30%) than with vaginal delivery (less than 5%)
c. Other risk factors include prolonged membrane rupture more than 12 hours, anemia, multiple vaginal examinations in labor, indigent patients

d. Diagnosis: temperature greater than 100.4° F on two occasions during the first 10 days postpartum, accompanied by uterine tenderness, foul lochia, and malaise
e. WBC count may or may not be helpful; many normal women will have WBC count greater than 20,000 following delivery
f. Fever less than 48 hours postpartum—suspect gram-positive streptococci
g. Fever more than 48 hours postpartum—suspect mixed anaerobic and gram-negative infection
h. Treatment (Any of the following drug regimens are succesful in 90% or more of cases):
   (1) High dose penicillin/ampicillin
   (2) Clindamycin plus gentamicin
   (3) Second- and third-generation cephalosporins
i. Prevention:
   (1) Handwashing by hospital personnel
   (2) Fewest possible vaginal examinations in labor
   (3) Remove all placenta and associated membranes
   (4) Prophylactic antibiotics have been shown to reduce the rate of endometritis in high-risk patients, e.g., those delivered by cesarean section—first-generation cephalosporin (cefazolin) is best choice
j. Prognosis:
   Usually excellent with prompt therapy; delay in diagnosis may lead to pelvic abscess
k. Complications—pelvic abscess:
   Septic pelvic thrombophlebitis bacterial heparinase leads to clots in pelvic vessels, with possible septic emboli; treat with heparin and antibiotics

Wound infections

a. Incidence 2% to 20% of cesarean births
b. Risk factors:
   Diabetes, obesity, poor nutrition, immunosuppressant therapy, long operative time, emergency surgery
c. Caused by endogenous flora from skin or genital tract
d. Diagnosis:
   (1) Wound erythema, induration, and finally suppuration with drainage
   (2) Fever, leukocytosis common
   (3) Same bacteriologic variation seen in endometritis: early, strep; late, mixed aerobe/anaerobe
   (4) Cultures helpful if initial therapy fails
e. Treatment: drainage!
   (1) Debridement of devitalized tissue
   (2) Antibiotics may help but are not sufficient without drainage
f. Prevention:
   (1) Minimize tissue trauma at surgery
   (2) Use nonreactive suture, e.g., synthetic absorbable
   (3) Drainage
   (4) Use secondary or delayed primary closure for contaminated wounds

Mastitis

Infection of the breast occurs almost exclusively in lactating women in two forms: *epidemic,* often acquired in the hospital and caused by *Staphylococcus aureus,* and *non-*

epidemic, usually acquired outside the hospital and caused by host flora, including *Staphylococcus* sp., and most often the result of incomplete evacuation of the breast.
a. Diagnosis:
   (1) In the epidemic form, hospital epidemiologic surveillance may be key; fever and localized tenderness occur 2-4 days postpartum. Abscess is common.
   (2) Nonepidemic mastitis also presents with fever, tenderness, and malaise. Abscess is uncommon.
b. Treatment:
   (1) Oral or parenteral semisynthetic penicillins, penicillinase-resistant drugs, or cephalosporins.
   (2) Continue nursing on the affected breast; cessation confers no advantage to the infant unless frank abscess is present and may make the infection more difficult to clear.
   (3) Abscess requires parenteral antibiotics and incision and drainage.
c. Prevention:
   (1) Nipple hygiene.
   (2) Active care of cracks and fissures; lanolin is most helpful.
   (3) Early diagnosis and prompt antibiotic therapy can prevent most abscesses.

HEMORRHAGE

Blood loss after vaginal and cesarean deliveries is approximately 500 and 1000 ml, respectively. Effective hemostasis depends on the physical constriction of uterine blood vessels by the myometrium. Excessive blood loss is usually related to failure of the myometrium to contract promptly or adequately after delivery. This is called *uterine atony* and is commonly associated with the following risk factors:
1. *Uterine overdistention,* e.g., multifetal gestation or polyhydramnios
2. *Prolonged* or *dysfunctional* labor
3. *Uterine relaxants,* e.g., halothane anesthetic
4. *Infection,* chorioamnionitis
5. Uterine fibroids
Other causes include: cervical or vaginal laceration, incomplete placental separation or retained placental fragments, uterine rupture, and generalized coagulopathy.
   Initial *evaluation* is aimed at simultaneously beginning treatment for uterine atony and excluding the less common but potentially more serious traumatic causes:
1. Explore vagina and cervix for lacerations.
2. Use bimanual uterine massage to compress the uterus and stimulate uterine contraction.
3. Administer intravenous oxytocin, 20 to 30 units/L of saline, at 200 to 500 ml/hour.
4. If there is no evidence of laceration and the oxytocin infusion plus massage fails to produce uterine contraction, then additional drugs should be tried:
   a. Ergotrate 0.2 mg IM followed by
   b. Prostaglandin 15 methyl F2 alpha, 0.25 mg IM every 1 to 2 hours.
Any evident cervical or vaginal lacerations obviously should be repaired. Adequate assistance for retraction and excellent lighting are essential to the success of this endeavor.
   If bleeding continues despite the above measures, the uterus should be carefully reexplored for retained placental fragments and for uterine lacerations extending into the myometrium. The latter may be remarkably difficult to detect. The endometrial surface should be gently scraped, or curetted, with a *large* curette to remove any additional

250   Chapter 19

placenta or membranes that might be impeding uterine contraction.

Persistent uterine hemorrhage requires aggressive fluid and blood component therapy followed by surgical management.

Surgical Management

1. Ligation of the ascending branch of the uterine arteries bilaterally.
2. Bilateral hypogastric artery ligation.
3. Ovarian vessel ligation.
4. Hysterectomy may be required when other, less drastic measures fail. Manual compression of the aorta below the renal arteries helps to prevent excessive blood loss while correcting volume and red cell deficits before beginning hysterectomy in this situation.

PUERPERAL DEPRESSION

Seventy percent of women experience some degree of transient tearfulness, anxiety, or restlessness commonly known as "the postpartum blues." As long as this syndrome is transient, shortlived, and resolves spontaneously, it may be viewed as a normal part of the childbearing experience. No therapy other than family support and good humor are needed.

However, it is important to distinguish the more serious *postpartum depression* from the "blues." This neurosis/psychosis may occur in as many as 10% of women, and is neither short-lived nor benign. It may recur with subsequent pregnancies and requires psychiatric consultation and therapy.

REVIEW QUESTIONS

1. True or False: At 2 weeks postpartum, the uterus has returned to the pelvic cavity and by 6 weeks, complete resolution and involution has taken place.
2. Which of the following most correctly represents the interval from delivery to the first menstruation in the nonlactating patient:
   a. 70-75 days (10-12 weeks)
   b. 190 days (27 weeks)
   c. 70 percent by 84 days (12 weeks) mean = 49-63 days (7-9 weeks)
   d. 70% by 252 days (36 weeks)
3. True or False: In response to perinatal loss, a normal resolution of grief generally occurs within 18 months.
4. Which of the following is not considered a risk factor for developing postpartum endometritis:
   a. Cesarean section
   b. Frequent vaginal examinations during labor
   c. Low socioeconomic status
   d. Vaginal trichomonas
5. True or False: "Postpartum blues" should be distinguished form "postpartum depression" because "blues" is benign, transient, a normal part of the childbearing experience, and requires no therapy other than family support.

ANSWERS

1. True
2. c
3. True
4. d
5. True

BIBLIOGRAPHY

1. American College of Obstetricians and Gynecologists: Pregnancy, work, and disability, Technical Bulletin no. 58, May 1980.
2. Bowes WA Jr: Postpartum care. In Gabbe SG, Niebyl JR, and Simpson JL, editors: Obstetrics: normal and problem pregnancies. New York: 1986, Churchill Livingstone, Inc.
3. Clark SL, Phelan JP, and Cotton DB: Critical care obstetrics, New York, 1987, Medical Economics Co., Inc., pp. 40, 41, 57.
4. Jennings B, and Edmundson M: The postpartum period: after confinement—The fourth trimester, Clin Obstet Gynecol 23:1093, 1980.
5. Kowalski K: Managing perinatal loss, Clin Obstet Gynecol 23:1113, 1980.
6. Monheit AG, Cousins L, and Resnik R: The puerperium: anatomic and physiologic readjustments, Clin Obstet Gynecol 23:973, 1980.
7. Neville MC, and Neifert MR: Lactation, physiology, nutrition, and breast feeding, New York, 1983, Plenum Press.
8. Resnik R: The puerperium. In Creasy RK, and Resnik R, editors: Maternal fetal medicine: principles and practice, Philadelphia, 1984, W.B. Saunders Co.
9. Ryding EL: Sexuality during and after pregnancy, Acta Obstet Gynecol Scand 63:679, 1984.
10. Villasanta U: Thromboembolic disease in pregnancy, Am J Obstet Gynecol 92:142, 1965.

Breast-Feeding

20

Lindsey K. Grossman

New mothers are often at a loss to know where to turn for help with breast-feeding. Physicians are often unsure about advice for the lactating mother because few have been adequately trained in anything beyond the physiology of lactation. It is reasonable to expect that pediatricians and family physicians are knowledgeable about breast-feeding, but it is often during pregnancy that the foundation for successful lactation is developed. The obstetrician is therefore in a key position to promote and foster breast-feeding. Each pregnant woman should be asked her plans for infant nutrition during the first trimester of pregnancy. Bottle-feeding can certainly provide adequate nutrition to the newborn, but there is now abundant evidence that breast-feeding is preferable for a variety of reasons.

ADVANTAGES OF BREAST-FEEDING

1. Immunologic*: Breast milk contains several immunologically active substances that have been shown to result in a decreased incidence of gastroenteritis, otitis media, and respiratory illness in breast-fed infants compared to bottle-fed infants. They include:
   a. Secretory IgA
   b. Bifidus factor—inhibits enteric pathogens
   c. Complement
   d. Leukocytes (macrophages, T and B lymphocytes, polymorphonuclear leukocytes)
   e. Milk lipids—inactivate pathogenic viruses
   f. Lysozyme
   g. Lactoferrin—inhibits enteric pathogens
2. Better nutrition: Breast milk contains less protein than formula, producing decreased renal solute load to the relatively immature kidney of the newborn. The fat in breast milk is more digestible, and calcium absorption is better because of a favorable ratio of calcium to phosphorus. Iron bioavailability is superior to that of formula as well. The composition of breast milk changes as the child grows so that infant nutrition is optimal throughout infancy. Additionally, there is a decreased prevalence of obesity in breast-fed infants, with potential life-long benefits.
3. Less expensive and more convenient.

---

*A decrease in the prevalence of eczema in the children of allergic parents has been observed when breast-feeding is employed, with an inverse correlation of allergic problems and duration of nursing.

4. Psychologic advantages: Mother-infant bonding is enhanced by nursing, which is something a mother can do for the infant that others cannot.
5. Physiologic advantages: Lactation leads to oxytocin production, with improved postpartum uterine involution.

POLICIES TO PROMOTE BREAST-FEEDING

In addition to actively encouraging breast-feeding, the obstetrician should examine the mother's breasts and nipples at the first prenatal visit and again during the first visit of the third trimester. This should be done because 1% to 2% of all women have inverted nipples that are believed to be caused by adhesions. The nipples of these women do not become erect during orgasm or tactile stimulation and will be impossible for the infant to latch onto after birth. If diagnosed sufficiently early (at least several weeks to months before delivery), the Hoffman technique can be used to break adhesions and release the nipple (see Fig. 20-1). The Hobbit nipple shell, which is worn within the woman's bra before delivery, can also be used as an adjunct.

The obstetrician can greatly facilitate a good start with breast-feeding by managing delivery with nursing in mind:

1. Use as little systemic anesthesia/analgesia as possible so that the baby will be wide-awake; an effect on the infant's ability to nurse after receiving barbiturates for sedation during labor has been shown to last for as long as 4 days after delivery.

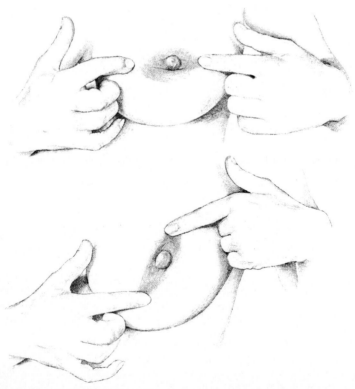

Fig. 20-1
Hoffman technique for inverted nipples.
From Messenger M.: The breastfeeding book, New York, 1982, Von Nostrand Reinhold Co.

2. Local anesthetics are rapidly cleared from the mother's serum, are not absorbed orally, and are therefore quite safe.
3. General anesthesia (including short-acting barbiturates and succinylcholine and narcotics) drugs are all rapidly cleared. Inhaled agents (such as halothane and nitrous oxide) are cleared by the mother's respiratory tree. By the time the mother is awake enough to nurse, her milk will be safe for her baby.
4. Allow early nursing in birthing/recovery room. The oxytocin released during sucking will assist in uterine involution and decrease bleeding. Additionally, this allows early bonding and a good initial nursing by taking advantage of the brand-new infant's "alert" period.

Hospital postpartum policies must be supportive of breast-feeding:
1. A 24-hour rooming-in policy allows free access to baby; a policy of no visitors outside the immediate family allows mother to rest and protects infant from infection.
2. Each mother should have frequent access to postpartum nurses who are experienced in and knowledgeable of appropriate breast-feeding initiation techniques.
   a. Multiple nursing positions, including football hold, madonna hold, and side-lying, and appropriate latch-on/detachment should be taught to prevent sore nipples (Fig. 20-2).
   b. Frequent, short feedings round-the-clock establish good supply (*supply-and-demand* physiology of lactation).
3. Infant feeding policies to include:
   a. *No* supplement of any kind. *No* pacifiers. Water supplements increase the incidence and magnitude of hyperbilirubinemia, and formula supplements decrease the infant's drive to nurse, which is necessary to stimulate good milk supply. Newborns may develop a strong attachment to artificial nipples over mother's *(nipple confusion),* making the transition to the breast difficult or impossible.
   b. Ad libitum feedings round-the-clock—the more the infant suckles, the more prolactin is produced and the more milk is available to the infant. Milk left in the breast for prolonged periods (i.e., overnight) inhibits milk production.
4. In cases in which early (less than 3 or 4 days postpartum) discharge is required or desired, home visitation by a knowledgeable nurse who can assist with early lactational difficulties is strongly suggested.

LACTATION FAILURE

It is probable that more than 95% of all cases of lactation failure are indeed caused by an inadequate supply of milk. With appropriate assistance in managing lactation, however, most of these women could have supplied adequate amounts of milk. Fig. 20-3 illustrates the "vicious cycle" of difficulties many women experience that ultimately lead to lactation failure; all of the difficulties should be easily prevented with prenatal and postpartum lactation counseling.

Organic causes do occur but are very uncommon. These include:
1. Retained placental fragments, which cause continued progesterone secretion that, in turn, causes inhibition of prolactin secretion
2. Drug ingestion (high-dose estrogen, ergot, bromocriptine)
3. Ingestion of excess vitamin B_6 (10 to 100 times RDA of 2.5 mg/day) has been proposed as a possible organic cause
4. Previous augmentation or reduction mammoplasty with disrupted innervation
5. Sheehan's syndrome/hypopituitarism (.01% to .02% of pregnant women)
6. Anatomic absence of glandular tissue (rare)
7. Nipple adhesions—1% to 2% of women (for discussion of nipple adhesions, see under Policies to Promote Breast-Feeding)

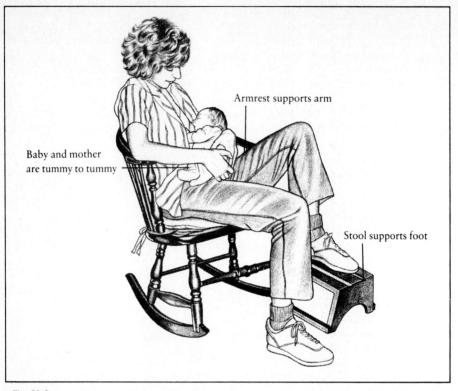

A

Fig. 20-2
Various breast-feeding positions decrease nipple soreness. **A,** Madonna hold. **B,** Side-lying. **C,** Football hold.
From Eiger MS, and Olds SW: The complete book of breast-feeding, New York, 1987, Workman Publishing Co Inc.

PRACTICAL POINTS FOR LACTATION MANAGEMENT

1. Supply and demand—mothers need to understand the importance of the supply-and-demand phenomenon on which lactation physiology is based. The more often (not the longer) a mother nurses, the more milk she will make. The breast is 80% to 90% emptied in approximately 7 to 10 minutes so longer nursing periods will only make her nipples more sore.
2. Sore nipples
   a. Causes
      (1) Inappropriate latch-on and/or detachment.
      (2) Use of only one nursing position.
      (3) Engorgement or inappropriate feeding schedules.
   b. Treatment
      (1) Air to the nipples and rest for the mother.
      (2) Topical lanolin is sometimes helpful.
      (3) Nipple shields are rarely helpful and may be harmful.
3. Let-down difficulties—inadequate stimulation for oxytocin release.
   a. Causes
      (1) Engorgement—baby unable to latch on.

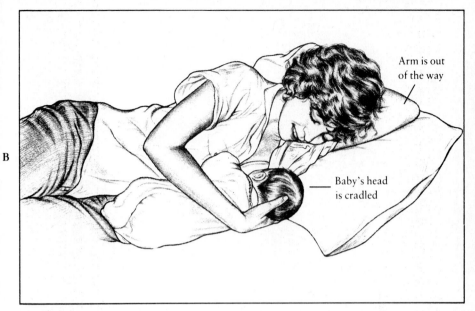

Fig. 20-2, **B**
For legend see opposite page.

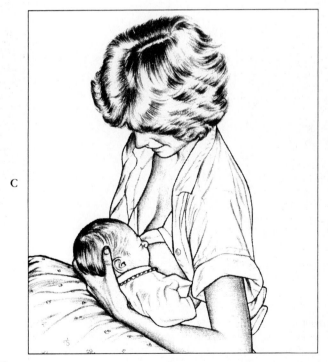

Fig. 20-2, **C**
For legend see opposite page.

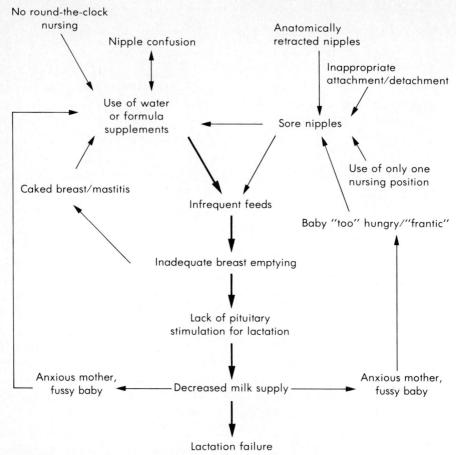

Fig. 20-3
Sequence of events leading to lactation failure.

    (2) Sore nipples—pain of sucking inhibits feedback to pituitary.
    (3) Baby is too eager (painful sucking) or too quiet (inadequate sucking stimulus).
    (4) Anxiety and/or fatigue of mother.
    (5) Baby may need to nurse for 3 to 4 minutes before let-down occurs; therefore nursing schedules that limit nursing to less than 7 to 10 minutes per breast are inappropriate.
  b. Treatment
    (1) Best managed clinically without synthetic oxytocin (Syntocinon) spray.
    (2) Treat for sore nipples if necessary.
    (3) Assist mother in relaxing; use light tactile stimulation to nipple.
4. Caked breast/mastitis—consider when mother reports a postpartum fever.
  a. Pathophysiology—related primarily to stasis, not bacteriology.
    (1) When free flow of milk out of the ductal system is inhibited, stasis of milk may cause inspissation of milk in a duct and back up with redness, warmth, and tenderness in a pie-shaped distribution in the breast. This is known as *caked breast*.

(2) When bacteria are introduced from the baby back through the ducts into this area of stasis, the perfect setup for infection begins, and *mastitis* occurs with generalized malaise and fever.

b. Treatment
  (1) Increase nursing on the affected side—do not decrease. The baby is not at risk of infection because the organisms involved invariably originated from the mother's skin and baby's nasopharyngeal flora.
  (2) Local compresses and rest for mother.
  (3) Antibiotics—choice is not critical. Be certain drug is safe for baby (see under Antibiotics).

Obstetricians must be prepared to actively encourage and support breast-feeding for the infants they deliver; this is the completion of the responsibility they have to assist the mother in assuring the healthiest start for her baby.

MATERNAL MEDICATIONS AND BREAST-FEEDING

When managing drug therapy for the lactating woman, remember that the breast is not a sieve—all substances given to the mother do not necessarily pass directly to the baby in the milk. The relative amount of a substance's concentration in the milk is expressed as the *milk/plasma ratio*. Usually the milk/plasma ratio is .005 to .05 for medium-sized drug particles. However, the actual dose of the drug in the breast milk also depends on the percent of the drug absorbed into the mother's serum, the relative distribution to the mother's serum, the mother's rate of clearance, and the volume of milk produced. Therefore the milk/plasma ratio is not the same as the percentage of the mother's dose received by the baby. Usually the percentage of the drug in milk is much lower than the milk/plasma ratio.

Certain practical considerations also vary the amount of the drug the baby receives:
1. Age of baby—the newborn still receiving colostrum receives a very low volume of milk and therefore very little drug. Likewise, the older, partially weaned baby also receives less milk and therefore less drug.
2. Timing of dose—avoid dosing schedules that will time peak plasma level of drug with maximal milk secretion (during and right after feeding). It may be best to dose mother 1 hour after feeding or at a time when baby feeds less (nighttime).
3. Choose drugs that are:
   a. Rapidly cleared from plasma.
   b. Protein-bound to plasma.
   c. Bound to large molecules.
   d. Acidic rather than basic.
4. Watch carefully for side effects in the infant whenever medication is administered to the mother.

TYPES OF MEDICATIONS
Analgesics
1. Acetylsalicylic acid (nonarthritic doses) and acetaminophen quite safe
2. Nonsteroidal antiinflammatory drugs are excreted into milk, but no adverse side effects have been shown
3. Narcotics excreted into milk in very low dose

Antibiotics
1. Most are safe, including gentamicin (cannot be absorbed from GI tract), ampicillin,

and cephalosporins
2. Some antibiotics to avoid if possible:
   a. Avoid sulfonamides during the first month of life (interfere with bilirubin conjugation)
   b. Avoid erythromycin and clindamycin (basic salts) if possible
   c. Avoid tetracycline, although little is absorbed by infant (interferes with neonatal tooth formation)
   d. Avoid chloramphenicol, although excreted in very low dose (idiosyncratic bone-marrow suppression)
   e. Metronidazole—probably best to give as single dose for vaginitis; pump and discard milk for 12 hours after dose has been administered

Anticonvulsants

1. Seizure control must be maintained
2. Drugs pass into breast milk, but side effects other than drowsiness in infants are uncommon, and a schedule calling for a single nighttime dose usually avoids the problem

Medication for Thyroid Disease

1. Thyroid disease is common in young women. Women with severe hypothyroidism may not establish lactation; women with hyperthyroidism may safely nurse (hormone does not cross into milk).
   a. Diagnostic scans—pump milk for 24 to 48 hours after scan and discard.
   b. Treatment
      (1) Replacement thyroid hormone is safe.
      (2) Iodides are rapidly excreted into milk and are contraindicated.
      (3) Propranolol is extensively used and is apparently safe.
      (4) Propylthiouracil is the most extensively used and apparently the safest thyroid treatment for lactating mothers. Monitor baby's thyroid function.
      (5) Therapeutic radioactive iodine can be excreted into milk for several weeks; use of it probably requires that the baby be weaned.

TREATMENT OF HYPERTENSION

1. Lactating hypertensive women may require considerably less medication than they did previously; pregnancy-induced hypertension will probably not require treatment during lactation
2. Apparently safe drug choices are:
   a. Methyldopa
   b. Hydralazine
   c. Spironolactone
3. There is some controversy about the use of propranolol, but it is probably safe
4. Clonidine, metoprolol (Lopressor), and atenolol (Tenormin) are apparently safe; captopril may be safest of all—its level in tested milk is extremely low
5. Thiazides decrease milk production even more effectively than estrogens in the immediate postpartum period and may interfere with bilirubin metabolism
6. Furosemide can cause dangerous fluid and electrolyte shifts in the infant
7. Reserpine should *not* be used because infant may experience nasal stuffiness, respiratory distress secondary to tracheobronchial secretions, and bradycardia
8. Magnesium sulfate is often used in treating eclampsia—the milk/plasma ratio is

rather high, but the concentration of magnesium in the breast milk of a mother receiving magnesium sulfate is less than that in Similac Special Care infant formula; the baby should be able to nurse

TREATMENT OF ASTHMA

1. Sympathomimetics, especially β-agonists—inhaled or systemic (e.g., metaproterenol and salbutamol)—are probably the preferred treatment over methylxanthines.
2. Methylxanthines—babies may be more susceptible to side effects, and the metabolism of these drugs in infants may be unpredictable. On the other hand, these drugs are often used in treating bronchospasm or apnea of prematurity in infants, so there is extensive experience in using them, and microtechniques for testing infant blood levels are widely available. Use short-acting theophylline/aminophylline preparations, time doses around feeding schedule if possible, and monitor baby's serum level.
3. Steroids—large molecules and low availability in milk and are therefore quite safe.

ANTICOAGULANTS

1. Heparin—very large protein, not excreted in breast milk, and not absorbed from GI tract.
2. Coumadin—low excretion into milk, if at all; give vitamin K to infant to be certain of avoiding bleeding problems in infant.

GI CATHARTICS

1. Milk of magnesia, mineral oil, stool softeners, bulk-forming laxatives, and suppositories are all quite safe.
2. Dihydroxyanthraquinone (Dorbane and Dorbantyl) are highly excreted into milk and can cause infant diarrhea and colicky pain.

ORAL CONTRACEPTIVES

1. Estrogen and progesterone are rather large molecules, so they are poorly excreted into milk. No side effects reported in infants exposed to them via breast milk, but the long-term effect is unknown. Overall, the best choice of contraception for the lactating woman is, if possible, a barrier method.
2. Pills containing estrogen may decrease milk supply and are not an appropriate alternative to a barrier method.
3. Progesterone "mini-pill" will not decrease milk supply and should be used when barrier contraception is not an option.

DRUGS THAT ARE PROBABLY CONTRAINDICATED

1. Atropine
2. Cimetidine
3. Lithium
4. Bromides
5. Iodides
6. Radioactive elements
7. Chronic use of ergot alkaloids

DRUGS THAT ARE ABSOLUTELY CONTRAINDICATED

1. Chemotherapeutic agents
2. Radioactive therapeutic agents

MOTHER'S MEDICAL CONDITION AND NURSING RECOMMENDATIONS

The most frequent medical problem lactating women experience is an intercurrent viral illness. Because the baby has, undoubtedly, already been exposed, the mother may continue to nurse, giving her baby the immunologic benefit of her milk. Other infections may pose a dilemma:

1. "Closed" infections, including UTI, and diagnosed bacterial infections that are being treated with antibiotics (mother afebrile)—baby may nurse
   a. Consider that a febrile reaction with engorgement may be the cause of a woman's postpartum fever
   b. Endometritis with fever can usually be considered to be in this category— mother should use good hand-washing technique and continue to nurse
2. Other serious bacterial infections (sepsis, pneumonia)—delay nursing until after 24 hours of appropriate antibiotics
3. Chronic hepatitis carrier—may nurse after appropriate postpartum prophylaxis with globulin and vaccine as recommended in the 1988 AAP Committee report (see bibliography)
   a. Currently active hepatitis—nursing is controversial; safe if hepatitis occurred in early pregnancy and is now resolved
4. Herpes viruses
   a. Herpes simplex
      (1) Breast-feeding is contraindicated only if an active lesion is present on mother's breast
      (2) Use good hand-washing technique if genital lesion is present
      (3) Do not kiss infant if active oral lesion is present
   b. CMV—safe to nurse but mother may not contribute to a milk bank
5. AIDS
   a. Most babies will have been exposed *in utero* if mother is HTLV−3+
   b. Little definitive data as yet regarding actual risk from breast-feeding alone
   c. Currently, if mother's serology is positive for AIDS, she should probably not nurse; this is, however, usually a moot point because few drug abusers will have reformed sufficiently to allow breast-feeding

REVIEW
QUESTIONS

1. Breast-feeding has been shown to afford the following immunologic benefits to the infant:
   a. Immunoglobulins and lymphocytes
   b. Decreased respiratory illness
   c. Decreased gastroenteritis
   d. Inactivates pathogenic viruses
   e. All of the above
2. Breast-feeding provides better nutrition for the baby than formula because breast milk contains:
   a. More protein
   b. Less fat and carbohydrates
   c. More digestible fat
   d. More iron
   e. All of the above
3. Infant intake of a drug administered to the lactating mother can often be minimized by:
   a. Dosing mother approximately 1 hour after nursing

b. Dosing mother approximately 1 hour before nursing
c. Administering a drug that has a high milk/plasma ratio
d. Administering a drug that is slowly cleared from mother's plasma
e. Administering a drug that is not protein bound

4. Which antibiotic is safe for the nursing mother?
   a. Erythromycin
   b. Gantrisin
   c. Gentamicin
   d. Chloramphenicol
   e. None of the above

5. Which antihypertensive is not safe for the nursing mother?
   a. Methyldopa
   b. Captopril
   c. Spironolactone
   d. Thiazides
   e. None of the above—all are safe for mother and baby

6. Which of the following are almost always contraindicated for the breast-feeding mother?
   a. Magnesium sulfate
   b. Cimetidine
   c. Heparin
   d. Coumadin
   e. Theophylline

7. Which condition contraindicates breast-feeding?
   a. UTI
   b. AIDS
   c. Genitial herpes
   d. b and c above
   e. None of the above

8. Most lactation failure is caused by:
   a. Infrequent nursing
   b. Nipple adhesions
   c. Retained placental fragments
   d. Anatomic absence of breast glandular tissue
   e. Previous cosmetic breast surgery

9. The most important aspect of therapy for mastitis is:
   a. Amoxicillin 250 mg tid
   b. Warm compresses
   c. Temporary cessation of breast-feeding on the involved side
   d. Pain relief
   e. Frequent nursing on the involved side

ANSWERS

1. e
2. c
3. a
4. c
5. d
6. b
7. b
8. a
9. e

BIBLIOGRAPHY

American Academy of Pediatrics: Report of the Committee on Infectious Disease, Elk Grove, Ill, 1988, The Academy.

Eiger MS, and Olds SW: The complete book of breast-feeding, New York, 1987, Workman Publishing Co Inc.

Goldfarb J, and Tibbetts E: Breast-feeding handbook: a practical reference for physicians, nurses and other health professionals, Hillside, NJ, 1980, Enslow Publishers.

Ladik CF, and Holzman IR: A guide to drug usage during breast-feeding, Pittsburgh, Magee Women's Hospital.

Lawrence RA: Breastfeeding: a guide for the medical profession, ed 2, St. Louis, 1985, The CV Mosby Co.

Lawrence RA: Breast-feeding: a symposium, Clin Perinatol 14(1):1, 1987.

Neville MC, and Neifert MR: Lactation: physiology, nutrition and breast-feeding, New York, 1983, Plenum Publishing Corp.

Contraception and Sterilization

21

William G. Dodds

The World Health Organization (WHO) has identified contraception as one of the most important issues facing the world today. Even in western societies, such as the United States, where zero population growth has been achieved for over a decade, the problem of teenage pregnancy remains large. It is the concern of all physicians to help people obtain proper information and access to contraception.

ORAL CONTRACEPTIVES

Oral contraceptives (OCs) are the second most frequently chosen method of contraception for use by reproductive-age females. It is estimated that 9 to 10 million American women are presently on OCs.

The amount of misunderstanding in the general population about OCs is significant. A 1985 Gallup Poll showed that three out of every four women interviewed believed OCs carried substantial health risks. One third believed OCs caused cancer. The Gallup Poll points out the need for physicians to be specific in discussing cancer and cardiovascular risks with all patients to alleviate unwarranted fears.

Composition of OCs

OCs contain estrogens and progestin components in combination. The estrogen is either mestranol or, more commonly, ethinyl estradiol. Mestranol is converted to ethinyl estradiol in the body. Differences in potency between mestranol and ethinyl estradiol are insignificant. Five different progestins are currently used in the different OC formulations:

1. Ethynodiol diacetate
2. Norethindrone
3. Norethindrone acetate
4. Norethynodrel
5. Norgestrel

No absolute scientific measure can compare potencies between different progestins in OCs. However, a relative progestin potency with respect to serum high-density lipoprotein (HDL) cholesterol changes is given in Table 21-1. The more potent progestins adversely lower serum HDL cholesterol. Decreases in HDL cholesterol have been associated with increased atherogenic risk.

Side Effects and Complications of OCs
Side effects

1. Breakthrough bleeding—usually subsides with first two to three cycles of use.
2. Amenorrhea—can change prescription to OC with higher estrogen or lower progestin.

Table 21-1   Relative progestin potency and HDL cholesterol changes

Progestin	Potency
Norethindrone	1
Norethindrone acetate	1
Ethynodiol diacetate	1
Norgestrel	5-10
Levonorgestrel	10-20

3. Breast tenderness—OCs usually decrease fibrocystic breast disease.
4. Chloasma.
5. Acne—often improved but occasionally worsened.
6. Nausea and vomiting—generally subsides within the first two to three cycles. Advise patient to take OC with food or at bedtime.
7. Weight gain—usually only transient gain of several pounds.
8. Depression.
9. Libido change—equal number of patients with increased libido as with decreased libido.

Major complications

1. Thrombosis—a relative risk for all OC users of 2.8 times the nonuser rate. Negligible increased risk in nonsmoking patients who are less than 35 years old and take OC preparations with 35 μg or less of ethinyl estradiol.
2. Myocardial infarction (MI)—actual risk of 1.9/100,000 women per year in 35- to 44-year-old OC users. No increased risk with OC preparations of 50 μg or less of ethinyl estradiol used by women who are less than 35 years old. Relative risk increases in nonsmokers over age 40 and in smokers at age 35. Patients with hyperlipidemia, hypertension, and diabetes are at increased risk for MI.
3. Stroke—relative risk of 3.1 times the nonuser risk rate or 41/100,000 OC users per year. No increased risk in nonsmoking patients who are 35 years old or younger. Smoking is associated with an increase in hemorrhagic stroke. Thrombotic stroke in an OC user is often heralded by migraine headache development.

OCs and oncogenicity

1. Breast cancer—*no* increased risk.
2. Ovarian cancer - 40% *reduction* over nonusers.
3. Endometrial cancer - 50% *reduction* over nonusers.
4. Cervical cancer—no study to date has examined OCs and cervical-cancer risk with controls for age of first coitus, sexual-partner number, and sexually transmitted diseases. When sexual activity differences alone are controlled, there is no significant statistical increase.

OC Management
Absolute contraindications

1. Undiagnosed abnormal genital bleeding
2. Estrogen-dependent cancer (e.g., breast cancer)
3. Known or suspected pregnancy
4. Thromboembolic disorder
5. Hepatic adenoma or acute hepatitis
6. Cerebral vascular disease

Table 21-2   Failure rate during first year of contraceptive use

Method	Lowest Observed Failure Rate (%)	Failure Rate in Typical Users (%)
Injectable progestin	0.25	0.25
Oral contraceptives	0.5	2
IUD	1.5	5
Condom	2	10
Diaphragm (with spermicide)	2	19
Sponge (with spermicide)	9-11	10-20
Foams, creams, jellies, and vaginal suppositories	3-5	18
Withdrawal	16	23
Rhythm	2-20	24
Chance (no method of birth control)	90	90

Relative contraindications

1. Smoker over age 35—many now consider this to be an absolute contraindication because of the known increase in cardiovascular-disease risk
2. Hyperlipidemia
3. Severe migraine history
4. Hypertension
5. Diabetes mellitus
6. Epilepsy
7. Sickle-cell disease—OC increases sickling of red blood cells

Careful evaluation and counseling of patients are required before OC initiation. Currently, many recommend a screening cholesterol and HDL cholesterol evaluation in all patients. A total cholesterol–to–HDL cholesterol ratio of 4.5 or less constitutes a lower risk of atheromatous heart disease.

OCs and Breast-feeding

The American Academy of Pediatrics has approved the use of OCs during breast-feeding. However, OCs can delay and decrease breast-milk production if begun before lactation is well established. Barrier contraceptives remain the best option for breast-feeding women.

BARRIER CONTRACEPTION

Barrier methods of contraception have recently increased in popularity because of the concern over sexually transmitted disease (STD). This is particularly true of condoms, which have a known protective benefit against chlamydia, gonorrhea, herpes, condyloma, and, most significantly, AIDS.

Contraceptive failure rates with all barrier methods depend to a large degree on patient age and consistency of use. Table 21-2 gives contraceptive failure rates in the first year of actual patient use.

INTRAUTERINE DEVICE

The intrauterine device (IUD) is a popular method of contraception, with over 50 million women using them worldwide. Presently, only two IUDs, the Progestasert, containing progesterone, and the Paragard, containing copper, are marketed in the United

States. For monogamous couples, the IUD can be an excellent contraceptive choice. Women need to be carefully screened for IUD usage because of the extensive list of contraindications for its use.

IUD Contraindications
Absolute contraindications

1. Pregnancy
2. Uterine cavity abnormalities
3. Uterine or cervical cancer or an unresolved Pap smear
4. Cervicitis
5. Abnormal genital bleeding of unknown etiology
6. Presence or history of:
   a. Sexually transmitted disease
   b. Pelvic inflammatory disease (PID)
   c. Ectopic pregnancy: IUDs prevent intrauterine pregnancy but do not prevent ectopic pregnancy—IUDs have been associated with an *increased* ectopic-pregnancy risk

Relative contraindications

1. Severe dysmenorrhea—IUDs can increase dysmenorrhea
2. Multiple sexual partners
3. Congenital or valvular heart disease
4. Nulliparity
5. Less than 18 years old

IUD insertion is performed in a sterile manner. The uterus is sounded to determine depth and cavity direction. An IUD is not inserted if the uterus is less than 6.5 cm or greater than 10 cm. After fundal insertion, a string is left projecting 3 cm from the external os. Because of the certainty that the patient will not be pregnant, the last 2 days of menstruation are the best time to insert the IUD. Users of IUDs are instructed to check for the string after each menstrual period. When the tail string is not easily identified by digital self-examination, a visit to the physician is required.

Missing IUD Tail String

1. Pelvic examination to confirm missing tail.
2. Pregnancy test—string can retract into enlarging pregnant uterus. The IUD should always be removed if the tail is present when pregnancy occurs. There is *less* chance of miscarriage if removed than if left in place. There is significant risk of infection, sepsis, septic shock, and/or preterm birth if an IUD cannot be removed during pregnancy.
3. Probe endocervix and uterus if pregnancy is ruled out.
4. Ultrasonography will usually locate the IUD.
5. Anteroposterior and lateral pelvic x-ray evaluation with uterine sound in uterine cavity to help localize IUD position.
6. Hysteroscopy may be required in difficult cases.

The IUD is associated with an increased risk of PID, especially in women with multiple sexual partners or a history of PID. Actinomyces PID is particularly associated with the IUD. Actinomyces on a Pap smear in an IUD user requires treatment with penicillin or ampicillin. IUD removal is recommended whenever PID is present.

STERILIZATION

Sterilization is the most frequently used method of contraception (Fig. 21-1). Approximately 1 million sterilizations are performed each year in the United States. Female

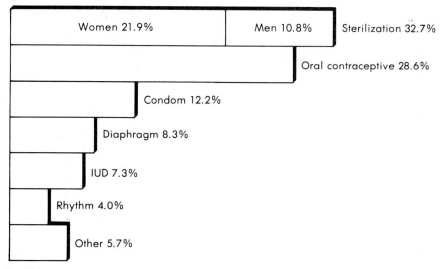

Fig. 21-1
Methods of contraception.

Table 21-3   Sterilization failure rates

Technique	No. of Pregnancies per 100 Women
Laparoscopy	
Ring	0.5
Filshie clip	0.1
Hulka clip	0.7
Unipolar coagulation	0.2
Bipolar coagulation	0.4
Minilaparotomy	
Pomeroy's operation or modified Pomeroy's operation	0.2
Fimbriectomy (Kroener)	0.2
Ring	0.3

sterilization techniques and failure rates are given in Table 21-3.

Women who are not obese and who have had no previous pelvic surgery or PID can be considered for laparoscopic sterilization under local anesthesia.

Sterilization in Men

Vasectomy is safer and less expensive than tubal ligation, albeit slightly less effective. Vasectomy is performed under local anesthesia. Pregnancy rates with vasectomy are less than 1%. Large epidemiologic studies have failed to show increased cardiovascular disease rates in men who have had vasectomies.

REVIEW
QUESTIONS

More than one correct answer is possible.

1. Which of the following are considered absolute contraindications to the use of oral contraceptive pills?
   a. Unexplained vaginal bleeding.
   b. History of hepatitis in the past.
   c. Previous deep venous thrombosis.
   d. Insulin-dependent diabetes.
2. Which of the following statements are true concerning women who are less than 35 years old and use birth control pills containing 35 μg or less of ethinyl estradiol?
   a. No change in ovarian-tumor risk.
   b. No increase in cardiovascular disease–related deaths.
   c. A fourfold increase in deep venous thrombosis.
   d. An approximately 50% decrease in uterine-cancer risk while on the birth control pill.
3. Contraindications for IUD use include:
   a. Documented history of pelvic inflammatory disease.
   b. Documented history of two previous gonorrhea infections without pelvic inflammatory disease.
   c. Cervicitis.
   d. Ventricular septal defect.

True or False

4. There is less chance of miscarriage if an IUD is removed in early pregnancy than if left in place.
5. A nonsmoking woman who is less than 35 years of age who uses a low-dose (less than 50 μg ethinyl estradiol) OC is at no increased risk of stroke or myocardial infarction.
6. Sickle-cell disease is a relative contraindication for OC use.

ANSWERS

1. a, c
2. b, d
3. a, b, c
4. T
5. T
6. T

BIBLIOGRAPHY

American College of Obstetricians and Gynecologists: Sterilization, Tech Bull 113, Washington, DC, 1988, The College.
Edelman DA, Berger GS, and Keith LK: Intrauterine devices and their complications, Boston, 1979, GK Hall & Co.
Massey FJ et al: Vasectomy and health: results from a large cohort study, JAMA 252:1023, 1984.
Ory HW, Forrest JD, and Lincoln R: Making choices—evaluating the health risks and benefits of birth control methods, New York, 1983, Guttmacher Institute.
Paul C, et al: Oral contraceptives and breast cancer: a national study, Br Med J 293:723, 1986.
Realini JP, and Goldzieher JW: Oral contraceptives and cardiovascular disease: a critique of the epidemiologic studies, Am J Obstet Gynecol 152:729, 1985.

Royal College of General Practitioners' oral contraceptive study: Incidence of arterial disease among oral contraceptive users, J R Coll Gen Pract 33:75, 1983.

Soderstrom RM: Sterilization failures and their causes, Am J Obstet Gynecol 152:395, 1985.

Struthers BJ: Pelvic inflammatory disease, intrauterine conception and conduct of epidemiologic studies, Adv Contracept 1:63, 1985.

Vessey MP, Lawless M, and Yeates D: Oral contraceptives and stroke: findings in a large prospective study, Br Med J 289:530, 1984.

Williams NB: Contraceptive technology 1986-1987, New York, 1986, Irvington Publishers.

Sexually Transmitted Diseases 22

Garth Essig

In dealing with patients with sexually transmitted diseases (STDs), one has to keep in mind that more than one disease may be present. The patient may or may not be aware that she has an STD. The treatment of STDs depends on the ability of the physician to diagnose. Since the treatment may be influenced by concurrent conditions, it is essential to have a complete history. For example, pregnancy and allergies to drugs might alter the therapeutic regimen.

GENERAL MANAGEMENT

In the course of management, be sure to ensure the patient's privacy, display a non-judgmental attitude, and be sure to look for a "second disease."
1. History
   a. Illnesses
   b. Allergies
   c. Medications (drugs)
      (1) Routes of use
      (2) Dosage
      (3) Dates of use
   d. Sexual history
   e. Last menstrual period
   f. Review of systems
2. Physical examination—as complete as possible
   a. Inspection
   b. Palpation
3. Laboratory
   a. Tests suggested by history and physical findings
   b. Specimen sites suggested by history and physical findings
      (1) Culture where
      (2) Culture or test for what
   c. a and b above also influenced by physician's index of suspicion

NORMAL VAGINAL ECOLOGY

Maintenance of normal pH is the primary function of the bacterial flora. Acidity can be altered physiologically by alkalinity of the following:
1. Excessive cervical mucus
2. Menses
3. Semen

Table 22-1   Normal vaginal ecology

	Anaerobes	Aerobes
Gram positive	**Cocci**	**Cocci**
	Peptococcus species 30%-64%	Group D streptococcus 34%
	Peptostreptococcus sp. 20%-45%	Group B streptococcus 5%-22%
		Staphylococcus epidermitis 41%-94%
		Staphylococcus aureus 5%
	Rods	**Rods**
	Clostridium sp. 1%-18%	Lactobacilli 50%-88%
	Lactobacillus sp. 10%-45%	Diphtheroids 31%-76%
	Eubacterium sp. 7%-30%	
Gram negative	**Cocci**	**Rods**
	Veillonella sp. 10%-15%	*E. coli* 9%-28%
		Klebsiella 4%
	Rods	*P. mirabilis* 4%
	Bacteroides fragilis 1%-5%	
	Bacteroides sp. 12%-30%	
	Fusobacterium sp. 7%-23%	

pH of Vaginal Secretions

In prepubertal females, the pH of vaginal secretions is normally between 6 and 8. During the reproductive years, the pH of vaginal secretions is normally between 3.5 and 4.5.

Origin of Normal Vaginal Secretion

The vaginal epithelium produces most of the vaginal secretion, predominately exfoliated cells, transudate, and necrobiosis of epithelial cells. The cervix and uterus produce mucus (glycoprotein and H_2O). The vulva contributes minimally to vaginal secretion from skenes, sweat, and sebaceous and Bartholin's glands.

VULVOVAGINITIS

Vulvovaginitis is so named because the symptoms of "vaginitis" (pain, pruritus) are caused by irritation of vulvar structures.

Etiology

Prevalence in 1000 consecutive patients with vulvovaginitis (Gardner) showed the following:
1. Gardnerella: 42.5%
2. Candidiasis: 37.3%
3. Trichomoniasis: 14.2%
4. HSV: 9.4%
5. Condylomata (HPV): 7.2%
6. Others: 3.7%

Signs and Symptoms

1. Increased volume of vaginal discharge
2. pH rise
3. Odor
4. Increased number of WBCs
5. Abnormal microflora

SPECIFIC ORGANISMS
Gardnerella vaginalis

1. Formerly called *hemophilus vaginitis*
2. A leading cause of vaginitis
3. Transmitted by sexual intercourse (one possibility, probably not only way)
4. Pathogenesis
   a. Large quantities of the organism adhere to epithelial cells (clue cells)
   b. Increased desquamation and thinning of epithelium
   c. pH rises (greater than 5) as result of anaerobic metabolism of amino acids (fishy odor)
   d. Facilitates anaerobic growth, may be its most pathogenic function
5. Diagnosis
   a. Smear—clue cells in absence of trichomonas
   b. Culture—Columbia, CNA, and human blood agar
   c. "Whiff test"—10% KOH to smear produces fishy odor
6. Treatment
   a. Metronidazole 2 g single dose *or* 500 mg twice daily for 7 days
   b. Sulfa vaginal cream twice daily for 10 days
   c. Ampicillin 500 mg every 6 hours for 7 days
   d. Tetracycline 500 mg every 6 hours for 7 days

Candidiasis

1. *C. albicans* predominates: 67% of vulvovaginitis cases
2. *Candida* of species found asymptomatically in 10% to 20% of nonpregnant patients and 40% of pregnant patients
3. Symptoms and signs: "curdy" discharge
4. Usually symptomatic just prior to menses: vulvar erythema seen on examination
5. Diagnosis
   a. 10% KOH to "thick" dry smear of vaginal discharge—hyphae seen under low-power microscopy
   b. Selective media: Sabourauds, Nickersons (24 to 48 hours)
6. Treatment (topical or vaginal—cream and/or suppository of Imidazole derivatives)
   a. Miconazole
   b. Clotrimazole
   c. Terconazole
   d. Butaconazole

Trichomoniasis

1. Species and site specific
   a. *T. vaginalis*—"genital"
   b. *T. tenax*—mouth
   c. *T. hominis*—GI tract

2. Pathogenesis
  a. *Trichomonas* organisms attach to epithelial cells and disrupt surface by desquamation—cytotoxins(?), mechanical(?)
  b. Vaginal epithelium thinned
  c. Anaerobes increase in number
  d. pH rises to more than 5
3. Symptoms and signs
  a. Dysuria, pruritus, fishy odor
  b. Erythema, edema, capillary prominence, microhemorrhage
  c. Outpouring of WBCs, amount reflects severity
4. Diagnosis
  a. Saline wet mount (swab saturated with vaginal secretion in normal saline)—*Trichomonas* organisms present, abundant WBCs, clue cells occasionally present
  b. Culture—Diamond, Kupferberg media
  c. Smear is reported to diagnose only 75% of cases
5. Treatment—single dose of metronidazole 2.0 g
  a. Failures occur with low zinc levels and also in presence of phenobarbital and phenytoin
  b. Treat asymptomatic individual also
  c. Clotrimazole cream has some trichomonacidal activity

Herpes Simplex Virus Types I and II (HSV-1, HSV-2)

1. HSV-2 more likely to be the cause of genital lesion but *not* exclusively; HSV-2 more virulent than HSV-1
2. Primary infection
  a. Lesions occur on vulva, vagina, or cervix, or on any combination of these sites associated with systemic symptoms such as fever, malaise
  b. Incubation period: 2 to 7 days
  c. Initial lesions are vesicles that rupture and shallow painful ulcers
  d. Begins lifetime association with the virus
3. Recurrent infection
  a. Lesions fewer in number and confined to one area
  b. Systemic symptoms lacking
  c. May shed virus from cervix without lesions, but titer of virus is significantly lower in this case than if lesions present
4. Clinical differences between primary and recurrent vulvovaginitis (from Monif)

Physical Findings	Primary	Recurrent
Number of lesions	Multiple	Scattered 1 to 3
Location of lesions	Tends to involve both labia and vagina	Limited involvement
Size of lesions	Tend to be larger than recurrent	Smaller than primary
Inguinal adenopathy	Present	Usually absent
Viremia	Occurs	Absent
Systemic symptoms (malaise, fever, etc.)	Present	Absent
Local symptoms (dysuria, pruritus, pain)	Present	Present
Specific antibody titers	Greater than fourfold increase between preinfection and postinfection	Usually no significant change

5. Treatment
   Acyclovir is the only effective treatment to date

Condyloma Acuminata (Human Papilloma Virus [HPV]):

Papova family of intranuclearly replicating DNA virus
1. In 1984, known HPV types numbered only 16; by the end of 1986, 41 types had been identified.
2. Condyloma acuminatum (venereal warts) types 6, 11.
3. Cervical dysplasia or intracellular neoplasia associated with HPV.
4. More than one type of HPV can cause a given lesion, and types may be grouped according to tissue tropism. For example, types 6, 11, 16, 18, and 31 are found not uncommonly together in external genital warts.
5. Evidence continues to mount implicating HPV as a carcinogen, or at least a cocarcinogen, in cancer of the cervix.
6. Typing of HPV cervical lesions, especially, is important to treatment and follow-up. Kits to do this are becoming available.
7. Treatment
   a. Podophyllin
   b. Trichloro-acetic acid
   c. 5-Fluorouracil
   d. Interferon injection into the lesion
   e. Excision
   f. Hot cautery
   g. Cryocautery
   h. Laser vaporization
   i. Autogenous vaccine

Chlamydia Trachomatis

1. Pathogenesis
   a. Gram-negative, intracellular parasites
   b. Infect metaplastic or columnar epithelium
   c. Elementary body attaches to lost cell and is phagocytized
   d. Multiplication occurs, host cell bursts, releasing more elementary bodies
   e. *Does not cause vaginitis* but does cause urethritis, cervicitis, and salpingitis in female
   f. Not uncommonly found in women who are *N. gonorrhea* positive
   g. Latency has been recognized in chlamydial infections (asymptomatic carriers) as common
   h. One of the causes of upper genital tract infection and infertility
2. Diagnosis
   a. Cytology identification of elementary bodies
   b. Culture—expensive, requires tissue culture but is definitive
   c. Non-culture tests such as monoclonal antibody tests (i.e., Chlamydazyme, Microtrak) are cheaper, 98% reliable
3. Treatment
   a. Doxycycline 100 mg twice daily for 7 days—first choice except in pregnancy
   b. Tetracycline 500 mg four times daily 7 days
   c. Erythromycin 250 mg four times daily 7 to 10 days

STD MANIFESTATIONS AND POSSIBLE ETIOLOGIES

Attempting to outline the possible STDs by anatomic location does not mean that a disease is confined to that area (i.e., the primary lesion of syphilis may occur on the face). The following cutaneous lesions can occur any place on the body.

1. Rash
   a. Syphilis, secondary (usually generalized)
   b. Mycotic–usually localized (candidiasis)
   c. Parasitic
      (1) Scabies
      (2) Crab louse
2. Ulcers
   a. Syphilis, primary (chancre)
   b. Herpes simplex (HSV)
   c. Chancroid (hemophilus ducrey)
   d. Lymphogranuloma venereum
   e. Donovanosis
3. Bumps
   a. Syphilis (condyloma lata)
   b. Condyloma acuminatum (HPV—human papilloma virus)
   c. Molluscum contagiosum
4. Lymphadenopathy—local and generalized
   a. AIDS (Acquired immune deficiency syndrome)
   b. Lymphogranuloma venereum
   c. Donovanosis
   d. Chancroid
   e. Herpes simplex—primary infection

Symptoms and Signs of STD by Anatomic Locations

Tables 22-2 through 22-7 describe the signs and symptoms of STDs in various anatomic locations.

PID (PELVIC INFLAMMATORY DISEASE)

Dr. Giles Monif refers to PID as standing for "pretty inadequate diagnosis." Because this term encompasses so much, it is best to be more precise in diagnosis. This not only aids in **establishing treatment goals,** but in prognosticating as well.

Better terms are endometritis-salpingitis (ES) and endometritis-salpingitis-peritonitis (ESP). Consider the following descriptions using gonorrhea as an example.

ES—Gonococcus ascends into the endometrial cavity and begins to involve the fallopian tubes (salpingitis).

ESP—The infectious process continues throughout the tubes and finally involves the peritoneum.

Table 22-2   Symptoms and signs of STDs in vulva.

Symptoms	Signs	Etiology
Pruritus Pain Discharge Bumps	Erythema Edema Rash	Mycotic (candidiasis) *Trichomonas* organisms
	Rash	Syphilis (secondary) Scabies Crab louse
	Ulcers	Herpes simplex (HSV) Syphilis (primary) Chancroid *Lymphogranuloma venereum* Donovanosis
	Bumps	*Condyloma acuminatum* (HPV) *Molluscum contagiosum* Syphilis, secondary *(Condyloma lata)*

Table 22-3   Symptoms and signs of STDs in vagina.

Symptoms	Signs	Etiology
Discharge Pain Dyspareunia Dysuria Bleeding Fever	Discharge Profuse Odorous (?) Abnormal flora	*Trichomonas* organisms *Gardnerella* organisms Mycotic (candidiasis) Chlamydia *N. gonorrhea*
	Plaque	Mycotic
	Erythema	*Trichomonas* organisms Mycotic (candidiasis) *Gardnerella* organisms
	Ulcer	Primary syphilis herpes simplex (HSV)
	Bumps	*Condyloma acuminatum* (HPV) *Condyloma lata* (secondary syphilis)

Table 22-4   Symptoms and signs of STDs in cervix.

Symptoms	Signs	Etiology
Pain: dysparunia Increased vaginal discharge Postcoital spotting Fever	Ulceration	Herpes simplex (HSV) Syphilis (1°)
	Abnormal Pap smear	Condyloma organisms (HPV) Herpes simplex (HSV)
	Warts	Condyloma organisms (HPV)

	Discharge from cervix:
	  Purulent
	  Mucopurulent
		Gonococcus
		Chlamydia

	Fever Leukocytosis Manipulation pain Elevated sedimentation rate Elevated pulse rate	Tubal Peritoneal involvement

Table 22-5   Symptoms and signs of STDs in uterus.

Symptoms	Signs	Etiology

Pain
Fever
Increased vaginal discharge
Dyspareunia
	Manipulation pain
	Discharge from cervix:
	  Purulent
	  Mucopurulent
	Fever
	Leukocytosis
	Elevated (sedimentation
	  rate)
	Elevated pulse rate
		N. gonorrhea
		Chlamydia organisms
		N. meningitis
		Group A beta-hemolytic
		  strepococcus
		Anaerobes

Table 22-6   Symptoms and signs of STDs in tubes.

Symptoms	Signs	Etiology
Pain Bloating Fever Nausea Vomiting	Peritoneal signs Rebound tenderness Abdominal distension Ileus Fever Elevated pulse rate Leukocytosis Elevated ESR Pelvic mass	Anaerobes Gonococcus Chlamydia N. meningitis Group A beta-hemolytic strepo- coccus

Table 22-7   Symptoms and signs of STDs in ovaries.

Symptoms	Signs	Etiology
Pain	Peritoneal signs	Anaerobes
Bloating	Abdominal distension	Gonococcus
Fever	Ileus	*Chlamydia* organisms
Nausea	Fever	*N. meningitis*
Vomiting	Elevated pulse rate	Group A beta-hemolytic strepo-
	Elevated ESR	coccus
	Leukocytosis	
	Pelvic mass	
	Hypotensive	

Pathogenesis of Infection

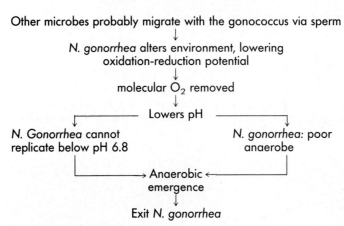

Other microbes probably migrate with the gonococcus via sperm

↓

N. gonorrhea alters environment, lowering oxidation-reduction potential

↓

molecular O_2 removed

↓

Lowers pH

N. Gonorrhea cannot replicate below pH 6.8   *N. gonorrhea*: poor anaerobe

→ Anaerobic ← emergence

↓

Exit *N. gonorrhea*

The same scenario can also be created by:
1. Group A beta-hemolytic streptococcus
2. *N. meningitis*
3. *Chlamydia trachomatous*

The therapeutic principle to keep in mind is that the above organisms, although pathogenic themselves, are facilitators to anaerobic infections. The longer the infection is present, the greater is the likelihood of anaerobic involvement. The likelihood of polymicrobial infection is so high that the therapy also must be polymicrobial. Because of the predominance of anaerobes in the vagina, one must never ignore the possibility of anaerobic involvement.

Diagnosis of E.S. and E.S.P.

1. Usually suggested by history
2. Physical findings
   a. Purulent endocervical discharge
   b. Pain on manipulation of cervix and uterus
   c. Fever
   d. Peritoneal signs
   (Clinical findings not constant)

3. Laboratory findings and studies
   a. Leukocytosis
   b. Elevated sedimentation rate
   c. Endocervical culture
      (1) *Neisseria* organisms—Thayer-Martin media
      (2) Anaerobes—culture not very helpful
      (3) *Chlamydia* organisms—culture; tests—MicroTrak, Chlamydazyme, etc.
   d. Culdocentesis
      (1) Contraindicated if mass in cul-de-sac or uterus retrodisplaced
      (2) Do if peritoneal signs present
      (3) Consider not doing if cannot culture for anaerobes
      (4) Prognosis is good if culdocentesis is negative for purulent material
   e. Laparoscopy—usually not necessary
   f. Serial pelvic ultrasound examinations

Therapeutic Staging and Treatment (After Monif)

1. Stage I: ES

Goal	Treatment
1. Eradicate infection 2. Prevent progression	1. Ampicillin 3.5 g and probenecid 1 g by mouth 2. Amoxicillin 3.0 g and probenecid 1 g by mouth 3. Procaine penicillin IM 4.8 million units plus probenecid 1 g by mouth 4. *Follow* with tetracycline 0.5 mg four times daily for 10 days *or* doxycycline 100 mg twice daily for 10 days. NOTE: Do not give to pregnant patients and those with group A streptococcus

2. Stage II: ESP

Goal	Treatment
Preserve structure and function of tube	1. Cefoxitin 2gm I.V. initially then 1-2gm q6 hours plus 2. Doxycycline 100 mg I.V. q12h until improvement, then 100 mg p.o. bid for 10 days (contraindicated in pregnancy and group A streptococcus)

3. Stage III: ESP plus tubo-ovarian complex

Goal	Treatment
Preserve ovaries	Triple antibiotics 1. Penicillin IV 5 million units every 4 hours 2. Clindamycin IV 600 mg every 4 hours until response, then 450 mg by mouth every 6 hours to complete 10 days of therapy 3. Aminoglycoside—tobramycin or gentamicin according to drug nomogram for 48 to 72 hours; watch for renal toxicity 4. Follow this with 10 days of tetracycline or doxycycline doxycycline 100 mg twice daily by mouth. Tetracycline or doxycycline 0.5 g four times daily, especially if culture or tests are positive for chlamydia

4. Stage IV: Rupture of tubo-ovarian complex
   (NOTE: Rupture is more common on the left side; ovary usually is site of rupture; once ovary is involved, risk of septic thrombophlebitis increases)

Goal	Treatment
Preserve life	1. *Antibiotics:* triple therapy, consider adding IV metronidazole 2. Compulsive IV fluid management; correct electrolyte imbalance; blood transfusion 3. Monitor central venous pressure 4. Consider infectious disease, consult 5. n-g suction 6. Intake and output 7. Minidose heparinization 8. See below

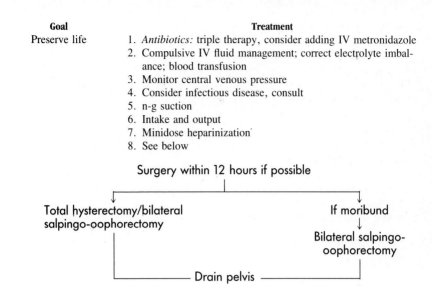

Surgery within 12 hours if possible

Total hysterectomy/bilateral salpingo-oophorectomy

If moribund

Bilateral salpingo-oophorectomy

Drain pelvis

ACQUIRED IMMUNE DEFICIENCY SYNDROME (AIDS)

The AIDS virus first infected humans 15 to 20 years ago (that is known from serologic testing). Before that time, the infection, if present, was not recognized. There is some evidence that the human immunodeficiency virus (HIV) that causes AIDS may have first caused the disease in central Africa before it was found elsewhere. One intriguing possibility is that this virus is a new pathogen.

It is a retrovirus, so named because of the unique enzyme it possesses called reverse transcriptase. This allows DNA to be transcribed from RNA, thus invading the lymphocyte—usually the human T4 "helper" lymphocyte—and imprints itself into the genome of the lymphocyte. The infected lymphocyte then begins to manufacture HIV virus. Since the T4 helper lymphocyte is the main organizer of the immune response, its impairment causes inability to respond to life-threatening infections and malignancies. The incidence of AIDS is increased in areas where ulcerative STDs (i.e., herpes, syphilis) are more prevalent. Breaks in the integument simply increase the risk of acquiring HIV infection.

Nomenclature

Original names of the retrovirus include the following:
1. Human T lymphotropic virus type III (HTLV-III)
2. Lymphadenopathy associated virus (LAV)
3. AIDS-related/associated virus (ARV)

The current and accepted term is human immunodeficiency virus (HIV). There have been 2 strains identified: HIV-I, and HIV-II.

Human Retroviruses*

1. Oncovirinae (RVA tumor virus group)
   HTLV-I
   HTLV-II—Human T-cell leukemia
   HTLV-V

*After "Basic Biology of HIV" in *Contemporary OB/Gyn*, 9/88

2. Spumavirinae (foamy virus group)—Human foamy virus
3. Lentivirinae (slow virus group)
   a. HIV-I (also HTLV-III, LAV-I, ARV)
   b. HIV-II (also HTLV-IV, LAV-2)

Transmission of the Virus

1. Sexual intercourse
   a. Anal
   b. Vaginal
2. Contaminated needles
   a. IV drug users
   b. Needle stick injuries
   c. Injections
3. Mother to child
   a. In utero
   b. At birth
   c. Breast milk and other secretions
4. Organ/tissue donation
   a. Semen
   b. Kidneys
   c. Skin, bone marrow, corneas, etc.

HIV in Body Fluids

Isolated	Implicated in Disease Transmission
Amniotic fluid	Blood
Blood	Breast milk
Breast milk	Semen
Cerebrospinal fluid	Vaginal secretions
Saliva	
Semen	
Tears	
Urine	
Vaginal secretions	

Natural History of HIV Infection

From the beginning of infection, there is gradual depletion in T4 helper lymphocytes. The immune response becomes increasingly impaired. Patients finally show anergy to skin testing that they had previously been reactive to.

Infection
↓
Persistent generalized lymphadenopathy (PGL)
↓
AIDS-related complex (ARC)
↓
AIDS

Common Causes of Persistent Generalized Lymphadenopathy

Condition	Diagnostic Tests
Infections	
Bacterial	Culture
Syphilis	Serologic tests
Brucellosis	Serologic tests
Viral	
Infectious mononucleosis	Paul-Bunnell
(Epstein-Barr virus)	
Cytomegalovirus	CMV cultures or antibody
Hepatitis B	Serology
Hepatitis A	Serology
Rubella	Serology
Parasites	
Toxoplasmosis	Serology
Tumors	
Lymphomas	Biopsy of lymph node
Leukemias	Bone marrow

AIDS-RELATED COMPLEX (ARC)

ARC is diagnosed in a patient who presents with any two or more signs or symptoms that have been present 3 months or longer and any two or more abnormal laboratory values.

Signs and Symptoms

1. Fever (temperature 38° C or greater)—intermittent or continuous
2. Weight loss: 10% or more
3. Lymph nodes: PGL
4. Diarrhea: intermittent or continuous
5. Fatigue that reduces physical activity
6. Night sweats

Laboratory Abnormalities

1. Lymphopenia, leukopenia
2. Thrombocytopenia
3. Anemia
4. Reduced ratio CD4 lymphocytes: CD8 lymphocytes (greater than 2 SD)
5. Reduced T-helper cells (greater than 2 SD)
6. Reduced blastogenesis in bone marrow
7. Raised gamma globulin
8. Cutaneous anergy

AIDS

Not everyone infected with HIV has developed AIDS. However, the longer the time of seroconversion, the greater the chance of progression to AIDS. The incubation period for this to happen is usually reported as from 2 to 5 years, as the T4 lymphocytes decline. It is not known what triggers the HIV from latency to activity.

The two main clinical manifestations of AIDS are tumors and opportunistic infections. Most patients in the United States present with *Pneumocystis carinii* pneumonia (64%), other opportunistic infections (22%), and Kaposi's sarcoma.

Laboratory Detection of HIV

1. Indirect methods
   a. Antibody
      (1) Enzyme-linked immunosorbent assay (ELISA)
      (2) Immunofluorescence assay (IFA)
      (3) Western blot immunopheresis
   b. Antigen
      (1) Capture ELISA
2. Direct methods
   a. Blot hybridization
   b. Fluorescent immunolabeling
   c. In situ hybridization
   d. Tissue culture

The test most used at this time for screening is an ELISA test, which detects antibodies to HIV core protein. Although the test is sensitive, it does have some slight false reactivity. Because of the gravity of a positive HIV test, the western blot (immunopheresis) test is used for confirmation with a proscribed reaction to multiple viral proteins, rather than only one, as in the case of the ELISA test.

Prevention

1. Do not share needles
2. Practice safe sex (risk increases with multiple partners)
3. No risk
   a. Solo masturbation
   b. Celibacy
4. Low risk
   a. Mutual masturbation
   b. "Dry" kissing
   c. Body rubbing
5. Medium risk
   a. Wet kissing
   b. Fellatio
   c. Anilingus
6. High risk
   a. Anal and vaginal sex (*may* be safe if rubber condom used)
   b. Fisting (insertion of hand or fist into rectum)
   c. Sharing sex toys
   d. Any sex that draws blood

Projections

Future course of the epidemic as estimated by the Public Health Services (1986) is as follows:

1. By the end of 1991, there will be more than 270,000 cases of AIDS, with more than 74,000 of those occurring in 1991 alone.
2. By the end of 1991, there will have been more than 179,000 deaths from AIDS, with 54,000 of those occurring in 1991 alone.
3. The vast majority of AIDS cases will continue to come from the currently recognized high-risk groups.
4. New AIDS cases in men and women acquired through heterosexual contact will increase from 1100 in 1986 to almost 7000 in 1991.
5. Pediatric AIDS cases will increase almost tenfold in the next 5 years, to more than 3000 cumulative by the end of 1991.

Health care providers must understand that there is a small but definite risk in caring for HIV-infected patients, particularly the AIDS patients. But, that risk can be essentially negated if universal precautions are observed in caring for *all* patients. The most dangerous patient is the undiagnosed HIV-infected individual. Mistakes in technique have already been fatal to health care workers. Printed below is a modified *universal precaution protocol* from the Centers for Disease Control (courtesy Fahey, Meeham and Henderson).

Universal Precautions to Prevent
Occupational/Nosocomial Transmission of HIV-1

- Hands should be washed before and after patient contact and after removing gloves
- Gloves are indicated when soiling of hands with blood or body fluids is likely (e.g., venipuncture)
- Masks and protective eyewear are not generally indicated but are necessary when performing procedures during which splashing or spraying of blood or body fluids is likely
- Masks and protective eyewear are not generally indicated but may be advisable for patients with undiagnosed pulmonary disease who are coughing, or for patients being treated with mechanical positive pressure who have copious or blood-streaked secretions
- Gowns are generally not indicated but should be worn if clothing is likely to be soiled with blood or body fluids
- Food service should be provided in regular tray service and served by hospital's usual food servers
- Private room is not usually indicated unless patient is too ill to use good hygiene or has another infection for which private room is indicated
- Articles contaminated with blood or body fluids should be bagged with isolation labels for decontamination and reprocessing
- Needles and syringes must be handled cautiously; used needles must not be recapped and must be placed in puncture-resistant container designated for this purpose
- Spills of blood or body fluids should be cleaned with dilute solution of sodium hypochlorite (bleach) and water; bleach solution should be no older than 24 hours

---

From Fahey et al.

REVIEW QUESTIONS

1. In normal vaginal ecology, the most predominant category of organism is:
   a. Aerobes
   b. Microaerophilic aerobes
   c. Anaerobes
   d. Microaerophilic anaerobes
   e. CMV
2. In treating acute salpingitis, it is best to treat as:
   a. Caused purely by *N. gonorrhea*
   b. Caused purely by *C. trachomatous*
   c. Caused purely by anaerobes
   d. Caused purely by aerobes
   e. Caused by polymicrobial infection

Both HSV-1 and HSV-2 can produce genital lesions. The primary infection is usually followed by recurrent infections which differ in the following way. (Match)

3. _____ Lesions smaller   a. Primary
4. _____ Viremia   b. Recurrent
5. _____ Systemic symptoms   c. None
6. _____ No significant antibody Titer change
7. _____ Large number of lesions
8. The human papilloma virus:
   a. Has been associated with abnormal Pap smears.
   b. May be a cause of chlamydia infections.
   c. Is found only in nonhuman mammals.
   d. Is a cause of AIDS.
   e. None of the above.
9. The human immunodeficiency virus (HIV) in infected persons has been found in essentially all body fluids, however, to date has been implicated in disease transmission in all except one of the following.
   a. Blood
   b. Saliva
   c. Breast milk
   d. Semen
   e. Vaginal secretions
10. The two main clinical manifestations of AIDS are tumors and infections. The most common presenting illness in the United States is:
    a. Kaposi's sarcoma
    b. Thrush
    c. PGL
    d. *Pneumocystis carnii* pneumonia
    e. CMV

ANSWERS

1. c.
2. e.
3. b.
4. a.
5. a.

6. b.
7. a.
8. a.
9. b.
10. d.

BIBLIOGRAPHY

Adler MW: ABC of AIDS, London, 1988, British Medical Journal.
Centers for Disease Control: STD treatment guidelines MMWR 34(45):1985.
Centers for Disease Control: Recommendations for prevention of HIV transmission in health care settings, MMWR 36(25):15-183, 1987.
Confronting AIDS, Directions for Public Health Care and Research, Washington, DC, 1986, National Academy Press.
Fahey BJ, Meehan PE, and Henderson DK: Infect Surg April 1988.
JAMA 255(13): April 4, 1986.
Monif GRG: Infectious diseases in obstetrics and gynecology, Philadelphia, 1982, Harper & Row, Publishers, Inc.
Reeve P: Clamydial infections, New York, 1987, Springer-Verlag, New York, Inc.
Science of AIDS, Sci Am October, 1988.

Vulvovaginitis

Frederick P. Zuspan

Infections in the lower female genital tract are some of the most common complications that a woman faces. The female genital tract—the vagina, cervix, uterus, and tubes—provides an ascending route for infection to the peritoneal cavity. Fortunately, there are natural barriers to infection in the genital tract, including the following:

1. The physical apposition of the vaginal walls in the perineum.
2. A low pH or vaginal acidity in the sexually mature female. This low pH acts to resist bacterial invaders.
3. Cervical mucus, which acts as a barrier to ascending infection.

Susceptibility to infection in the vagina is proportional to thickness of vaginal epithelium, the amount of glycogen present, the number of lactobacilli present, and acidity or pH (Table 23-1).

The presence or absence of symptoms in the vulvovaginal-cervical area is related to the nerve supply to these particular structures. The cervix can be cauterized and biopsied with minimal discomfort, whereas dilation of the cervix creates severe pain. The vagina can easily house a diaphragm or pessary with no discomfort to the patient because it contains relatively few nerve endings. On the other hand, the vulva has many nerve endings, so a patient with vulvitis is most likely to be symptomatic. A patient with cervicitis or pure vaginitis, because of the less abundant nerve supply to these structures, is usually asymptomatic except for leukorrhea. Because of the variation in sensory nerve supply to the vagina, cervix, and vulva, pathogenic conditions or organisms found in an asymptomatic patient should be treated.

DIAGNOSTIC TOOLS

Discussions of the most commonly used tools to diagnose vulvovaginitis follow.

pH Paper

pH paper is an excellent screening tool that should be used at each gynecologic examination. If the pH is less than 4.5, it is unlikely that a vaginal infection exists.

Table 23-1 Susceptibility to vaginal infections

Age	Vaginal Epithelium	Glycogen	Lactobacilli	pH
Newborn	Max. thickness	Present	Few	Alkaline
1 month	Min. thickness	Absent	Very few	Alkaline
Prepuberty	Min. thickness	Absent	Very few	Alkaline
Puberty	Thickened	Present	Plentiful	Acid
Pregnancy	Thickened	Highest	Most plentiful	Acid
Post-menopausal	Thin	Absent	Very few	Alkaline

Saline Wet Prep

All patients who complain of vulvovaginal infections should have a saline wet prep. Safranin dye 1% will identify and show clue cells, bacteria, and other organisms easily. These take the slightly red stain and are therefore easy to identify. One drop of this solution is mixed on the slide with the wet prep solution. Additionally, potassium hydroxide is added to another portion of the slide or on another slide to the wet prep solution, and the odor is noted. If putrescine is emitted, the presence of *gardnerella vaginalis* is suspected. The potassium hydroxide lyses cells and facilitates the diagnosis of candidiasis by demonstrating hyphae and yeast buds.

Additional Microscopic Examination

The microscopic examination should also include a check for the presence or absence of normal Döderlein's bacilli and the amount of the bacteria present. A high pH reading (i.e., above 5.0) is often associated with an absence of or a decrease of Döderlein's bacilli. Additionally, the degree of estrogenation of vaginal cells is evaluated to determine whether or not they are cornified or that basal cells are present. Dysplasia can also be detected by this method by recognizing abnormal nuclei in vaginal and cervical cells.

Visual Inspection

Visual inspection is probably the most common diagnostic method. The findings from visual inspection should alert the physician to utilize other techniques i.e., pH and saline wet prep. Diagnosis on visual inspection can often be made more likely than for herpes, condyloma, and yeast.

Colposcopy

Colposcopy is an essential procedure in confirming a diagnosis of condyloma acuminata of the cervix and dysplasia. The aceto-white reaction that appears on the cervix after the application of acetic acid is diagnostic, and diagnosis can then be confirmed by a pathologist by examining biopsy specimens by identifying the koilocytosis.

SPECIFIC VULVOVAGINAL-CERVICAL INFECTIONS

The infections of the lower genital tract may be asymptomatic or associated with increased leukorrhea, an odor to the secretions of the vagina, pruritus, and swelling or redness of the vulva. When these signs or symptoms are elicited in the history and physical examination, suspect lower genital tract infections that are commonly the cause of these signs and symptoms. However, remember that the patient with an infection of the lower genital tract may have no symptoms. It is unusual for a patient to have isolated vulvitis without associated vaginitis; exceptions to this statement include the presence of *candida sp., herpes sp., and condyloma acuminata.*

Table 23-2 enumerates the signs and symptoms and associates each with the specific lower genital tract disease.

A strip of pH paper can be touched to the lower third of the vagina and used as a screening test to see whether or not abnormal pathogens are present in the vagina. The low pH of 3.5 to 4.5 normally seen in the vagina identifies the presence of an adequate amount of lactobacillus, which produce organic acids to maintain this pH. It is unlikely that a vaginal infection exists if the pH is in the normal acid range.

Table 23-2   Vulva and vagina

Organism	Redness	Pruritus	Swelling	Pain	Fishy Odor	Leukorrhea	pH
Candida	+	+	±	0	0	Cottage cheese	5.0-6.5
Trichomonas	0	+	−	0	0	Frothy	5.8-6.3
Gardnerella vaginalis	0	0	0	0	+	± to +	5.0-5.8
Chlamydia	0	0	0	0	0	0	3.5-5.0
Herpes	±	0	±	+	0	0	3.5-4.5
Condyloma acuminatum	0	0	±	0	0	0	3.5-5.0

The normal pH is 3.5 to 4.5 after puberty and before menopause.

Candidiasis

What to look for and think about

1. Itching vulva.
2. Burning and red vulva; may have dysuria.
3. Discharge most often cottage cheese–like and thick.
4. Peeling of discharge from vagina may cause punctate hemorrhage.
5. Candidiasis is the most common lower vaginal tract infection in the pregnant female (10%).
6. Think of diabetes if recurrent.
7. Reinfection most likely comes from the gastrointestinal tract; Cultures of rectal swabs are usually positive for candida.
8. Pregnancy is associated with recurrent *Candida* infection since there is a higher glycogen content in vaginal cells. The receptors in cytosol of *Candida* are for estrogen and progesterone, which stimulate proliferation and influence vaginal cell adherence. Symptomatic *Candida* vulvovaginitis is present in at least 10% of pregnant women.
9. Oral contraceptives, especially those high in estrogens, promote colonization of *Candida*.
10. Antibiotic therapy, especially with tetracyclines, ampicillin and cephalosphorines, promotes a carriage rate of 10% to 30% 2 to 3 weeks after therapy. They appreciably decrease the lactobacillus count.
11. Immunocompromised or suppressed patients are prone to develop *Candida* infections.

What to do

Diagnosis should made by culture (Nickerson's media), but more simply can be made by saline wet prep identifying pseudohyphae and buds after a drop of KOH on the slide to lyse cells. The pH of the vagina is usually 5.5 to 6.5.

Acute vulvitis can be handled by swabbing the vagina with saline or betadine and then painting the vulva and vagina with aqueous gentian violet (1%) for immediate relief.

Clotrimazole vaginal tablets 500 mg can be inserted once with a cure rate of better than 80% (Table 23-3). Other forms of therapy include use of miconazole nitrate (Monistat Dual Pack with cream and 3-day suppository). Nystatin (Mycostatin) vaginal suppositories may be used once at bedtime for 14 nights.

Candida infections are easy to treat, but the relapse rate approached 25% in one study (Table 23-4).

Table 23-3 Clotrimazole

	500 mg Single	100 mg × 6 Days
Wet film neg. 1 week	93%	92%
Culture neg. 1 week	89%	85%
Wet film neg. 4 weeks	83%	87%
Culture neg. 4 weeks	82%	85%

In case of recurrent vulvovaginitis, consider the possibility of diabetes and obtain a formal glucose tolerance test after 3 days of carbohydrate loading.

If the male partner is affected, clotrimazole cream 1% can be used; the patient may also find this helpful in relieving her symptomatic vulvitis.

Recalcitrant *Candida* (now called *Candida*-related complex, or CRC)

In cases of recalcitrant candida, most likely the reinfection is coming from the gastrointestinal tract. An antiyeast (low carbohydrate) diet is now available and should be implemented along with long-term high dose oral Nystatin therapy. This regimen utilizes two Nystatin tablets qid for 7 days, then three tablets qid for 7 days, then four tablets qid for 7 days, and finally two tablets qid for 2 months. These patients have oral candidiasis in 30% of cases and rectal candidiasis in almost 100% of cases prior to this long-term therapy. Use of an antiyeast diet is essential to help prevent recurrences.

Trichomoniasis
What to look for

The patient with trichomoniasis may have no symptoms, but most often there is some pruritus. The vulva may be inflamed, and there may be a burning sensation. Often there is a frothy, nonodorous discharge. The urethra may also be involved with associated kidney-upper bladder (KUB) symptoms. Petechiae are seen on the cervix in 25% to 30% of cases.

What to do

Make a specific diagnosis by a saline wet smear of vaginal secretions, identifying a motile parasite with flagelli. The pH of the vagina is usually between 5.8 and 6.3.

Therapy is aimed at both the male and female, utilizing metronidazole 250 mg tablets to be taken 3 times a day for 10 days for each person. An alternate means of therapy would be to give 2 g of metronidazole at one time and then repeating this in 14 days for both the male and female. Single-dose therapy results in 78% cure rate, whereas 7-day therapy results in an 88% cure rate. However, more gastrointestinal symptoms are seen with high-dose therapy.

Haemophilus Vaginalis
What to look for

This may well be the most common vaginal infection. The major complaint is a foul, fishy odor from the vagina. There may also be a frothy grey leukorrhea.

What to do

Make a specific diagnosis using a saline wet prep and look for "clue bodies." A drop of potassium hydroxide on the slide will emit a putrescine odor and result in a positive

Table 23-4 Treatment of *Candida*

Drug	Treatment Regimen	Relapse Rate (at 35 days)
Nystatin	Two pessaries per night for 15 nights	25%
Amphotericin B	One pessary per night for 15 nights	24%
Nystatin	One pessary per night for 6 nights	29%
Nystatin	Two pessaries per night for 15 nights plus oral four times day for 10 days	24%
Amphotericin B	One pessary per night for 15 nights plus oral nystatin	21%
Liconazole		25%
Econazole		25%
Clotrimazole	500 mg single	26%
Isoconazole	Two 300 mg tablets	22%

Table 23-5 Other forms of therapy for *haemophilus vaginalis* infections

Therapy	Dose
Metronidazole	500 mg bid for 7 days
Ampicillin	500 mg qid for 7 days
Amoxicillin	500 mg qid for 7 days
Cephradine	500 mg qid for 7 days

sniff test. A culture can be done, but this is usually not necessary. The pH of the vagina is somewhere between 5.0 and 5.8.

Therapy is for both male and female using metronidazole 2 g (four 500 mg tablets) at one time and then repeating this regimen 14 days later (Table 23-5). Additionally, Triple Sulfa Cream may be used for a period of 10 days, using an applicator-full at bedtime. Recurrence is common, and treatment should be repeated.

An alternate treatment would be to use ampicillin 250 mg four times a day for 10 days. The disadvantage of this therapy is that the ampicillin usually eliminates the normal flora of the vagina (i.e., lactobacillus), and the overgrowth of the vagina may then be *Candida sp*. Hence, if ampicillin or another broad-spectrum antibiotic is used, nystatin (Mycostatin) vaginal suppositories should be used during therapy for at least 5 days later at bedtime.

Chlamydia
What to look for

Chlamydial infections should be suspected if the patient complains of lower abdominal discomfort and has a history of a sexual partner with chlamydial infection. Diagnosis can be made by cultures of the cervix (Table 23-6). Suspicion of a chlamydial infection may first be identified on a Pap smear, with a culture then done to confirm the

Table 23-6   Identification of *Chlamydia*

Test	Sensitivity (%)	Specificity (%)	Positive predictive value (%)	Negative predictive value (%)
Papanicolaou	54	71	33	85
Immunofluorescent stain smears	94	99	98	98
Immunofluorescent stain spec.	92	99	98	98

diagnosis. A green, purulent discharge from the cervix (not the vagina) may be the only symptom.

What to do

Chlamydial infections respond to oral tetracycline or doxycycline therapy for 10 days of therapy. Erythromycin may be used for pregnant patients since both of the above are contraindicated after 12 weeks of gestation.

Herpes virus Type II
What to look for

Painful vesicles on the vulva or cervix usually appear 3 to 10 days after exposure. The vesicles may be filled with clear fluid, but once opened they become secondarily infected and lose that appearance.

Herpes Simplex Type I or II

Etiology

Incubation period: 3 to 10 days
Viral shedding: lasts 1 to 2 weeks
   25% infections are type I
   75% infections are type II
Recurrence: 50% of cases

Identification

Tissue culture using primary rabbit kidney cells sensitive only to herpes virus.
   40% positive in 24 hours
   82% positive at 48 hours
   15% positive after 48 hours
   Cultureset—sensitivities of 6% to 72% compared with culture

What to do

Make a positive diagnosis by viral culture; the results should be returned between 24 and 48 hours. Serologic confirmation is of limited value because a positive titer may be present if an infection has been present in the past. A Pap smear will show intranuclear inclusions; however, the Pap smear may only suggest herpes virus infection and is not diagnostic.

Until the advent of acyclovir, various forms of therapy were used without much benefit except for treating secondary infection. Acyclovir ointment should be used for a period of 5 to 7 days, with the patient applying the ointment 7 times per day. Recurrence is less likely if the diagnosis is made on first infection and acyclovir ointment is used. In severe and more generalized infections, oral acyclovir may be needed; therapy is for 10 to 14 days (250 mg qid). There may be associated adenopathy, and in severe cases this may create enough problems for the patient that a Foley catheter is necessary.

The patient is contagious in the 24 to 36 hours before the outbreak of the vesicles and for the first several days the vesicles are present. Corticoid therapy is contraindicated.

For the pregnant patient, once a positive culture is obtained, cultures should be done on a weekly basis after 34 weeks of gestation to determine whether or not there is infection of the vulva and vagina. If infection is present within 7 days of the expected date of onset of labor, a cesarean section is usually done.

Condyloma Acuminatum
What to look for

Diagnosis of condyloma acumination is made by gross inspection of a wartlike projection on the vulva, vagina, or cervix. If doubt exists, a biopsy is appropriate. The patient usually discovers the lesion herself and seeks help.

What to do

The extent of the lesion dictates therapy. If less than 6 condyloma are present on the vulva, treatment in the absence of pregnancy is usually application of podophyllin (25%) in tincture of benzoin solution. This is applied on a weekly basis, and often after several applications the condyloma regress.

An alternate form of therapy is use of trichloroacetic acid. The advantage of this therapy is that the patient can treat herself two to three times a week; however, it is painful on the vulva. Trichloroacetic acid therapy can be used if the patient is pregnant.

If the patient has extensive condyloma, consider hospitalization and electrocautery or laser therapy. In 80% of cases, if a female has condyloma, then the male partner will also have condyloma even though they may be microscopic. Hence, a consultation with a urologist is essential. 5-Fluorouracil cream has been used on both the male and female in recalcitrant cases.

Condyloma Acuminatum of the Cervix
What to look for

Often nothing is seen by the naked eye, and the diagnosis is made by the cytologist on a Pap smear. Condyloma acuminatum of the cervix may be associated with dysplasia and warrants further investigation with colposcopy, endocervical curettage, and biopsy for specific tissue diagnosis. Currently, tissue typing is investigative but should become a reality in the near future.

Human Papillomavirus (there are more than 55 types at present) has the potential of causing the following:

Type	Lesion
6a-f	Condylomata acuminata
	CIN I, II, III
	VIN I, II, III
11a, b	Condylomata acuminata
	CIN I, II, III
16	Condylomata acuminata
	CIN I, II, III
	VIN I, II, III
	Bowenoid papulosis
	Carcinoma cervix
18	Carcinoma cervix
31	CIN
	Carcinoma cervix
33	Bowenoid papulosis
	CIN
	Carcinoma cervix
34	Bowenoid papulosis
35	CIN
	Carcinoma cervix

(Types 16, 18, 31, 33 and 35 currently are significant.)

What to do

Several forms of therapy can be used for these acetal white changes in the surface epithelium of the cervix. The easiest and least expensive is to paint the cervix with trichloroacetic acid on a monthly basis at least two times. Then repeat the Pap smear in 3 to 4 months. More than 80% of these lesions can be handled in this simplified manner.

Another form of therapy is the use of a laser, which can be done on an outpatient basis. However, it is more expensive and time-consuming and yields approximately the same results. Again, it is important to send the male partner to a urologist for microscopic evaluation of the glans penis and the shaft of the penis. If condyloma are present therapy should be undertaken.

Some investigators have utilized 5-fluorouracil as a cream to prevent recurrence, but this often causes a major reaction in the female. Recent studies indicate that up to 25% of sexually active females may have asymptomatic condyloma, and these are most likely sexually transmitted. However, individuals can acquire this disease without sexual transmission.

Cervicitis
What to look for

Cervicitis is often a misnomer, because the most common reason for cervicitis is usually an eversion of the glandular epithelium moving out on the cervix. This is seen in women who have had a baby and in women who take oral contraceptives. Their complaint is often increased leukorrhea, and laser, cryotherapy, or cautery of this area will cure the problem.

Chlamydial and gonorrheal infections should be suspected and cultures should confirm or deny their presence and indicate the appropriate therapy.

LONG-TERM CONSIDERATIONS

Women who have repeated bouts of vaginal infections require careful work up and consideration. The object of therapy to prevent vaginitis is to instruct the woman that if she takes broad-spectrum antibiotics that she should at the same time use some type of an antiyeast vaginal preparation, either a cream or more easily a vaginal suppository such as nystatin, nightly during the antibiotic therapy and for at least 5 days thereafter.

The theme of treatment of vaginitis is preventing the infection (such as after antibiotic therapy) and instructing the patient that if she has sufficient number of Doderlein's bacilli in her vagina, her chances of infection are less. Doderlein's bacilli are available in the form of acidophilus tablets to be taken 1 tablet 4 times per day. Also, the patient should be encouraged to eat yogurt with active bacteria present (at least three cup-fulls per week).

The patient should not use a douche, because it does nothing more than wash out the medication, and often it will alter the bacterial flora.

REVIEW
QUESTIONS

More than one correct answer is possible.
1. Which of the following are correct statements in regard to vaginitis?
    a. The pH of vaginal secretions is 3.5 to 4.0.
    b. There is a decrease in Döderlein's baccilus.
    c. A saline wet prep of vaginal secretions is not helpful.
    d. Vaginal cultures are the most appropriate method for diagnosis.
    e. Douching is usually recommended.
2. Natural barriers that prevent ascending infection in the female reproductive tract are:
    a. Low pH of vaginal secretions
    b. Physical apposition of vaginal walls
    c. Cervical mucus
    d. Cleanliness of vulva
3. Which is the most common infection in the lower reproductive tract during the reproductive years?
    a. *Candida albicans*
    b. *Gardnerella vaginalis*
    c. Gonorrhea
    d. Chlamydia
    e. Herpes
4. The human papillomavirus may cause which of the following?
    a. Carcinoma of the cervix
    b. Severe dysplasia
    c. Bowenoid papulosis
    d. Atypical cells
    e. All of the above

ANSWERS

1. b
2. a, b, c
3. a
4. e

BIBLIOGRAPHY

Binns B et al: Screening for chlamydia trachomatous infection in a pregnancy counseling clinic, Am J Obstet Gynecol 159:1144, 1988.

Loendersloot EW et al: Efficacy and tolerability of single-dose versus six-day treatment of candidal vulvovaginitis with vaginal tablets of clotrimazole, Am J Obstet Gynecol 152:953, 1985.

Sobol SD: Epidemiology and pathogenesis of recurrent vulvovaginal candidiasis, Am J Obstet Gynecol 152:924, 1985.

Sweet R: Importance of differential diagnosis in acute vaginitis, Am J Obstet Gynecol 152:921, 1985.

Witkin S, Hirsch J, and Ledger WJ: A macrophage defect in women with recurrent candida vaginitis and its reversal by prostaglandin inhibitors, Am J Obstet Gynecol 155:790, 1986.

Endometriosis

Jeffrey Goldberg

Endometriosis, the presence of extrauterine endometrial glands and stroma, is one of the most common and least understood gynecologic conditions. Despite a great deal of published literature and active research, confusion and controversy shroud its demographics, pathogenesis, natural history, and optimal therapeutic management.

INCIDENCE

In the general population of reproductive-age women, the true incidence of endometriosis is unknown but is estimated to be 5% to 15%. There does not appear to be a racial predisposition, as was previously believed. The incidence in women undergoing surgery for infertility evaluation and treatment is 30% to 50%. A 7% occurrence is found in first-degree relatives, suggesting a polygenetic, multifactorial mode of inheritance.

ETIOLOGY

Several mechanisms have been proposed, but no single theory can satisfactorily account for the anatomic distribution of endometriosis.

1. Retrograde menstruation—this theory best explains the predominance of disease in the dependent portions of the pelvis (Fig. 24-1) and the high incidence in patients with menstrual outflow obstruction. Because retrograde menstruation has been noted to occur in 90% of women, some other, as of yet undetermined, predisposing factor must be contributory.
2. Celomic metaplasia—this accounts for the rare finding of endometriosis in the pleural cavity. In addition, celomic metaplasia may be induced after irritation by menstrual debris from retrograde flow.
3. Lymphatic and hematogenous dissemination—endometriosis has been documented in the lymphatics and veins that drain the uterus. This could explain the very rare occurrence of endometriotic implants at distant sites, such as the umbilicus, lung, kidney, or nasopharynx. In addition, endometriosis may be seeded in abdominal and vaginal incisions.

PATHOPHYSIOLOGY

Endometriotic implants respond like normal endometrium to hormonal stimulation, with cyclic bleeding into the tissue. Accumulation of this blood produces the classic "powder-burn" lesions and "chocolate-fluid" filled endometriomas. Endometriosis incites an inflammatory reaction that leads to adhesion formation and the characteristic stellate scars. When the pelvic anatomy is significantly distorted by endometriomas and pelvic adhesions, the impediment to fertility is obvious; however, the mechanism

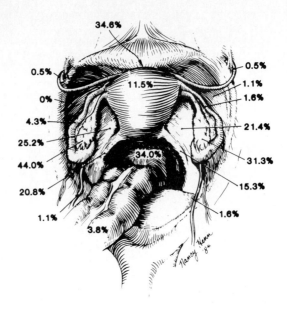

Fig. 24-1
Anatomic locations of endometriosis implants in 182 consecutive infertility patients found to have
endometriosis by laparoscopy. The rates shown indicate percentage of all patients with implants in a
given location.
(From Jenkins S et al: Obstet Gynecol 67:335, 1986. Reprinted with permission from the American College
of Obstetricians and Gynecologists.)

of reduced fertility with minimal or mild disease is not known. Further, it must be
questioned whether minimal or mild disease hinders fertility at all because recent studies have demonstrated no improvement in pregnancy rates with conservative surgery or
danazol administration versus expectant management.

The following findings, alone or in combination, may be contributory:
1. Increased peritoneal fluid.
2. Increased peritoneal macrophages with increased phagocytosis of sperm.
3. Increased concentrations of prostaglandins in peritoneal fluid. May also explain
   pelvic pain symptoms.
4. Altered fallopian tube motility and impaired oocyte pick-up.
5. A possible association with luteinized unruptured follicle syndrome, luteal phase
   defect, and hyperprolactinemia.
6. Abnormal immunologic response to endometrial and ovarian tissues.

EVALUATION

The most frequent initial complaints of patients with endometriosis are pelvic pain and
infertility. The pain usually manifests as dysmenorrhea, often with dyspareunia. No
correlation exists between the severity of the pain and the extent of the disease. Menstrual dysfunction does not appear to increase with endometriosis. More recent studies
seem to refute the earlier claims of an association between endometriosis and an increased risk of spontaneous abortion. The following findings on bimanual examination
are suggestive of endometriosis: fixed uterine retroversion, tender nodularity and/or
thickening of the rectovaginal septum and/or uterosacral ligaments, and adnexal
masses. Pelvic ultrasonography is a useful adjunct for differentiating a cystic adnexal

mass, which is consistent with an endometrioma, from a solid neoplasm. Nevertheless, a definitive diagnosis can be made only by direct inspection of the entire pelvic cavity with laparotomy or laparoscopy. Laparoscopy should always be performed using a double-puncture technique to ensure complete visualization of the under surface of both ovaries. Endometriotic implants are classically blue-black or brown powder burns but may be red cream, white, or clear. If the diagnosis is in doubt, a biopsy of the lesion should be performed, and the lesion should be examined histologically for the presence of endometrial glands and stroma.

A monoclonal antibody assay is available for *CA-125,* a cell-surface antigen on derivatives of celomic epithelium. CA-125 levels are elevated in approximately 50% of women with moderate or severe endometriosis. It can be used as a marker to evaluate therapeutic success and recurrence; however, the sensitivity of the assay is too low to be useful for routine screening.

CLASSIFICATION

Several classification systems have been devised to facilitate uniformity in reporting the results of clinical trials. The extent of the endometriosis should always be documented and the results maintained as a permanent part of the patient's record. Keep in mind, however, that these staging systems were arbitrarily formulated and that the disease stage does not necessarily correlate with the prognosis for fertility. The classification system that is currently in vogue is the American Fertility Society Revised Classification of Endometriosis (Fig. 24-2).

TREATMENT

For relief of pain, nearly all medical and surgical modalities are very effective. Many questions exist regarding the treatment of an infertile woman with endometriosis: Does hormonal or surgical therapy offer any advantage over expectant management in minimal or mild disease? If hormonal therapy is selected, which agent and what dose should be used and how long should therapy continue? When should surgery be performed, what procedure should be used and does preoperative and/or postoperative hormonal therapy improve pregnancy rates? The answers to these questions remain unresolved.

1. Expectant management—*expectant management* does not mean doing nothing. Rather, it means that all other treatable infertility factors are corrected while withholding specific therapy for endometriosis. Recent reports suggest that for minimal or mild disease, no improvement in pregnancy rates occurs with danazol administration or conservative surgery versus expectant management. Expectant management is not recommended for patients with moderate or severe disease or with pain.

2. Hormonal therapy—several agents are available that, through different mechanisms, lead to atrophy of the endometriotic implants by depriving them of hormonal support. Because the disease tends to recur after hormonal therapy, hormonal therapy should be considered suppressive rather than curative.

   a. Oral contraceptives (pseudopregnancy)—the observation that endometriosis seems to improve or resolve after pregnancy led to the use of progestin-dominant oral contraceptives. Oral contraceptives are probably best suited for young patients with pain and for the limitation of the progression of endometriosis when immediate fertility is not desired. Any formulation should be effective when administered daily for at least 6 months.

   b. Progestins—oral medroxyprogesterone acetate 10 mg tid for at least 3 months results in pregnancy rates comparable to those achieved with danazol, with the

Peritoneum	Endometriosis	<1 cm	1-3 cm	>3 cm
	Superficial	1	2	4
	Deep	2	4	6
Ovary	R Superficial	1	2	4
	Deep	4	16	20
	L Superficial	1	2	4
	Deep	4	16	20
	Posterior cul-de-sac obliteration	Partial		Complete
		4		40
Ovary	Adhesions	< ⅓ enclosure	⅓-⅔ enclosure	> ⅔ enclosure
	R Filmy	1	2	4
	Dense	4	8	16
	L Filmy	1	2	4
	Dense	4	8	16
Tube	R Filmy	1	2	4
	Dense	4*	8*	16
	L Filmy	1	2	4
	Dense	4*	8*	16

*If the fimbriated end of the fallopian tube is completely enclosed, change the point assignment to 16.

Stage I (minimal) — 1-5
Stage II (mild) — 6-15
Stage III (moderate) — 16-40
Stage IV (severe) — >40
Total _____

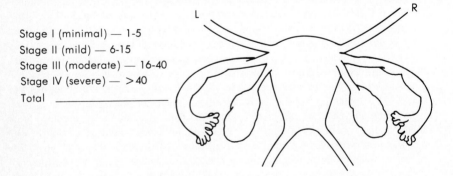

Fig. 24-2
Classification of endometriosis.

Table 24-1 Side effects of danazol

Side Effect	800 mg (71 patients) (%)	400 mg (119 patients) (%)
Weight gain	79	87
Muscle cramps	52	60
Decreased breast size	48	58
Flushing	42	55
Oily skin/hair	37	50
Depression	32	60
Acne	27	46
Hirsutism	21	29
Deepening of voice	7	15
Skin rash	8	10

Modified from Buttram VC, Jr et al: Fertil Steril 43:353, 1985.

advantages of reduced cost and side effects. Breakthrough bleeding and depression are the most common side effects. Because it causes prolonged amenorrhea, intramuscular medroxyprogesterone acetate (Depo-Provera) (150 mg approximately every other month) is not recommended for patients who may be interested in achieving pregnancy.

c. Danazol (pseudomenopause)—the isoxazol derivative of 17α-ethinyl testosterone produces a high androgen–low estrogen milieu through a variety of actions. Debate still continues regarding the optimal dose of danazol. A starting dose of 200 to 300 mg bid is reasonable. Therapy is initiated on day 1 of menses and continued for approximately 6 months. The dose should be increased by 200 mg per day if amenorrhea does not occur. Approximately 80% of patients experience side effects, although drug discontinuation is necessary in only 10%. Because progestins and gonadotropin-releasing hormone (GnRH) analogs have equal efficacy with fewer side effects, danazol is losing ground as the mainstay of hormonal therapy for endometriosis (Table 24-1).

d. GnRH analogs (medical oophorectomy)—numerous GnRH agonists have been developed that cause gonadotropin suppression by pituitary down regulation. These agents are administered daily via the intranasal or subcutaneous routes. Depo forms and GnRH antagonists are on the horizon. A large multicenter study recently found no difference in pregnancy rates or the reduction in visible disease between women who used danazol and women who used intranasal Nafarelin. The GnRH group had few side effects other than hypoestrogenism, and GnRH agonists did not induce the deleterious changes in lipoprotein levels that danazol did.

3. Surgical therapy—surgery is indicated in cases with adhesive disease or endometriomas larger than 1 cm because hormonal therapy is ineffective.

a. Laparoscopy—though scientific support is lacking, laser vaporization at the time of diagnostic laparoscopy is generally favored in cases of minimal and mild endometriosis and in some cases of moderate endometriosis. In addition, ablation of the uterosacral ligaments often ameliorates central pelvic pain. The laser does not offer better outcome rates than those of electrofulguration, but the precision of the laser adds a greater margin of safety when treating disease that overlies vital structures.

b. Conservative surgery—this refers to the restoration of normal pelvic anatomy by lysis of adhesions and the removal of visible endometriosis by excision, fulguration, or vaporization. Uterosacral ligament resection or ablation or presacral neurectomy should be considered in the symptomatic patient. The value of D & C, uterine suspension, and postoperative hormonal therapy in addition to surgery is still a subject of debate. Hormonal therapy initiated approximately 3 months before surgery may facilitate the operative procedure by softening the endometriotic implants and reducing inflammation. A preoperative IVP or bowel preparation should be performed if ureteral or intestinal involvement is known or suspected.

c. Radical surgery—if fertility is no longer desired, the definitive procedure for treating endometriosis is a total abdominal hysterectomy with bilateral salpingo-oophorectomy and excision or destruction of all visible disease. Preserving an uninvolved ovary or providing postoperative estrogen replacement therapy seems to add a very small risk of activating residual disease.

4. Other—pregnancy rates after in vitro fertilization or gamete intrafallopian transfer for women with minimal to moderate endometriosis are similar to those of women with pure tubal factors. Pregnancy rates for women with severe disease are poor.

ADENOMYOSIS

Adenomyosis is the invasion of endometrial tissue within the myometrium. It may be focal but is more commonly diffuse. Unlike endometriosis, adenomyosis usually is not hormonally responsive. Its peak incidence of 10% to 20% characteristically occurs in parous women in the fourth and fifth decades of life. Typical symptoms are progressive menorrhagia and secondary dysmenorrhea. However, the majority of patients are asymptomatic. On pelvic examination, a tender, symmetrically enlarged uterus suggests adenomyosis. The definitive diagnosis can only be made histologically and is often an incidental finding in the hysterectomy specimen. Because the diagnosis of adenomyosis is difficult to make preoperatively, hysterectomy is indicated solely on the basis of the patient's symptomatology.

REVIEW
QUESTIONS

Choose the best treatment modality from the following list for each patient. Answers may be used once, more than once, or not at all.

   a. Expectant management
   b. Oral contraceptives
   c. Conservative surgery
   d. Total abdominal hysterectomy and bilateral salpingo-oophorectomy
   e. Depo-Provera

1. An 18-year-old single female with pain symptoms. Does not desire to conceive in the near future.
2. A 24-year-old married woman with primary infertility and mild endometriosis on diagnostic laparoscopy.
3. A 32-year-old woman with primary infertility and moderate to severe endometriosis on diagnostic laparoscopy.
4. A 20-year-old married woman with a 3-cm endometrioma. She does not desire immediate fertility.
5. A 37-year-old woman Para 3003 with chronic pelvic pain and a 4-cm endometrioma.

True or False

6. The severity of pain correlates with the extent of the disease.
7. CA-125 is useful in making the diagnosis of endometriosis.
8. Eighty percent of patients on danazol experience side effects.
9. Use of the laser in conservative surgery improves pregnancy rates.
10. Adenomyosis is most common during the fourth and fifth decades of life.
11. The diagnosis of endometriosis should be confirmed by double-puncture laparoscopy.
12. Endometriosis is inherited as a multifactorial, polygenetic trait.

Multiple Choice

More than one correct answer is possible.
13. Infertility in minimal or mild endometriosis may be caused by:
    a. Increased peritoneal-fluid prostaglandin levels.
    b. Altered fallopian tube motility and oocyte pick-up.
    c. Luteinized unruptured follicle syndrome.
    d. Occlusion of the tubal lumen.
14. The following symptoms are suggestive of endometriosis:
    a. Dyspareunia
    b. Menometrorrhagia
    c. Dysmenorrhea
    d. Spontaneous abortion

ANSWERS

1. b
2. a
3. c
4. c
5. d
6. False
7. False
8. True
9. False
10. True
11. True
12. True
13. a, b, c
14. a, c

BIBLIOGRAPHY

Bayer SR et al: Efficacy of danazol treatment for minimal endometriosis in infertile women, J Reprod Med 33:179, 1988.
Buttram VC, Jr, Reiter RC, and Ward S: Treatment of endometriosis with danazol: report of a 6-year prospective study, Fertil Steril 43:353, 1985.
Haney AF, editor: Pathophysiology of the infertility associated with endometriosis, Semin Reprod Endocr 6:239, 1988.
Henzl MR et al: Administration of nasal Nafarelin as compared with oral danazol for endometriosis, N Engl J Med 318:485, 1988.
Jenkins S, Olive DL, and Haney AH: Endometriosis: pathogenic implications of the anatomic distribution, Obstet Gynecol 67:335, 1986.

Olive DL, and Haney AH: Endometriosis-associated infertility: a critical review of therapeutic approaches, Obstet Gynecol Surv 41:538, 1986.

Schmidt CL: Endometriosis: a reappraisal of pathogenesis and treatment, Fertil Steril 44:157, 1985.

Speroff L, Glass RH, and Kase NG: Endometriosis and infertility. In Clinical gynecologic endocrinology and infertility, ed 4, Baltimore, 1989, Williams & Wilkins.

Williams TJ: Endometriosis. In Mattingly RF, and Thompson JD, editors: Te Linde's operative gynecology, ed 6, Philadelphia, 1985, JB Lippincott Co.

Pelvic Masses in the Obstetric and Gynecologic Patient

Michael Blumenfeld
Frederick P. Zuspan

Pelvic masses in obstetric and gynecologic patients can arise from a variety of pelvic and abdominal structures. This chapter provides an overview of diagnosis and management of the patient with a pelvic mass. Leiomyomas and ovarian cysts, the most common pelvic masses, are outlined extensively in this chapter, while other etiologies are further expanded upon elsewhere in this book.

DIAGNOSIS

Many pelvic masses are totally asymptomatic and may be diagnosed incidentally on a routine pelvic examination, an x-ray examination, or ultrasonography. A concise history and careful general physical examination often provides information necessary for the differential diagnosis. Laboratory evaluation and diagnostic imaging can help confirm the diagnosis and in selecting medical or surgical options used for therapy.

The differential diagnosis of the pelvic mass can be subdivided with respect to the three stages of the female life cycle: prepubescent, reproductive, and postmenopausal. The cornerstone of all diagnostic regimens is the history, and it is especially important if pain is a dominant feature of the illness. The age and life-style of the patient are important in arriving at the appropriate diagnosis. Malignant masses are more often found in older women, whereas functional cysts, benign neoplasms, and complex masses caused by infection predominate in younger patients.

History

1. Age: A pelvic mass in a menstruating woman may have less significance than one in a postmenopausal woman. In the adolescent and the premenarchal girl, a pelvic mass may indicate a significant problem.
2. Chief complaint: Is the mass symptomatic? Is the symptom acute or chronic? Has it altered her life-style in any way?
3. Gynecologic history
   a. Menses: Age at menarche, cycle, flow, changes, or irregularities, and associated pain.
   b. Infection: Sexually transmitted diseases, history of pelvic inflammatory disease, history of tubal or ovarian abscess, significant and recurrent vaginitis, multiple sexual partners.
   c. Sexual history: Activity, dyspareunia, dysfunction, foreign bodies, history of sexual abuse.
   d. Urogenital history: Urinary stress incontinence, hematuria, dysuria, frequency, recurrent urinary tract infections, pyelonephritis.

   e. Endocrine system
     (1) Systemic: Weight changes, fatigue, temperature intolerance, skin changes, tremors, palpitations, insomnia, breast discharge, hair changes, change in libido.
     (2) Puberty: Sequence of changes, menarche, thelarche, pubarche, adrenarche.
   f. Menopause: History of postmenopausal bleeding, abdominal distension, bloating, hot flushes, sexual dysfunction, osteoporosis, relaxed pelvic floor symptoms.
   g. Previous gynecologic surgery: If at all possible, try to obtain the surgical pathology and the operative report.
   h. History of birth control: Use of IUD, oral contraceptives, barrier methods of contraception, failures.
   i. Obstetric history
     (1) Number of pregnancies, number of births
     (2) Number of abortions—elective or spontaneous (first or second trimester)
     (3) Living children
     (4) Obstetric procedures: forceps, vacuum, cesarean section (indication)
     (5) Complications: postpartum hemorrhage, coagulopathy, infection, trauma, incompetent cervix
   j. Medical: Illnesses including recent infection, hospitalizations, medications—over-the-counter and prescription.
   k. Past social history: Alcohol, tobacco and drug consumption, recreational drug use, travel, history of physical or sexual abuse.
   l. Family history: History of gynecologic malignancy and breast malignancy.
   m. Review of systems.
   n. Pain: If pain is a factor, details should be obtained as to whether or not it is associated with menses, defecation, urination, intercourse, provoked by activity, relieved with rest, etc.

Physical Examination

All patients should undergo a *complete* physical examination. The pelvic and the rectal-vaginal examination obviously are the most significant in this case. The examination should be done with the patient in a relaxed setting and in a proper position on the examining table. The examination should include the following:

1. Blood pressure, height, weight, all vital signs
2. Skin should be observed for acne, dryness, and lesions
3. Hair patterns—especially facial, pubic, balding
4. HEENT should include gross visual field examination and eye ground examination
5. Neck: Thyroid, presence or absence of goiter, presence or absence of adenopathy (supraclavicular)
6. Lymphatics: Adenopathy—especially supraclavicular, axillary, and inguinal
7. Breast: General systematic examination including teaching of self-breast examination; masses, tenderness, nipple discharge—Tanner staging of breast development may be useful in adolescent patients
8. Abdominal examination: Includes inspection for scars, stria, protuberances, distension, and symmetry
9. Auscultation of the abdomen
10. Percussion and palpation of abdomen: Tympanic versus solid sounds with palpation indicating point tenderness masses, ascites with fluid wave, guarding, rebound, rigidity, enlarged spleen and liver
11. Back examination: To rule out scoliosis, equal level of hips on standing, as well

as point tenderness lateral to the vertical axis of the spine
12. Pelvic examination:
  a. Inspection of the external genitalia, including the mons pubis, hair distribution, clitoris with evidence of enlargement, labia majora and minora, evidence of trauma, hematoma, pigment changes, edema, lesions.
  b. Introitus: Hymen intact, thick or scarred.
  c. Vagina: Discharge, rugae, moisture, congenital anomalies, pH should be done on secretions in the lower one third of the vagina and should be no higher than 4.5 (preferable range 3.5 to 4.5); otherwise, suspect an infection.
  d. Relaxations of the vaginal vault indicating a cystocele, rectocele, cysto-ureth-rocele and enterocele.
  e. Cervix: Ectropion lesions, DES changes with hooding, adenosis, bleeding, viscosity of cervical mucus.
  f. Uterus: Position, pain on cervical motion, point tenderness, prolapse.
  g. Bimanual examination:
    (1) Remember that stool in the rectum or a full and overly distended bladder will compromise the examination. The patient should empty her bladder and bowels prior to the examination if possible.
    (2) The gravid uterus, once it is beyond 14 weeks of gestation, precludes a reasonable examination of the adnexa. The obese patient who needs to be evaluated often may have a compromised examination, and imaging techniques may be required, especially with vaginal transducer sonogram.
    (3) The bimanual examination should include palpation of the vagina for tenderness and masses, the cervix for masses and fixation, movement, motion tenderness, and point tenderness to touch. The uterus should be noted for size, position, whether it is anteverted or retroverted, mobile or fixed, smooth or irregular, tender or prolapsed.
    (4) Adnexa: The ovary and tubes should be evaluated carefully with gentle palpation. Ovaries should be evaluated for size, mobility, consistency, and tenderness. The postmenopausal ovary is usually 1.5 by 1.5 centimeters or less in size and therefore not usually palpable.
    (5) Fallopian tubes: Evaluate for presence of masses, including ectopic pregnancy, hydrosalpinx or pyosalpinx. Thickening can often be detected, and tenderness is not uncommon.
    (6) A persistently enlarged bladder may indicate neuropathy with a neurogenic bladder. Point tenderness over the bladder often will signal a urinary tract infection.
    (7) Rectal-vaginal-abdominal examination: This should not be omitted. If the uterus is retrocessed or retroverted, this is a critical examination to determine size, position, and consistency. Endometriosis with scarring or thickening can be palpated on the sacro-uterine ligaments posterior to the cervix.
    (8) In the young female, especially one who has not had intercourse, a rectal-abdominal examination is usually tolerated easily by the patient and will provide adequate information. If unsatisfactory, an examination under anesthesia may be necessary.

Laboratory Assessment

After assessment of the patient by history and physical, a differential diagnosis should emerge that will lead to laboratory and ancillary testing and imaging to confirm the diagnosis. Tests that may be useful include the following:

1. Serum qualitative beta-HCG: A pregnancy test should be done when evaluating a woman between the ages of 10 and 50 years with a pelvic mass. A corpus luteum of pregnancy, ectopic gestation, and theca lutein cysts seen in gestational trophoblastic disease are all causes of adnexal masses associated with a positive beta HCG.
2. A blood profile should include a CBC with differential and erythrocyte sedimentation rate to evaluate the possibility of infection.
3. Vaginal and cervical examinations should include pH assay (above 4.5 indicates possibility of vaginosis, which can be confirmed by a wet prep, gram stain, and/or cultures).
4. STD cultures for chlamydia and gonorrhea.
5. A Papanicolaou smear should be done on all women regardless of age. This will provide information for hormonal evaluation and microbiology, as well as abnormalities of neoplasia.
6. Endocrine studies should be selective and based upon a provisional diagnosis.
   a. Follicle-stimulating and LH hormones: If FSH is greater than 40, menopause or ovarian failure is most likely.
   b. Estrogen, progesterone.
   c. Testosterone.
   d. Prolactin for pituitary assessment.
   e. DHEAS for adrenal gland function.
   f. Thyroid function tests.
7. Tumor markers (associate tumor): alpha-fetoprotein (endodermal sinus tumor); CA 125 (epithelial ovarian tumors); testosterone (Sertoli-Leydig); estrogen, progesterone (granulosa cell tumor); beta-hCG (germ cell tumors); LDH (dysgerminoma).
8. Quantitative Beta hCG if GTD is suspected.
9. Urinalysis and studies: Casts, culture, sensitivity, white blood cells—rule out pelvic kidney by use of intravenous pyelogram and palpation.

Ancillary Diagnostic Procedures that May be Useful

1. Culdocentesis—May be useful for:
   a. Culture of cul-de-sac secretions
   b. Gram stain for the presence of pelvic inflammatory disease (PID)
   c. The presence of serous or serosanguinous fluid indicating the possibility of a ruptured ovarian cyst or an ectopic pregnancy
2. Sigmoidoscopy and cystoscopy:
   a. Rule out specific lesions
   b. Diverticulitis and diverticulosis
3. Laparoscopy
   a. Permits a reasonably specific diagnosis
   b. Facilitates biopsies to confirm tentative diagnoses
   c. Performance of video pelviscopy for therapy

Imaging Procedures
Ultrasound

Ultrasound imaging of the pelvis can be an informative investigational tool. If need be, it can be done at the bedside or in the examining room following the examination.

The vaginal transducer is becoming a routine part of the gynecologic examination. It has many advantages over the abdominal transducer. One advantage is in the obese patient, in whom abdominal imaging may be compromised by excessive adipose tissue. Also, a full bladder is not required for transvaginal sonography, which makes for much less discomfort for the patient. The vaginal transducer examination is shorter and more definitive, in some cases using higher resolution probes closer to the mass in question. It is excellent for the diagnosis of adnexal masses and may become a superb ancillary tool in the evaluation of postmenopausal patients.

1. Assessment can be made of intrauterine pregnancy versus ectopic pregnancy, since the fetal sac can be seen inside or often outside of the uterus.
2. Gestational trophoblastic disease within the uterus gives a "snowstorm" appearance.
3. A pelvic mass can be determined to be either cystic, septated, solid, or complex.
4. Myomas can be determined to be intramural, subserosal, or intramyometrial, with or without degenerative changes.
5. The interior surface of the uterine cavity can be evaluated (e.g., for endometrial thickness) in hyperplasia, or uterine septum, or submucous fibroid.
6. Intraperitoneal fluid in the cul-de-sac can be detected, as can hydrosalpinx and hydroureter.
7. Urogenital pathologic processes can be ruled out by determining the presence of hydroureter, stones, pelvic kidney, and duplicated urinary tract symptoms.

Radiologic evaluation

1. Flat plate of abdomen: With an acute abdomen, bowel obstruction or perforation with air-fluid levels, abnormal gas pattern or free air. If the patient has a dermoid, a calcified structure such as teeth and bone may be seen deep in the pelvis.
2. Chest x-ray: Helpful in identifying pleural effusions associated with pelvic malignancies or benign ovarian tumors (Meigs syndrome).
3. Upper gastrointestinal study and barium enema: This is helpful to rule out malignancies and is especially helpful to rule out Crohn's disease.
4. Mammography: If a pelvic mass is present, utilize mammography to assist in ruling out a primary in the breast with metastasis to the ovary. Also, follow guidelines set by ACS, ACOG for screening.
5. CT scan: Detailed anatomy can be identified. If carcinoma is suspected, it is important to see whether or not there is metastatic disease. It is useful to determine the existence of intraabdominal abscess versus serous fluid. One of its values is the assessment of lymph adenopathy, especially aortic adenopathy prior to a major surgical procedure. The CT scan can be helpful in the obese patient when abdominal ultrasound is compromised and a transvaginal transducer is not available. Also, a CT-guided biopsy may avoid a major surgical procedure.
6. MRI: It is as helpful as a CT scan; however, it is not yet used very frequently in gynecologic disease. It may be useful in pregnancy because radiation is not a factor.

DIFFERENTIAL DIAGNOSIS
Premenarche

Before menarche, it is rare to have a physiologic cause for enlargement of an organ or development of a mass in the pelvis. This means that if a mass is present, it requires a careful assessment. Investigations and treatment should not be delayed by observation because most will be related to a dermoid or germ cell tumor. The young child has a small pelvis, and usually symptoms relate to abdominal pelvic pathology and not to pelvic pathologic processes per se.

The following outline will acquaint the reader with the various forms of pathologic processes that can be present in the premenarchal female.

Pelvic masses in the prepubertal female

1. Neoplasm (Ovarian)
   a. Germ cell tumors
      (1) Teratoma—may either be mature or immature with solid or cystic components.
      (2) Dysgerminoma
      (3) Endodermal sinus tumor
      (4) Choriocarcinoma
      (5) Embryonal cell carcinoma
      (6) Polyembryoma
      (7) Mixed tumors
   b. Gonadal blastoma—rare in this age group
   c. Epithelial ovarian tumor—rare
   d. Gonadal stromal tumor—rare (granulosa cell tumor)
   e. Other
      (1) Sarcoma botryoides (vagina, cervix)
      (2) Presacral teratoma
      (3) Lymphomas
      (4) Neuroblastoma
2. Congenital abnormalities
   a. Pelvic kidney (incidence 1 in 600)
   b. Uterine anomalies (bicornuate uterus, didelphys)
   c. Vaginal septum
3. Functional ovarian cysts (all rare in this age group)
   a. Follicular cyst
   b. Germinal inclusion cyst
   c. Paraovarian cyst
   Neonatal follicular cysts may occur secondary to maternal hormonal environment and may be seen before birth by ultrasound; they usually resolve spontaneously after delivery.

Reproductive Age Group

During the reproductive part of the female life cycle, the majority of findings occur because of cyclic hormonal stimulation causing physiologic or pathophysiologic changes in ovarian tissue. Pregnancy must always be considered in the initial evaluation of patients in this age group. Follicular or corpus luteum cysts and pathologic complications of these account for the majority of the etiologies. Infectious exposure is also common during these years, which may result in hydrosalpinx or tubal-ovarian abscesses.

   Masses that occur during the reproductive years include the following:
1. Congenital—see above
2. Functional cysts: These are most common in the reproductive years; the most common cause of adnexal masses; usually asymptomatic
   a. Follicular cysts
      (1) 20% to 50% of cysts
      (2) Can be from excessive pituitary stimulation or iatrogenic stimulation with clomiphene or HMG
      (3) Can be up to 6 to 8 cm in size

    (4) Can be incidentally found in routine pelvic examination, or patient may present with acute pelvic pain secondary to rupture, torsion or hemorrhage

    (5) Usually regresses after two to three cycles, spontaneously or may regress with hormonal suppression

    (6) If cysts rupture, clear or serosanguinous fluid on culdocentesis may be diagnostic

  b. Corpus luteum cysts

    (1) Result after ovulation, secondary to excessive hemorrhage into the cystic cavity, which remains

    (2) Less than or equal to 6 to 8 cm

    (3) Serosanguinous fluid

    (4) Usually regress after two or three cycles

  c. Theca-lutein cyst

    (1) Occasionally seen in normal pregnancies

    (2) Often accompanies trophoblastic disease or hyperplacentosis in patients with diabetes, multiple gestations

    (3) Rapid growth up to 15 cm, with widespread luteinization of ovary

    (4) Polycystic

    (5) Usually spontaneous regression when stimulation is removed; this takes place over 3 to 4 months or more

    (6) Can rupture or undergo torsion and create acute abdominal pain

3. Endometriomas (chocolate cyst)

  a. Present with signs or symptoms of endometriosis (see Chapter 24 regarding endometriosis for details)

  b. Secondary to cyclic menstrual bleeding into the cyst lined by endometrial-like tissue on the ovary

  c. Usually less than 10 to 12 cm with enlargement over several months

  d. Immobile and often scarred

4. Paraovarian cysts

  a. Account for 10% of adnexal masses

  b. Remnants of Wolffian duct

  c. Benign cysts, usually unilocular

  d. Can reach very large size up to 20 cm, but usually do not torse

  e. Have a mass effect, displacing the uterus

  f. Surgical removal is necessary to differentiate them from other neoplasms

  g. If reproductive function is an issue, the tube should be saved, if at all possible

5. Hydatid of Morgagni

  a. Small pedunculated cysts of Müllerian origin found at distal end of fallopian tube

6. Polycystic ovaries—Stein-Leventhal syndrome; hypothalamic pituitary ovarian axis dysfunction

  a. Typical patient is obese and hirsute-appearing, with history of irregular menses and infertility secondary to anovulation

  b. Ovaries enlarged with numerous cysts, and ovarian capsule is thickened, with a glistening whitish appearance

7. Leiomyomas-see below

Myomas

Myomas are defined as benign tumors of muscle cell origin. They have various amounts of fibrous tissue, possibly secondary to degeneration. They are common in 20% of all females over 35 years of age; specifically, they are more frequent in black women than white, occurring in 1 in 2 of the black female population and 1 in 4 of the white female population.

The majority of myomas are asymptomatic. They vary in size from microscopic to large multinodular masses that can weigh up to 50 pounds. Myomas are rarely occur before puberty and they undergo atrophy after menopause.

Etiology

Myomas are considered to originate from a single muscle cell, or otherwise monoclonal cell. Two theories regarding the etiology of myomas are as follows:
1. Persistent small embryonic rest cells
2. Smooth muscle cells of the blood vessels

The growth in myomas is probably hormonally stimulated. They seem to be responsive to hormones and have estrogen receptors, but heterogeneity in response to estrogen is present.

Pathology

Myomas are classified depending on growth.
1. Intramural: The vast majority remain within the myometrium
2. Subserosal:
    a. May become pedunculated
    b. May become parasitic either to the omentum or parametrium or other peritoneal structures
3. Submucosal: 5% to 10%; if pedunculated, may also present as a polyp
4. Cervical (1% to 5%)

Myomas are rarely solitary. They show slow growth or no growth after menopause (i.e., they atrophy). It is important to note that growth after menopause, especially rapid growth, is suggestive of either a leiomyosarcoma or a misdiagnosed ovarian carcinoma.

Clinical symptoms

1. Overall
    a. Most are asymptomatic
    b. One in three patients experience pain
    c. One in three patients experience abnormal vaginal bleeding
    d. May also experience urinary disturbances, constipation, pregnancy-related problems associated with abortion, infertility, or dystocia.
2. Submucous leiomyomas
    a. Most are clinically symptomatic
        (1) Menorrhagia occurs from abnormally stretched vessels or from increased surface area
        (2) Anemia secondary to increased blood loss
        (3) Infection, especially with pedunculated leiomyomas
        (4) Dysmenorrhea
        (5) Pelvic pain
        (6) Hemorrhage
        (7) Rare uterine inversion
        (8) Infertility—recurrent abortion with distorted uterine cavity
3. Intramural leiomyomas
    a. Most frequent
    b. Enlarged uterine cavity
    c. Associated with menorrhagia, infertility, pressure symptoms, and abdominal mass
4. Subserosal leiomyomas
    a. Often asymptomatic

   b. May present as abdominal mass
   c. If leiomyoma is pedunculated, patient is at risk to undergo torsion and may present with acute abdominal pain
   d. Rupture of large surface area vessel may result in severe internal hemorrhage
5. Cervical leiomyomas
   Cervical leiomyomas, as noted, are uncommon but may present with bleeding, infection, dyspareunia, infertility or dystocia. Pressure on the urogenital system may also be a complaint.

Complications

1. Histologic transformation or degeneration may occur with relatively poor vascular supply at the pedicle and continued growth, which subsequently surpasses the vascular supply
   a. Carneous infarction or red degeneration: most acute; typically in second trimester of pregnancy due to ischemic necrosis after rapid growth in pregnancy; usually large tumors; pain severe; localized peritoneal irritation. With chronic reduction in blood supply, tissue will undergo further degeneration
   Therapy: conservative management; analgesic therapy; avoid myomectomy in pregnancy because of significant risk of hemorrhage
   b. Hyaline degeneration (mildest)
   c. Cystic
   d. Fatty
   e. Myxomatous (15%)
   f. Calcification (10%)
   g. Malignant—rapid growth (less than .7%)
   h. Necrotic
2. Infection
3. Urologic problems secondary to effect from large fibroids
   a. Acute retention
   b. Dysuria
   c. Repeated UTIs
   d. Hydronephrosis
   e. Hydroureter
   f. Pyelonephritis
4. "Metastasis"
   a. Omentum
   b. Peritoneal cavity
5. Intravenous leiomyomatosis—rare; invade venous channel
6. Associated with pregnancy
   a. Red degeneration (see above)
   b. Abortion
   c. Premature labor
   d. Unstable lie
   e. Dystocia: Labor—dysfunctional uterine activity; delivery—obstructive
   f. Postpartum hemorrhage without infection
   g. Uterine inversion

Masses related to pregnancy

1. Uterus, in an intrauterine pregnancy
2. Enlarged corpus luteum in the first trimester—very common
3. Ectopic pregnancy—see Chapter 2

4. Ovarian cyst or neoplasm with pregnancy—most are benign, but 2% to 4% are malignant; most common types are dermoids and serous or mucinous cystadenomas

Masses secondary to infection (see Chapter 23 for PID)

Infection may produce a pelvic mass **acutely** during an active episode of pelvic inflammatory disease. The mass may be a pelvic abscess or tubo-ovarian abscess (TOA), involving the fallopian tube, ovary, broad ligament, uterus, and nearby omentum or bowel. These will often require surgical excision and drainage but can sometimes be treated with aggressive antibiotic therapy with success. The residual scarred area in the pelvis may later accumulate fluid, becoming a **postinflammatory** cyst or mass, which is also called a hydrosalpinx if it occupies the lumen of the tube. This mass is **chronic** and may present months or years after an acute episode of pelvic infection.

Miscellaneous pelvic masses in reproductive-age women

1. Distended bladder—usually due to neurogenic disorder or entrapped uterus
2. Appendiceal abscess
3. Epiploic appendagitis—torsion or infarction of epiploic appendage
4. Vascular or lymphatic hemangioma of the pelvis

Postmenopausal Women

During this period of the female life cycle, any mass or abnormal bleeding must be considered secondary to a neoplastic process until proved otherwise. Aggressive investigation is needed for these patients. Nongynecologic pathologic processes may also present during these years as an apparent pelvic mass.

1. Ovary
   a. Epithelial tumors, GCT, stromal tumors
   b. Functional cysts should not occur in the menopausal woman (see Chapter 32)
2. Uterus—endometrial carcinoma or sarcomas (see Chapter 35)
3. Fallopian tube—rare carcinoma
4. Urogenital—bladder divertiuclum, bladder carcinoma
5. Infection abscess from diverticulum, Crohn's disease, or tubovarian abscess
6. Gastrointestinal—diverticula, appendiceal abscess, Crohn's abscess
7. Vascular—abdominal aneurysm, pelvic hemangioma
8. Metastatic disease—Krukenberg tumor; site of primary is most commonly in breast or colon

MANAGEMENT

After completing the history and physical, a decision must be made to develop a working diagnosis. Other investigational tests need to be ordered to develop the working diagnosis. Management should be based on five strategic options:

1. Observation
2. Medical pharmacotherapy
3. Surgical therapy
4. Radiation therapy
5. Combinations of the above

Based on these five options, the final plan can be established in a sequential manner. The guidelines should be based on the life cycle of the female. A few of the following considerations can always be kept in mind, but there are exceptions to all generalizations, which are as follows:

1. It is rare to have a functional cyst prior to menarche.
2. It is rare to have a functional cyst after menopause.
3. Any mass or abnormal bleeding after menopause should be considered a carcinoma till proven otherwise.
4. Make sure a woman in her reproductive years is not pregnant before an extensive workup is ordered.
5. Any mass in excess of 8 cm in any age group should be evaluated surgically by laparoscopy or laparotomy.
6. Any solid mass probably should be surgically evaluated by laparotomy.

Therapy

Follicular/luteal cyst

1. If incidental finding is a cyst less than 6 to 8 cm, follow conservatively and observe for spontaneous regression over 1 to 2 months.
2. If cyst is symptomatic or persists or enlarges, proceed with laparoscopy; if aspirated, fluid should be sent for cytologic examination.
3. Ultrasonography is helpful in the differential diagnosis.
4. Ovarian hormonal suppression may be helpful with functional cyst, as well as hypothalamus-pituitary axis regulation.

Endometriomas or chocolate cysts

Therapy consists of surgical and pharmacologic approaches. See Chapter 24 regarding therapy.

Parovarian cysts

Surgical removal is usually indicated. If a conservative approach is desired, the tube can be dissected off and left because it will usually resume its normal size.

Hydatid of Morgagni

This does not need to be removed.

Polycystic ovaries

See Chapters 27 and 28.

Ovarian neoplasms

Please refer to Chapter 35.

Myomas

After a certain diagnosis is made, the therapy varies, depending on the patient's age, parity, and plans for childbearing. One should treat anemia, if present, with ferrous sulfate or transfusion, and treatment of infection, if present, should of course occur with antibiotics, fluids, and possibly surgery.

1. Options
   a. Conservative therapy with close observation and follow-up every 4 to 6 months: if minimal symptoms, small tumors, in pregnancy, or postmenopausal with small fibroid not increasing in size.
   b. Pharmacologic: hormonal therapy; GnRh analogs; antiprostaglandins.
   c. Surgery: Myomectomy versus hysterectomy—indications for myomectomy are previous repetitive abortions; longstanding infertility; persistent abnormal bleeding; pain or pressure; rapidly expanding pelvic mass; enlargement of asympto-

matic myoma to more than 8 cm in a female who has not completed childbearing.

Contraindications to myomectomy are important and include pregnancy; advanced adnexal disease; malignancy; and when myomectomy would result in a nonfunctional endometrial cavity. Remember, there is a high recurrence rate with myomectomy (5% to 25%).

Hysterectomy: Severe symptoms; considerable size (greater than 12 weeks); childbearing complete; rapid growth.

  d. Combination therapy: GnRh analogs used to decrease size, then surgery.

REVIEW QUESTIONS

1. A 26-year-old white female presents to the emergency room with acute pain in her left pelvis. She denies nausea, vomiting, or constipation. She has regular cycles—her last menstrual period was 2 weeks ago. The only medicine she is on is a triphasic oral contraceptive. Her white cell count is 9.2 and her hemoglobin is 12.8. You suspect she has:
   a. A ruptured ovarian cyst—mittelschmerz
   b. Torsion of a functional ovarian cyst
   c. Possible ruptured appendix
   d. Intermittent torsion of a benign mature teratoma
2. Your next test(s) to be ordered are (may be more than one correct answer):
   a. Flat plate of the abdomen
   b. Beta-hCG
   c. Ultrasonography of the pelvis
   d. CT scan
3. On flat plate, you find that she has a calcification in her midpelvic area. Ultrasonography shows a 5 cm mass in her posterior cul-de-sac. Your plan is:
   a. Culdocentesis to look for evidence of a ruptured cyst or blood
   b. Single puncture laparoscope for definitive diagnosis and therapy
   c. Analgesic therapy and serial examination with laboratory tests
   d. Exploratory laparotomy with Pfanenstiel's skin incision
4. A 55-year-old white female, G4 P4, with a known past history of a fibroid uterus about 8 weeks in size, now presents with complaints of pelvic pain. She has had no menses for 5 years. Work-up reveals that her uterus is now about 10 to 12 weeks in size. Scan is consistent with a uterus with a normal cavity, but multiple fibroids are present. Your plan is:
   a. Offer hormonal suppression with GnRH analogs and hope that her leiomyomas are responsive.
   b. Prescribe a 2-week trial of nonsteroidal antiinflammatory agents to relieve the pain.
   c. Do an in-office endometrial biopsy. If positive for malignant cells, refer to gynecologic oncologist.
   d. Schedule her for a complete metastatic work-up and admit her to the hospital as soon as possible for definitive surgery.
5. A 26-year-old female, G0 P0, is noted on routine examination to have a 5 cm cyst. Ultrasonography shows a 5 cm unilocular cyst on the left ovary. Your management would consist of:
   a. Exploratory laparotomy and possible LSO.
   b. Laparoscopy and aspiration of the cyst for cytology.

   c. In-office transvaginal aspiration of the ovarian cyst under direct ultrasound guidance.

   d. Serial observations and examinations over the next 6 to 8 weeks with possible ovarian suppression with oral hormonal therapy.

6. A 7-year-old white female presents to the emergency room with her mother. Her mother states that she has had vaginal bleeding for the past 3 days. On examination, you note that she has breast development at Tanner stage II. She also has sparse pubic hair and labial development with slight pigmentation. Abdominal and rectal-vaginal exam note a 6 cm mass in the midline. Your work-up and plan include (may be more than one correct answer):

   a. Laboratory analysis including E_2, progesterone, beta-hCG, and Ca-125.

   b. Transabdominal ultrasonography of the pelvis or CT imaging.

   c. Exploratory laparotomy and definitive surgery based on findings.

   d. Family center counseling regarding diagnosis and management.

7. A 32-year-old black female, G4 P2 Ab1, at 32 weeks gestation, presents with intense abdominal pain for the third time in 3 weeks. Ultrasonography shows a 5 cm mass on the anterior aspect of her uterine wall consistent with a uterine fibroid. She is afebrile, and the fetus is 1700 g. Fetal well-being is documented. You should:

   a. Admit the patient, place an IV line and treat with analgesic therapy for pain followed by 24 hours of steroid therapy to induce lung maturity with subsequent delivery of the fetus by induction.

   b. Admit the patient, do an amniocentesis. If fetal lungs are immature, take to operating room for a quick myomectomy. Prophylaxis with magnesium sulfate for prevention of preterm labor.

   c. Admit and treat with IV narcotics or p.o. analgesics. Assure patient that pain is probably secondary to degeneration of uterine fibroid and will improve with time.

   d. Admit patient. If fetal lungs are mature, do cesarean section followed by hysterectomy for uterine fibroids.

ANSWERS

1. d
2. a, b, and c
3. d
4. d
5. d
6. a, b, c, and d
7. c

BIBLIOGRAPHY

Droegemueller W, Herbst AL, Mishell DR, and Stenchever MA: Comprehensive gynecology, St. Louis, 1987, The CV Mosby Company.

Jones HW, Wentz AC, Burnett LS, and Novak S: Textbook of gynecology, ed 11, Philadelphia, 1988, Williams & Wilkins Co.

Havens C, Sullivan ND, and Tilton P: Manual of outpatient gynecology, Boston, 1986, Little, Brown & Co.

Varma, TR: Manual of gynaecology, London, 1986, Churchill Livingstone, Ltd.

Gompel C, and Silverberg SG: *Pathology in gynecology and obstetrics,* ed 3, Philadelphia, 1985, JB Lippincott Co.

Gabbe SG, Niebyl JR, and Simpson JC. *Obstetrics: normal and problem pregnancies,* New York, 1986, Churchill Livingstone, Inc.

Management of the Abnormal Pap Smear

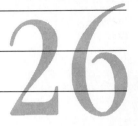

Christopher Copeland

The availability of cervical cytology and, more recently, colposcopy have greatly aided gynecologists in preventing cervical cancer. Once the leading cause of cancer mortality among women, this disease is now considered preventable with regular cervical cytologic evaluation and ranks a distant third to ovarian and endometrial cancers in mortality from gynecologic malignancies. However, this decrease in the incidence of invasive cervical cancer has been mirrored by a phenomenal increase in cases of premalignant cervical disease. **Cervical dysplasia** is a common finding on cervical cytologic evaluation. Approximately 7% to 10% of the Pap smears read in most major medical centers now show signs of **human papilloma virus** (HPV, condyloma acuminata, venereal warts), thought to be the major oncogen causing cervical cancer.

ETIOLOGY
Epidemiology of Cervical Dysplasia and Carcinoma

1. Early age of first sexual intercourse.
2. Early age of first birth.
3. Multiple sexual partners.
4. Low socioeconomic status.

Data collected from thousands of patients over several years has led to the belief that cervical cancer is caused by a sexually transmitted factor, most likely of viral etiology. Animal models have been produced that confirm this theory both in vitro and in vivo. Initial efforts centered on herpes virus type 2 as the oncogen triggering malignant change in the squamous epithelium of the cervix. However, these early studies failed to generate any correlation between the two entities. Subsequently, a significant pool of data has strongly linked HPV, specifically **HPV 16 and 18,** to all degrees of dysplasia and cervical carcinoma (Table 26-1).

Table 26-1 Strength of association between HPV infection and cervical neoplasia

Method	Intraepithelial Neoplasia (%)	Cervical Cancer (%)	Matched Controls (%)	Relative Risk
Histology	88	95	12.5	7×
Serology	60	93	15	10×
DNA hybrid	95	89	—	7×

From Reid R: Colpos Gynecol Laser Surg 1(1):3, 1984.

ANATOMY OF THE CERVIX
Benign

1. Squamocolumnar (S-C) junction. Meeting of the squamous and columnar cells of the exocervix and endocervix, respectively.
2. Squamous metaplasia. Repair process whereby columnar epithelium is gradually replaced by squamous epithelium by activation of a reserve cell. This natural process leads to the gradual ascent of the S-C junction into the endocervical canal with advancing age.
3. Transformation zone. Area of squamous metaplasia that has replaced native columnar epithelium.

Pathologic

1. Atypical cells, with or without inflammation. Cytologic description that defies clear delineation because of obscured cellular detail (i.e., vaginal infections or cervical trauma and repair).
2. Cervical intraepithelial neoplasia (CIN, dysplasia). True cellular abnormalities that meet specific cytologic characteristics (i.e., chromatin clumping, increased nuclear/cytoplasmic ratio, hyperchromatic nucleus, and prominent nucleoli) for premalignant conditions. Epithelial thickness dictates whether lesions are designated as CIN I (mild dysplasia), CIN II (moderate dysplasia), or CIN III (severe dysplasia).
3. Carcinoma in situ. Full-thickness dysplasia believed to correlate with CIN III.
4. Microinvasive squamous cell carcinoma of the cervix. Invasion of malignant cells to $\leq$ 3 mm below the basement membrane.
5. Invasive carcinoma of the cervix. Invasion of malignant cells to $\geq$ 3 mm below the basement membrane.

EVALUATION OF THE CERVIX

Pap smear cytologic screening followed by appropriate colposcopic evaluation in the case of an abnormal screen result detects more than 99% of premalignant conditions of the cervix.

Sampling Techniques

The patient, clinician, and laboratory personnel all determine the accuracy of cytologic screening. Although wide variations in accuracy have been described, most authorities would agree that a 20% false-negative rate is not uncommon. These inaccuracies result primarily from sampling error by the clinician, screening error, or interpretation error by the laboratory. This degree of error, involving even reputable clinicians, emphasizes two critical tenets in evaluating the cervix by cytology:
1. Yearly cytologic evaluation is recommended for all women who have commenced sexual activity.
2. A reputable laboratory that gives consistent, accountable cytologic evaluations and direct discourse between the clinician and cytologist should be used.

Colposcopy

Colposcopy is the process of viewing the cervix through a mounted microscope that magnifies the cervix by 15 to 20 times. Known colposcopic details are used to determine the size, location, and degree of abnormality of a dysplastic lesion. Reid (see bibliography) has described four distinct colposcopic parameters that, when used together, correctly predict the degree of dysplasia in a specific lesion.

1. Acetowhite epithelium. The cervix is washed with 4% acetic acid, and both HPV lesions and dysplastic lesions will appear white against native squamous or columnar epithelium.
2. Vascular atypia. Classic colposcopic teaching describes several vascular patterns associated with dysplastic lesions.
   a. Punctation.
   b. Mosaicism.
   c. Abnormal vessels.
3. Surface contour. Irregular lesion borders are most commonly seen in HPV and low-grade CIN lesions, whereas straight, rolled borders are consistent with high-grade CIN lesions or carcinoma in situ (CIS).
4. Iodine staining (Lugol's solution). Mild staining is seen with low-grade CIN and HPV lesions, and no staining is seen with high-grade CIN lesions and CIS. Iodine is picked up by glycogen in the cytoplasm and therefore is not picked up by dysplastic cells with high nuclear/cytoplasmic ratios.

Once a lesion has been delineated in the exocervix, appropriate biopsies are obtained from those areas with the most abnormal colposcopic characteristics. An endocervical curettage is also obtained in all cases to evaluate the possibility of dysplasia in the endocervix.

THERAPY FOR HPV INFECTION

Much controversy exists about the risk of cancer for those with HPV infections of the cervix. Approximately 70% of these lesions will regress spontaneously, but until commercial tissue typing becomes available, all individuals with evidence of persistent HPV should be treated as if they had cervical dysplasia. Recent reports have commented on the effectiveness of 70% trichloroacetic acid in treating cervical condyloma, with a response rate of 85%.

Cryotherapy

1. Use of liquid nitrogen and Jovle-Thompson effect to achieve extremely low temperatures ($-70°$ C).
2. Use of 3-minute freeze, 5-minute thaw, 3-minute freeze (3-5-3) technique.
3. Cure rates of 90% for low-grade CIN.
4. Initial failure rate of 15% to 30% for high-grade CIN; cure rate of 90% with repeat colposcopy, biopsy, and cryosurgery.
5. Office procedure.
6. Side effects include cramping during procedure and watery discharge for $\pm$ 2 weeks.
7. Regression of S-C junction into the endocervix. Difficult to follow colposcopically.

CO_2 Laser

Table 26-2 displays differences between cold knife conization and laser conization.
1. High wattage (40 to 60 watts) and large spot size to vaporize tissue.
2. Cure rate of 90% for both low- and high-grade CIN lesions.
3. Vaporization to a depth of 5 mm is critical.
4. Office procedure.
5. Side effects include slight pain during procedure and bloody discharge for $\pm$ 2 weeks.
6. Exceptional healing, with visible S-C junction and characteristic endocervical "button."

Table 26-2   Cold knife versus laser conization

Parameter	Cold Knife Cone	Laser Cone
Blood loss	50 to 500 ml	Minimal
Follow-up	Loss of S-C junction	Endocervical button
Margins	Clean margins	Possible distortion secondary to thermal effect

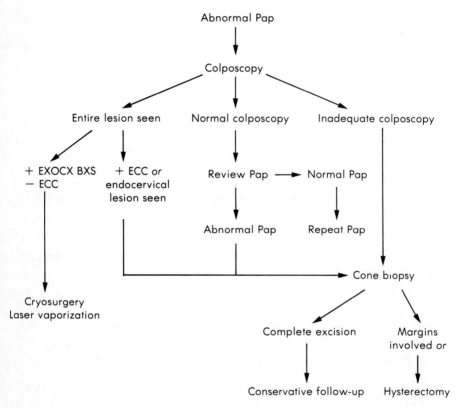

Fig. 26-1
Abnormal Pap smear management.

Table 26-3   Recurrence and progression of carcinoma in situ by initial therapy

Therapy for CIS	Recurrence (%)	Invasive Cancer (%)
Cone	2.3	0.9
Hysterectomy	1.3	1.5
		Long-term
		followup

From Kolstad P and Klem V: Obstet Gynecol 48:125, 1976.

Cone Biopsy

1. Indications.
   a. Dysplasia in the endocervical canal.
   b. Positive endocervical curettage.
   c. Pap smear/colposcopy discrepancy with the Pap smear results suggesting more significant disease than demonstrated on biopsy.
   d. Inadequate colposcopy.
   e. Pap smear evaluation states "suggestive of microinvasion" or "cannot rule out invasion."
2. Outpatient surgery.
3. General anesthesia.
4. Success rate of 95%.
5. Tumor positive cone margins at the exocervix can be followed conservatively. Cure rates of 80% have been documented.

Hysterectomy

The use of hysterectomy for treating high-grade CIN should be reserved for those with other gynecologic pathologic conditions (e.g., pelvic prolapse, stress urinary incontinence, or uterine leiomyomas).

SUMMARY

Management of the patient with an abnormal pap smear is summarized in the algorithm in Fig. 26-1.

REVIEW QUESTIONS

More than one correct answer is possible.
1. Which of the following cytologic findings are considered abnormal and require colposcopic evaluation?
   a. Squamous metaplasia
   b. CIN II
   c. Atypical cells with inflammation
   d. Dysplasia and condyloma
2. Appropriate therapy for CIN I of the exocervix would be:
   a. Cryosurgery
   b. Cone biopsy
   c. Laser vaporization
   d. Hysterectomy

3. Which of the following have been associated with an increased incidence of cervical cancer?
   a. Early first sexual encounter
   b. Early age at the delivery of first child
   c. Multiple sexual partners
   d. *Candida* infections
4. Which of the following would require cone biopsy for diagnosis and/or therapy?
   a. Pap smear evaluation stating "cannot rule out microinvasion"
   b. Colposcopically directed biopsy stating "invasive squamous cell carcinoma"
   c. Inadequate colposcopy
   d. CIN II of the exocervix
5. Which of the following HPV serotypes have been associated with the development of invasive squamous cell carcinoma of the cervix?
   a. HPV 11
   b. HPV 18
   c. HPV 6
   d. HPV 16
6. Colposcopic changes on the cervix that require directed biopsy are:
   a. Punctation
   b. Mosaicism
   c. Acetowhite changes
   d. Staining with (Lugol's) iodine solution

ANSWERS

1. b, d
2. a, c
3. a, b, c
4. a, c
5. b, d
6. a, b, c

BIBLIOGRAPHY

Morrow CP, and Townsend DE: Synopsis of gynecologic oncology, New York, 1987, John Wiley & Sons, Inc., pp. 1-44 (esp. pp. 28-38).
Burke L: Colposcopy. In Nichols DH, and Evrard JR: Ambulatory gynecology, Philadelphia, 1985, Harper & Row, Inc., Publishers, pp. 317-327.
Reid R: Colpos Gynecol Laser Surg 1(1):3, 1984.
Spirtos NM, Schlaerth JB, d'Ablaing G, and Morrow CP: A critical evaluation of the endocervical curettage, Obstet Gynecol 70:729-733, 1987.

Abnormal Uterine Bleeding

Chad Friedman

Abnormal uterine bleeding is a common gynecologic problem in all age groups. Etiologies vary from those that spontaneously resolve without significant morbidity to those that are life threatening, requiring very active intervention. The diagnosis is strongly dependent upon the patient's stage of reproductive function, though the difficulties of assigning reproductive stage based on chronologic age must be borne in mind.

The normal menstrual period occurs every 24 to 36 days, is of 3 to 7 days in duration, and in most cases can be predicted, based on a complex of premenstrual symptomatology (including cramps, moodiness, and breast tenderness). Menstrual blood loss averages 33 ml per cycle, with a range of 20 to 80 ml. Although consistency in the amount of blood loss is reported by most women, in the absence of extremes of bleeding, there have been few studies showing a correlation between the perception of blood loss and the actual blood loss. Thus, complaints of menorrhagia (heavy menstrual bleeding) must be considered in terms of social acceptability to the patient as well as medical significance (e.g., anemia as documented by a hemoglobin or hematocrit). The traditional pad count often reflects social acceptability as much or more so than actual blood loss.

This chapter presents the causes and treatment of abnormal uterine-vaginal bleeding, based upon different stages of reproductive function. Emphasis is placed on making the correct diagnosis rather than empiric treatments, such as estrogen therapy or D & C. However, one flow chart is included, which may be of benefit for management of severe uterine hemorrhage in order to stabilize the patient. Ideally, in most situations a more directed evaluation and treatment plan can be instigated that is based on a thoughtful history and physical examination.

BLEEDING IN CHILDHOOD AND ADOLESCENCE

Bleeding from the reproductive tract in childhood is uncommon. Although the causes are many, as shown in Table 27-1, trauma, sexual abuse, and foreign bodies should always be ruled out. Bleeding in adolescents is more commonly of endocrine origin, but sexual trauma should also be considered (Table 27-2).

REPRODUCTIVE AGE

The key decision to make in evaluating a patient in the reproductive age group with abnormal uterine bleeding is if the patient is anovulatory, ovulatory, or possibly pregnant. Given the multitude of pregnancy tests available, it is imperative that the physician always consider the possibility of pregnancy. Differentiation of ovulatory from anovulatory states cannot always be made with ease based on history and physical ex-

Table 27-1   Abnormal bleeding in infancy and childhood

Cause	Clinical Presentation	Management
Newborn		
Withdrawal of endogenous steroids	Scanty bleeding; limited duration	No treatment
Childhood		
Genital trauma	Physical findings consistent with history; nonrecurrent	Sutures if necessary
Sexual abuse	Inappropriate parental concern; inappropriate child behavior; patulous hymen	Documentation; cultures for sexually transmitted diseases; notification of appropriate agencies
Foreign body	Associated with vaginitis	Removal and examination, generally with anesthesia
Sarcoma botryoides	Erythematous, polypoid, vaginal lesion	Biopsy; chemotherapy; surgery
Abdominal and ovarian neoplasm (granulosa cell, choriocarcinoma, Sertoli Leydig cell, theca cell tumors, hepatoblastomas, adrenal tumors, Peutz-Jeghers syndrome)	Abdominal mass common; other signs of estrogen production (e.g., breast development, advanced bone age); high estradiol; low FSH; possibly elevated hCG	Document mass (ultrasonography, CT scan); surgery
Precocious puberty (idiopathic, McCune-Albright syndrome, LH-secreting adenoma, hamartomas, neurofibromatosis, hypothyroidism)	Before age 8, associated with other signs of puberty (e.g., thelarche, pubarche, advanced bone age); elevated estrogens and normal or elevated gonadotropins for age	Rule out CNS lesions; consider treatment with gonadotropin-releasing hormone agonist
Follicular cyst	1-2 cm clear cyst on ultrasonogram; prepubertal LH response to gonadotropin-releasing factor (GnRF)	Observe and if persists, aspirate or laparoscopy
Iatrogenic	Historic use of estrogen cream or use of estrogen-containing pills; low gonadotropin; possibly high estrone/low estradiol ratio	Discontinue use

Table 27-2   Abnormal bleeding in adolescence

Cause	Clinical Presentation	Management
Coagulation defect (Von Willebrand's disease, idiopathic thrombocytopenia, leukemia)	Profuse bleeding during first year of menarche; abnormal bleeding time, prothrombin time or partial thromboplastin time	Hematology consultation; consider oral contraceptives
Hypothalamic immaturity	Cyclic or acyclic heavy or light bleeding; generally without premenstrual symptoms; restricted to first year after menarche	Resolves after hypothalamic maturation and ovulatory function; conjugated estrogen 2.5-10 mg per day for 25 days and medroxyprogesterone 10 mg on days 19-25 may be used for symptomatic relief; dose of estrogen may be increased every 2 days until bleeding ceases, up to a dose of 10 mg per day
Chronic anovulation	Excessive, irregular bleeding, often preceded by oligomenorrhea; abundant cervical mucus present if not bleeding; absence of premenstrual symptoms	Cyclic medroxyprogesterone 10 mg per day for 14 days every 6 weeks in the absence of spontaneous menses; oral contraceptives
Sexual trauma	Acute profuse bleeding; history of sexual abuse; semen possibly present	Screen for sexually transmitted diseases; consider contraception and counseling
Bicolus hemihematocolpos	Intermenstrual spotting; dysmenorrhea; vaginal mass	Septum resection; evaluate for renal agenesis

amination. Therefore very liberal use of endometrial biopsies should be made, not only to rule out malignancy, which is rare, but also to confirm the clinical diagnosis (Table 27-3).

A last note of caution: clinical states often are not pure. For example, many patients with polycystic ovarian disease may ovulate sporadically (i.e., one or two times per year). Therefore do not ignore the possibility of pregnancy or the possibility of an endometrial biopsy showing secretory endometrium in a patient with classic polycystic ovarian disease.

MENOPAUSAL AND POSTMENOPAUSAL BLEEDING

The majority of women in the menopausal and postmenopausal age group, like those in the reproductive-age group, will respond to hormonal manipulation to correct their bleeding disorder. However, because of the increased prevalence of malignancy within

Table 27-3   Abnormal bleeding in the reproductive years

Cause	Clinical Presentation	Management
Anovulatory bleeding	History of oligomenorrhea; irregular variable bleeding; absence of premenstrual symptoms; obesity; copious cervical mucus if not bleeding; endometrial biopsy showing proliferative endometrium or benign glandular hyperplasia	If not actively bleeding, medroxyprogesterone 10 mg daily for 10 days; if actively bleeding, megestrol 40 mg bid for 14 days, or oral contraceptive 1 tablet 2 times/day for 10 days, or conjugated estrogen 5-10 mg daily for 14 days with Provera 10 mg daily for the last 7 days
	Biopsy shows atypical hyperplasia	Megestrol 40 mg bid for 3 months; rebiopsy off treatment—if normal, then cyclic progestin treatment
	Biopsy shows endometrial carcinoma	Surgery

NOTE: Underlying diseases causing anovulation should be sought (such as polycystic ovarian disease, hyperprolactinemia, and hypothyroidism). Treatment following the withdrawal bleeding induced by the progestins should be directed at correcting the anovulation (e.g., treatment of hyperprolactinemia, hypothyroidism, or obesity) or establishing chronic cyclic progestin withdrawal bleeding (e.g., oral contraceptive therapy or medroxyprogesterone 10 mg daily for 14 days each month). Failure to respond to hormonal treatment within 3 to 4 days should be evaluated by hysteroscopy and D & C. Polyps, endometritis, and endometrial carcinoma occur in anovulatory women at least as commonly as in ovulatory women.

Ovulatory Bleeding

Midcycle bleeding	Recurrent and restricted to periovulatory period and consistent with estrogen fall before ovulation; use basal body temperature to confirm timing	Reassurance or conjugated estrogen 1.25 mg daily for 3-4 days starting the day before onset of midcycle bleeding
Endometritis	Irregular bleeding throughout cycle; uterus tender; endometrial biopsy shows leukocyte infiltrate or plasma cells	Rule out gonorrhea or chlamydia; antibiotics— most commonly doxycycline 100 mg daily for 14 days
Polyps	Irregular bleeding throughout cycle; biopsy often uninformative	Hysteroscopy; polypectomy
Leiomyoma	Metrorrhagia, though more commonly menorrhagia; uterus often irregular in contour; diagnosis of submucous fibroid generally confirmed by hys-	Resection or excision via hysteroscope or laparotomy; gonadotropin-releasing hormone agonist may be used to temporize, allow correc-

Table 27-3   Abnormal bleeding in the reproductive years—cont'd

Cause	Clinical Presentation	Management
	teroscopy or hysterosalpingogram	tion of anemia (e.g., iron treatment), and simplify surgery; hysterectomy
Halbans syndrome (persistent corpus luteum)	Irregular bleeding often accompanied by ovarian cyst; biopsy—secretory or dyssynchronous endometrium; bleeding may worsen postcoital	Generally resolves spontaneously; may try gonadotropin-releasing hormone agonist
Cervical carcinoma	Gross cervical lesion; colposcopic lesion; Pap abnormal	Biopsy any gross cervical lesion; surgery; radiation treatment as appropriate
Cervicitis	Bleeding commonly postcoital; irregular spotting; Pap inflammatory changes	Screen and treat any sexually transmitted diseases; colposcopy; if nonneoplastic and cultures negative, cryosurgery or laser
Endometriosis	Bleeding commonly premenstrual; associated dysmenorrhea; abnormal pelvic exam (e.g., nodulation, thickening, adnexal mass); confirm by laparoscopy	Danazol or gonadotropin-releasing hormone agonist; surgery
Adenomyosis	Heavy cyclic bleeding; boggy tender uterus; dysmenorrhea	Hysterectomy; endometrial ablation?; danazol?; antiprostaglandins
Coagulation defects (Von Willebrand's disease, lupus erythematosus, idiopathic thrombocytopenic purpura, leukemia, factor 13 deficiency, renal failure, anticoagulants)	Menorrhagia; ecchymosis; abnormal prothrombin time and partial thromboplastin time; low platelet count; abnormal bleeding time	Hematologic consultation; cyclic oral contraceptives; GnRF agonist for temporary treatment or megestrol 80-160 mg daily; endometrial ablation?; avoidance of antiprostaglandins; iron replacement
Iatrogenic agents		
Spironolactone	Irregular bleeding	Decrease dose to 100 mg daily; add oral contraceptives
Erratic oral contraceptive use	Irregular bleeding	Education
Anticoagulant therapy	Heavy menstrual bleeding	Chronic progestin therapy (megestrol 80 mg daily); gonadotropin-releasing hormone agonist
Excessive antiprostaglandin therapy	Heavy menstrual bleeding	Decrease intake

Continued.

Table 27-3 Abnormal bleeding in the reproductive years—cont'd

Cause	Clinical Presentation	Management
Depo-Provera	Irregular bleeding	Conjugated estrogen 1.25 mg daily until bleeding stops
Uterine arteriovenous (A-V) fistulas	Very heavy menstrual bleeding, probably requiring transfusions; document by arteriogram	Embolization of A-V fistula; hysterectomy
Pregnancy complications	See Chapters 2 and 10	—
Oral contraceptive bleeding problem	See Chapter 21	—
Vaginal trauma	Acute onset; localized bleeding site	Surgical repair; consider evaluation for foreign body (x-ray or ultrasonography)
Perimenopausal bleeding	Commonly seen in older patients; vasomotor symptoms occasionally; upper range noncastrate FSH	Endometrial biopsy a must; conjugated estrogen 1.25-2.5 mg daily with cyclic progestin for 14 days (e.g., medroxyprogesterone 5-10 mg daily; later decrease estrogen dose

NOTE: Higher doses of estrogen than the standard menopausal replacement are recommended. This may suppress endogenous ovulatory function, which might result in unpredictable intermenstrual bleeding.

Premature ovarian failure and autoimmune oophoritis can present as perimenopausal bleeding in truly reproductive-age females.

the older population, it is imperative that the physician rule out malignancy as a cause for uterine or vaginal bleeding. With rare exceptions, the evaluation should consist of a vaginal and cervical Pap smear, biopsy of any suspicious lesion, endometrial sampling, and a very careful pelvic examination (Table 27-4). Consideration should also be given to performing a breast and rectal examination at the time of the visit. Persistence of unexplained bleeding will warrant surgical evaluation.

MANAGEMENT OF SEVERE UTEROVAGINAL HEMORRHAGE

Although rare, patients may present with such severe genital bleeding that treatment is required before an appropriate evaluation can be performed. The flow chart in Fig. 27-1 (p. 27-8) can be used in such situations, though its use should be restricted to those situations. Note that only in this setting is parenteral estrogen therapy recommended. Any benefits of parenteral estrogen over oral estrogen are, to date, unsubstantiated.

1. Obtain history and perform physical examination, start IV, and obtain blood for complete blood cell count and differential, platelets, prothrombin time, partial thromboplastin time, hCG, type and crossmatch, and electrolytes.
2. Infuse lactated Ringer's solution.
3. Vaginal examination, evacuate clots, and obtain endometrial sample if bleeding from uterus.
4. Transfuse as necessary. Consider military antishock trousers.

Table 27-4   Abnormal bleeding in the menopausal/postmenopausal woman

Cause	Clinical Presentation	Management
Atrophic bleeding		
Vulvar, vaginal, urethral	Atrophic changes source of bleeding; often atrophic endometrium on biopsy	Estrogen and progestin therapy
Endometrial	Atrophic genital changes; atrophic endometrium	Cyclic estrogen and progestin therapy; failure to promptly respond warrants further evaluation (e.g., hysteroscopy, D & C, possible laparotomy)
Endometrial hyperplasia (not on hormonal replacement)	Biopsy shows cystic hyperplasia	Cyclic medroxyprogesterone 10 mg daily for 14 days each month until without withdrawal bleeding
	Biopsy shows benign glandular hyperplasia	Cyclic medroxyprogesterone 10 mg daily for 14 days each month; rule out granulosa cell tumor (e.g., serum estradiol and ultrasonography)
	Biopsy shows atypical glandular hyperplasia	Hysterectomy; megestrol 40 mg bid for 3 months if poor surgical candidate; repeat biopsy off treatment followed by cyclic progestin therapy forever
Endometrial polyps	Unresponsive bleeding to preceding hormonal treatments; endometrial biopsy often shows atrophic changes, proliferative endometrium, or hyperplasia	Hysteroscopy; D & C
Carcinoma or sarcoma	Detected by appropriate biopsy of vulva, vagina, cervix, or endometrium or by documentation of adnexal mass by pelvic examination, ultrasonography, or MRI	Surgery

Continued.

Table 27-4 Abnormal bleeding in the menopausal/postmenopausal woman—cont'd

Cause	Clinical Presentation	Management
Bleeding on hormonal replacement therapy		
Predictable bleeding on cyclic estrogen and progestin	Occurs after withdrawal of progestin	Balance nuisance of bleeding vs. symptomatic needs; assure usage of progestin for 14 days; possibly decrease estrogen or switch to continuous estrogen
Late bleeding on cyclic estrogen and progestin	Bleeds shortly before withdrawing progestin	Endometrial biopsy—if benign, increase dose of progestin
Erratic bleeding on cyclic estrogen and progestin	—	Hysteroscopy; D & C; treatment dependent on pathologic findings
Erratic bleeding on continuous estrogen and progestin	Common during first few months of therapy	Treatment dependent on findings of endometrial biopsy and other evaluation

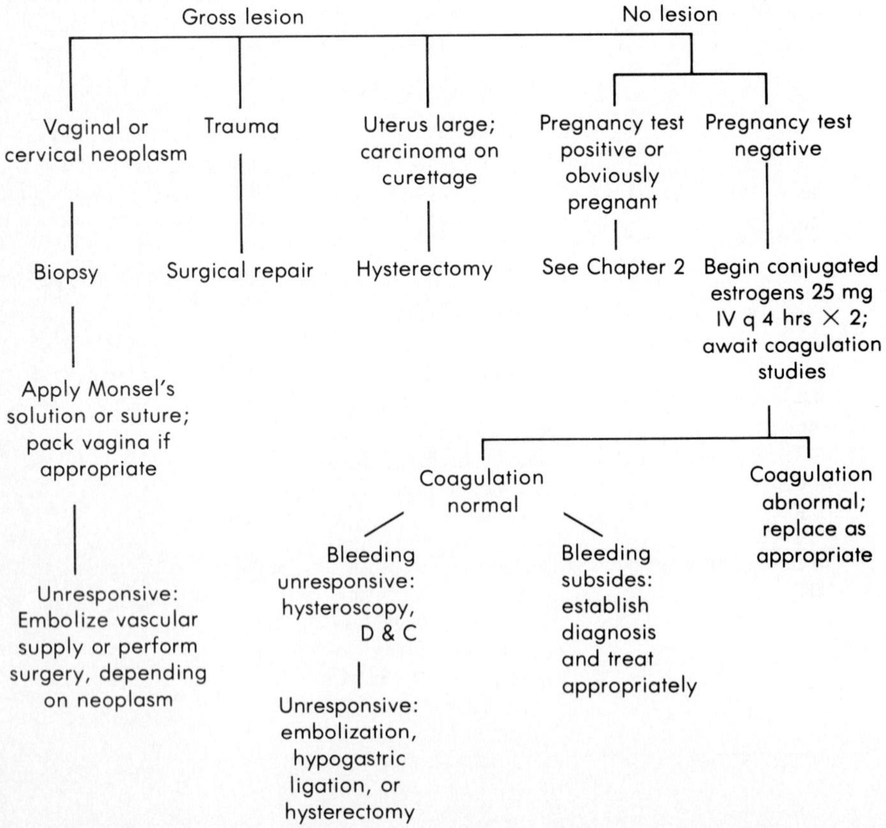

Fig. 27-1
Management of severe uterovaginal hemorrhage.

REVIEW
QUESTIONS

1. Von Willebrand's disease is most likely to have which of the following:
   a. Menorrhagia
   b. Metrorrhagia
   c. Polymenorrhea
   d. Oligomenorrhea
2. Prolonged anovulation (i.e., 6 months) in a 19-year-old female followed by a 1-week history of prolonged heavy vaginal bleeding is most consistent with:
   a. Ectopic pregnancy
   b. Anovulatory bleeding
   c. Cervical cancer
   d. Blood dyscrasia
3. A 14-year-old female is seen 8 months following menarche. Complaints include severe progressive dysmenorrhea (menses every 29 days), chronic intermenstrual blood-tinged discharge, and urinary retention. The most likely diagnosis is:
   a. Hypothalamic immaturity
   b. Sexual trauma
   c. Bicolus hemihematocolpos
   d. Idiopathic thrombocytopenic purpura
4. A 21-year-old female is being treated for idiopathic hirsutism with spironolactone 200 mg daily. Over the past 2 months, her periods have become irregular and excessively heavy. The most likely cause is:
   a. Endometriosis
   b. Leiomyoma
   c. Endometritis
   d. Iatrogenic menstrual dysfunction
5. A 33-year-old female presents with a history of frequent erratic vaginal bleeding. She has a long history of oligomenorrhea. A red crater lesion is seen on her cervix. The most appropriate diagnostic procedure is:
   a. Do a Pap smear
   b. See if the bleeding responds to estrogen and progestin therapy
   c. Obtain a biopsy of the cervical lesion
   d. Laparoscopy, hysteroscopy
6. A 5-year-old female is seen for vaginal bleeding. A careful examination in the knee-chest position reveals a patulous hymen (diameter of 1 cm). Condyloma is noted on the labia. You should:
   a. Treat with erythromycin or doxycycline
   b. Obtain an ultrasonogram of the pelvis
   c. Report your suspicion of child abuse to a government agency
   d. Treat with a GnRF agonist

ANSWERS

1. a.
2. b.
3. c.

4. d
5. c
6. c

BIBLIOGRAPHY

March CM, Hoffman DI, and Lobo RA: Dysfunctional uterine bleeding. In Mishell DR, and Davajan V, editors: Infertility, contraception, and reproduction, Oradel, NJ, 1986, Medical Economics Books.

Richards-Kustan CJ, and Kase NG: Diagnosis and management of perimenopausal and post-menopausal bleeding, Obstet Gynecol Clin North Am 14:169, 1987.

Styne DM, and Grumbach MM: Puberty in the male and female. In Yen SSC, and Jaffe RB, editors: Reproductive endocrinology, physiology, pathophysiology, and clinical management, Philadelphia, 1986, WB Saunders Co.

Amenorrhea

28

Jeffrey M. Goldberg

Amenorrhea may be classified as primary or secondary. *Primary amenorrhea* is defined as failure to menstruate by age 16. Evaluation is also advised if no secondary sexual characteristics have appeared by age 14 or if 3 or more years have passed since thelarche (breast development) without menarche. *Secondary amenorrhea* is defined as the cessation of menses for a duration of 3 or more cycles or a total of 6 months or more.

PATHOPHYSIOLOGY

Disruption of normal physiologic function at any of the following levels may cause amenorrhea (see box on p. 28–2).

1. Hypothalamus: Neuroendocrine integrative function and pulsatile release of gonadotropin-releasing hormone (GnRH).
2. Pituitary: Intact feedback mechanisms and secretion of the gonadotropins, FSH and LH, in response to GnRH.
3. Ovary: Presence of follicles with enzymatic machinery to produce estrogen and progesterone after gonadotropin stimulation.
4. Outflow tract: Endometrium responsive to estrogen, and progesterone and patency from uterus to vaginal introitus.

HISTORY

The history will yield important clues to the correct diagnosis.

Gynecologic History

1. Pubertal development: growth rate, age at thelarche, adrenarche
2. Detailed menstrual history
   a. Age at menarche
   b. Cycle interval, duration and amount of flow
   c. Cyclic symptoms
   d. Last normal menses
   e. Abnormalities such as irregular cycles, intermenstrual bleeding, or excessively heavy or light flow
3. Pregnancy history
   a. Lactation
   b. Postpartum bleeding
   c. Curettage for miscarriage
4. Contraception
   a. Oral contraception
   b. IUD
   c. Medroxyprogesterone acetate (Depo-Provera)

Causes of Amenorrhea

Physiologic
Prepuberty
Pregnancy
Lactation
Menopause

Hypothalamic
Stress
Weight change, e.g.,
    anorexia nervosa
Exercise induced
Pseudocyesis
Delayed puberty
Kallmann's syndrome
CNS lesions, e.g.,
    craniopharyngioma
Meningitis/
    encephalitis
"Hypothalamic dys-
    function"

Pituitary
Empty-sella syndrome
Hypopituitary: Shee-
    han's syndrome,
    Simmonds' syn-
    drome, sarcoidosis,
    radiation, isolated
    gonadotropin defi-
    ciency
Tumors
Hyperprolactinemia

Ovary
Gonadal dysgenesis,
    e.g., Turner's syn-
    drome
Premature ovarian
    failure:
    autoimmune; infec-
    tious, e.g., mumps;
    radiation; idiopathic
Resistant-ovary
    (Savage) syndrome
True or pseudo her-
    maphroditism: de-
    fect in testosterone
    production, andro-
    gen insensitivity,
    testicular dysgenesis
17α - hydroxylase
    deficiency
Tumors: estrogen and/
    or androgen secret-
    ing
Polycystic ovary syn-
    drome (PCOS)

Outlet Tract
Asherman's syndrome
Endometritis, e.g.,
    tuberculosis
Müllerian agenesis,
    Rokitansky-Küster-
    Hauser syndrome
Cervical agenesis/
    stenosis
Transverse vaginal
    septum
Imperforate hymen

Other
Adrenal disease, e.g.,
    insufficiency, Cush-
    ing's syndrome,
    congenital adrenal
    hyperplasia
Hyperthyroidism or
    hypothyroidism
Chronic disease, e.g.,
    liver, renal
Drugs, e.g., post-pill
    amenorrhea, ste-
    roids, opioids, tri-
    cyclic anti-
    depressants

5. Surgical history
   a. D & C
   b. Conization

General and Endocrine History

1. Stress, weight change, exercise
2. Acne, hirsutism
3. Heat/cold intolerance, hot flushes
4. Galactorrhea
5. Headache, visual change, anosmia
6. Acute or chronic illness
7. Infectious disorders: TB, mumps
8. Autoimmune diseases
9. Medications

PHYSICAL EXAMINATION

The physical examination, together with a thorough history, will lead to the correct diagnosis or at least greatly limit the differential diagnosis.

General Examination

1. Height, weight, body habitus, arm span
2. Vital signs
3. Skin—color, dry/oily/acne/hirsutism
4. Pubic and axillary hair
5. Visual fields, olfactory function
6. Thyroid size and consistency
7. Breast development, galactorrhea

Pelvic Examination

1. External genitalia: pubertal development, clitoral size, inguinal hernia, imperforate hymen.
2. Speculum examination: vaginal septum, cervical patency, vaginal maturation index, and cervical mucus—the in-office clue to estrogen status.
3. Bimanual examination: uterine size, adnexal mass, ovarian size.

LABORATORY EVALUATION

It is far too common to see women with amenorrhea or disordered menses subjected to a battery of tests, many of which are unnecessary in these cases. The laboratory should be used to confirm or exclude diagnoses that are suspected largely on the basis of the history and physical examination. The most significant contribution the laboratory can make is the *exclusion of pregnancy,* which is always a possibility in the reproductive-age female, regardless of history and physical findings. Pelvic ultrasonography should be considered. Important tests for *primary* amenorrhea include FSH, LH, prolactin, thyroid-stimulating hormone (TSH), karyotype, and bone age. In *secondary* amenorrhea, prolactin, TSH, and progestin challenge tests are necessary once pregnancy has been ruled out. Other tests may be necessary as shown in Figs. 28-1 to 28-3.

TREATMENT

Also see Figs. 28-1 to 28-3.
1. Estrogen replacement therapy: To establish and/or maintain secondary sexual characteristics and to prevent osteoporosis. A widely used regimen is Premarin 1.25 mg po qd days 1 to 25 and Provera 10 mg po qd days 16 to 25.
2. Adrenal replacement: Refer to medical endocrinologist.

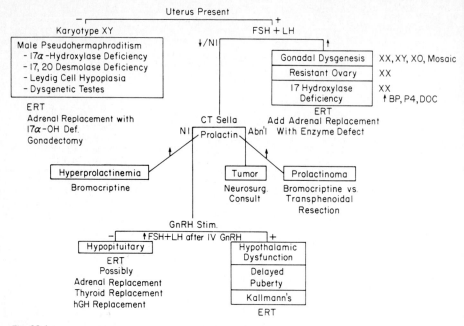

Fig. 28-1
Primary amenorrhea: absent secondary sexual development.

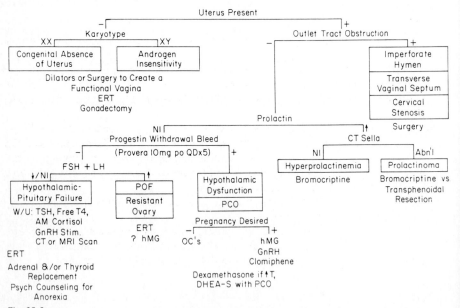

Fig. 28-2
Primary amenorrhea: secondary sexual development present.

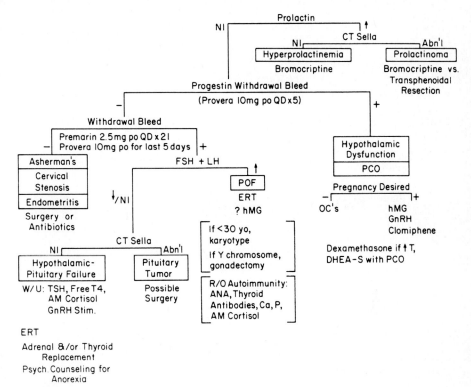

Fig. 28-3
Secondary amenorrhea.

3. Thyroid replacement: Synthroid 100 μg po qd. Adjust dose to keep TSH in normal range.
4. Bromocriptine: Begin with 2.5 mg po qhs. May increase up to 7.5 mg in split doses to suppress prolactin to normal range.
5. Oral contraceptives: Use a low-dose combination pill, i.e., 35 μg or less of ethinyl estradiol.
6. Human menopausal gonadotropins (hMGs): Each ampule contains 75 U FSH and 75 U LH. Daily intramuscular (IM) injections begin on day 3 and continue to follicle maturity; daily dose is based on ultrasonography and E_2 monitoring. 5000 U hCG given IM to simulate LH surge and trigger ovulation approximately 36 hours later. Refer to reproductive endocrinologist.
7. GnRH: Given IV/SQ in pulsatile fashion via a portable infusion pump. Refer to reproductive endocrinologist.
8. Clomiphene citrate: Starting dose is 50 mg po qd × 5, beginning on days 3 to 5. Increase by 50 mg each cycle, up to 200 mg, until ovulation is initiated.
9. Dexamethasone: 0.5 mg po qhs to suppress adrenal androgen secretion.

REVIEW
QUESTIONS

More than one correct answer is possible.
1. A 16-year-old girl presents with primary amenorrhea and absent secondary sexual development. Physical examination reveals a blind-ending vagina with no palpable uterus. BP is elevated. The gonadotropins are in the menopausal range. The most

likely diagnosis is:
a. Testicular feminization
b. Congenital absence of the uterus
c. 11β-hydroxylase deficiency
d. 17-hydroxylase deficiency (karyotype XY)
e. 21-hydroxylase deficiency

2. Elevated gonadotropins with primary amenorrhea are consistent with all of the following *except:*
a. Gonadal dysgenesis
b. Resistant ovary
c. 17-hydroxylase deficiency
d. Premature ovarian failure
e. Hyperprolactinemia

3. Absence of progestin withdrawal bleeding in secondary amenorrhea is consistent with:
a. Premature ovarian failure
b. Sheehan's syndrome
c. Asherman's syndrome
d. Polycystic ovary syndrome

4. Treatment for testicular feminization should include:
a. Androgen replacement
b. Gonadectomy
c. Creation of a neovagina
d. Estrogen replacement therapy

5. Initial workup for primary amenorrhea should include:
a. FSH/LH
b. Bone age
c. Karyotype
d. CT of the sella

6. Acceptable symptomatic treatments for polycystic ovary syndrome include:
a. Clomiphene citrate
b. Human menopausal gonadotropins
c. Oral contraceptives
d. Gonadotropin-releasing hormone

ANSWERS

1. d
2. e
3. a, b, c
4. b, c, d
5. a, b, c
6. a, b, c, d

BIBLIOGRAPHY

Aiman J, and Smentek C: Premature ovarian failure, Obstet Gynecol 66:9, 1985.
Mashchak C et al: Clinical and laboratory evaluation of patients with primary amenorrhea, Obstet Gynecol 57:715, 1981.
Schenker J, and Margalioth E: Intrauterine adhesions: an updated appraisal, Fertil Steril 37:593, 1982.
Speroff L, Glass R, and Case N: Clinical gynecologic endocrinology and infertility, Baltimore, 1989, Williams & Wilkins.
Wentz A, and Jones G: Prognosis in primary amenorrhea, Fertil Steril 29:614, 1978.

Evaluation of the Infertile Couple

29

Moon Kim

The term *infertility* implies the inability to become fertile. The couple (husband and wife) must be considered as a unit when evaluating their infertile condition. The diagnosis of infertility is made when pregnancy does not occur after a year of sexual intercourse without contraception. It is a relative term when applied to a couple, and in some situations it merely means reduced fertility or subfertility. The term *primary infertility* means that the couple has never conceived, and *secondary infertility* is applied to a couple developing an infertility problem after having had at least one previous conception.

In evaluating the infertile couple, various factors that may not affect a person's general health but do affect his or her reproductive abilities must be considered. The physician's awareness of the importance of the couple as a unit is essential in successfully evaluating and helping the couple through the often frustrating and painful experience of numerous tests and treatment. Frequent counseling and compassionate understanding by the physician and nurses will inspire the couple to cooperate and accept the outcome of treatment more readily even if no conception occurs.

INCIDENCE OF INFERTILITY

Although the exact incidence of infertility in any given population is unknown, it has been estimated that 10% to 15% of all married couples in the United States are infertile. Human fertility is influenced by many factors, such as ages of the couple, duration and frequency of sexual intercourse, and emotional factors. Currently available data indicate that fertility declines as the ages of the husband and wife advance (Tables 29-1 and 29-2).

Table 29-1 Female fertility as a function of age: conception results in artificial insemination of donor sperm

Conception Rates	Percent Achieving Conception			
	25 yrs	26 to 30 yrs	31 to 35 yrs	35 yrs
Mean rate per cycle	11	10.5	9.1	6.5
Cumulative rate after 12 cycles	73	74.1	61.5	53.6

Modified from Schwartz D et al: N Engl J Med 306:404, 1982.

Table 29-2 Expected fertility rates of fertile married women not using contraception

Age Groups	Percent Conceiving in 12 Months
20 to 24 yrs	86
25 to 29 yrs	78
30 to 34 yrs	63
35 to 39 yrs	52

Modified from Hendershot, GE, et al: Fam Plan Perspect 14:287, 1982.

Table 29-3 Incidence of infertility factors

Factors	Percent of Incidence
Male factor	35 to 40
Female factors	
Tubal factor	25 to 30
Ovulatory factor	10 to 15
Cervical factor	10 to 15
Other factors	5
Unexplained	5 to 10

FACTORS AFFECTING THE INFERTILE COUPLE

Besides some biologic factors such as ages and sexual life of the couple, various physical factors causing infertility must be considered. Although the exact incidence of each factor effecting infertility can not be determined, Table 29-3 shows the approximate incidence of various factors.

Many couples have more than one factor contributing to their infertility. Therefore it is important to thoroughly evaluate the couple to achieve conception. The basic evaluation of the infertile couple should include both (1) a complete review of history and physical examination, and (2) an evaluation of each infertility factor.

HISTORY AND EXAMINATION OF THE COUPLE

It is important to interview the couple at the initial visit, if possible. The initial interview and counseling give the couple a sense of working as a unit, rather than as individuals, and give them some ideas as to what future tests and counseling will entail. Like any new patient, the infertile couple should undergo a complete history review. The following list contains general information to be elicited at the initial visit.

1. Present illness: ages of the couple, duration of marriage and infertility, past history of contraceptive use, and results of previous studies.
2. Menstrual and obstetric history: irregular menses and obstetric complications.
3. Review of past history: history of pelvic infection, pelvic surgery and ruptured appendicitis, and endocrine diseases.
4. Other information such as sexual history (e.g., frequency, ejaculatory difficulty, and use of any lubricant), exercise, and weight loss or gain.

The initial examination should include a complete general and gynecologic examination for all female patients, and urological examination for husbands if needed. At the conclusion of the initial interview and examination the couple should be assured that all necessary tests will be done as rapidly and thoroughly as possible. The reasons for each test and how each is done should be explained to the couple. It is also important to explain the basics of human reproductive biology and the prognosis of various infertility factors.

BASIC DIAGNOSTIC TESTS

Numerous new diagnostic tests have been developed in the recent past, many of which are too complicated and may not offer any practical benefit to the patients. The physician must decide what tests can help the couple in clinical management of their infertility. The basic tests should include evaluation of the (1) male factor, (2) cervical factor, (3) tubal and uterine factors, (4) ovulatory factors, and (5) others if indicated. In addition, a complete blood count, blood typing, a Pap smear, a rubella antibody titer, and a fasting blood sugar test should be ordered. Inform the couple that these tests must be scheduled at appropriate times in relation to her ovulation.

Evaluation of Male Factor

One of the basic premises of successful fertility is that the husband must provide a sufficient number of healthy motile spermatozoa. The semen analysis is the single most important test in evaluating the male factor. The lack of standards in defining fertility or infertility in terms of sperm count, motility, and morphology has resulted in controversy over correct evaluation of the male factor. The commonly used criteria of normality for a semen sample are shown in Table 29-4.

The specimen should be collected after at least 2 days of sexual abstinence. Because of the well-known fluctuation in sperm count in an individual, 2 semen samples collected at least 2 weeks apart should be evaluated. See Table 29-5 for definitions of terms used in semen analysis.

Evaluation of Cervical Factor

The cervical canal is the first path in the female reproductive tract that spermatozoa must pass through to achieve fertilization. The endocervical epithelium produces a mucus secretion, stimulated by the rising level of estrogens near ovulation, to allow

Table 29-4   Normal semen analysis

Factor	Normal Value
Volume	2.0 ml
pH	7.2 to 7.8
Sperm concentration	20×10^6/ml
Total sperm count	40×10^6
Motility	At least 50% of spermatozoa with forward progression within 60 minutes after collection
Fructose	+

Modified from the WHO Laboratory Manual, 1987.

Table 29-5   Nomenclature for common semen variables

Term	Definition
Normospermia	Normal ejaculate (defined in Table 29-4)
Oligospermia	Sperm count lower than 20×10^5/ml
Asthenospermia	Fewer than 50% of spermatozoa with forward progression
Azoospermia	No spermatozoa in the ejaculate
Aspermia	No ejaculate

sperm migration, or penetration. This secretion has the following properties: (1) facilitates sperm penetration at or near time of ovulation, (2) protects sperm from the acid
environment of the vagina, (3) has a filtering effect, (4) serves as a possible sperm
reservoir, and (5) serves as a site for possible capacitation of sperm.

Evaluating sperm survival in the cervix following coitus is an important test in evaluating the cervical factor. The test was initially described by Sims in 1866 and Huhner
in 1913 and is thus called the Sims-Huhner postcoital test. Although its prognostic
value is somewhat controversial, this test is the only test that evaluates sperm-mucus
interaction in vivo. A favorable test result suggests (1) appropriate timing of the test
(near ovulation), (2) good quality of cervical mucus, (3) appropriate coital technique,
(4) probable absence of hostile factors in mucus (i.e., sperm antibody or low pH) and
in upper reproductive tract, and (5) probably normal sperm quality. However, although
the correlation between semen analysis and postcoital test is high, the postcoital test
can not replace semen analysis.

1. Postcoital test (Sims-Huhner test).
   a. Schedule the test as closely as possible to the time of presumed ovulation (i.e.,
      days 12 to 14 in women having a 28-day menstrual cycle).
   b. Advise the couple to have coitus after 2 to 3 days of sexual abstinence.
   c. Collect cervical mucus from the canal by gentle aspiration with a tuberculin sy-
      ringe (without needle) about 2 to 9 hours after coitus.
   d. Place the mucus sample on glass slide, protect with a cover glass, and examine
      under the microscope ($400\times$ magnification).
   e. Evaluate the quality of mucus (i.e., for ferning, cellularity, and spinnbarkeit).
2. Interpretation of the postcoital test.
   a. Greater than 10 sperm with directional movement within high-power field (HPF)
      of microscope—good.
   b. Total of 5 to 10 motile sperm within HPF—fair.
   c. Less than 5 motile sperm within HPF—poor.
   d. Sperm with shaking motion suggest possible presence of sperm antibody.
3. Causes of abnormal results of the postcoital tests.
   a. Abnormal semen quality.
   b. Incorrect timing of test in relation to ovulation time.
   c. Abnormal mucus secretion.
   d. Presence of sperm antibody.
   e. Inproper coital exposure (e.g., hypospadias, premature ejaculation, or ejacula-
      tion outside the vagina).

An abnormal test must be confirmed by repeating the test. Examining the vaginal
pool specimen for the presence or absence of sperm when performing the cervical mucus test is also recommended.

Evaluation of Tubal and Uterine Factors

The fallopian tube provides a channel for the transport of sperm and then the fertilized
oocyte. The tube does have important functions other than as a transport path. It provides for ovum pick up by the fimbria, its ciliary motion and muscular contractions
promote gamete transport, and its secretory activity provides nourishment for the fertilized gamete. The uterus is the site of a normal pregnancy and must be anatomically
normal for the growth of the fetus. Any pathologic condition compromising a normal
uterine cavity (e.g., septate uterus, intrauterine synechia, or submucous fibroid) should
be evaluated.

For evaluation of the tubal and uterine factors, hysterosalpingography (HSG), laparoscopy, and hysteroscopy can be performed. Tubal CO_2 insufflation (Rubin test), once a common procedure, has been abandoned because of frequent false findings.

1. HSG. This is the basic technique of evaluating tubal patency and the contour of the uterus (see upper box). An iodine-contrast media (either water-soluble or oil-based) is injected into the uterine cavity through a cannula that traverses the cervical canal. The filling of the uterine cavity and the tube(s) and the spillage of contrast media into the peritoneal cavity are observed on a fluoroscopic monitoring screen. In most instances only 1 film is taken for documentation, and less than 10 ml of the contrast media are needed.

   Several studies have shown that the incidence of pregnancy increases after HSG, suggesting some therapeutic benefit. Therefore it should be performed in all infertile patients unless it is contraindicated.

2. Laparoscopy. Laparoscopy is the most effective technique for evaluating peritoneal factors (e.g., tubal adhesions and endometriosis), fimbrial status, and patency of the tube (see lower box). This diagnostic procedure is usually performed under general anesthesia and requires distension of the peritoneal cavity (pneumoperitoneum) with CO_2 or N_2O. Through a small periumbilical incision, a laparoscope (0.5 to 1.1 cm diameter) is inserted to visualize pelvic organs directly. Usually, a second punc-

---

Hysterosalpingography

Schedule Time

Midfollicular phase after menstrual flow ceases (i.e., days 7 to 9 of a 28-day menstrual cycle).

Advantages

Simple, outpatient procedure.

Evaluation and documentation of uterine cavity, tubal patency and caliber, and uterotubal junction.

Evaluation of the site of occlusion if any.

Contraindications

Known allergy to iodine or active pelvic infection, including severe cervicitis or vaginitis.

Indications for Diagnostic Laparoscopy

Unexplained infertility after complete basic evaluation.

Abnormal hysterosalpingogram.

Anovulatory patients not conceiving after 6 ovulatory cycles after induction of ovulation.

History of PID, use of IUDs, or clinical evidence of endometriosis.

Preoperative evaluation for tubal surgery.

Before treatment with human menopausal gonadotropins.

ture is made suprapubically so that a probe can be used to mobilize the ovaries, tubes, and bowels for better evaluation. Chromotubation using a marker dye (i.e., indigo carmine or methylene blue) can show the tubal patency.

Although laparoscopy is an essential technique in evaluating the pathologic condition of the pelvis, it should be performed after weighing the advantages against its potential complications. Such complications, although rare with experienced examiners, include bowel perforation, bleeding, retroperitoneal hematoma, infection, problems resulting from pneumoperitoneum, and anesthesia-related complications. In general, it should be deferred until all other basic evaluations are completed.

3. Hysteroscopy. Hysteroscopy is an endoscopic examination of the uterine cavity. It is usually performed either to confirm the findings of the HSG or to therapeutically correct an intrauterine pathologic condition. To distend the uterine cavity for hysteroscopy, high molecular–weight dextran, water, or CO_2 can be used. Although hysteroscopy is indicated as a primary method of evaluating the uterine cavity in patients who are allergic to iodine-contrast medium, the routine use of hysteroscopy to diagnose a uterine factor in the presence of normal HSG results is in question (see accompanying box).

Currently, physicians are limited to determining the patency of the tube in evaluating tubal factors because evaluation of other important tubal functions is not yet possible. HSG and laparoscopy should not be considered competitive; each fulfills a unique role, thus they are complementary.

Hysteroscopy in Infertility

Indications

Abnormal HSG findings of uterine cavity (e.g., synechiae, submucous fibroid, polyp, or septate uterus).
Allergy to iodine.
Technical inability to do HSG (e.g., cervical stenosis or unable to tolerate HSG).

Contraindications

Active pelvic infection.
Profuse bleeding.

Evaluation of Ovulatory Factor

The function of ovulation and the quality of luteal function must be evaluated carefully. Three methods are commonly used for this evaluation: (1) basal body temperature (BBT) recordings, (2) determination of serum progesterone levels, and (3) endometrial biopsy. In addition, other hormonal evaluations (i.e., prolactin, TSH, and androgens) may be necessary. It should be remembered that these tests offer only presumptive evidence of ovulation.

1. BBT. The BBT must be measured daily, before any physical activity occurs, and recorded (Fig. 29-1). During the proliferative phase of the menstrual cycle, the BBT is usually below 98° F. Following ovulation, progesterone is secreted from the corpus luteum and is thermogenic, thus resulting in a rise of BBT (0.5° to 1° F). Although BBT recordings can not determine the exact time of ovulation, the physician can estimate the approximate time of ovulation and the length of the luteal

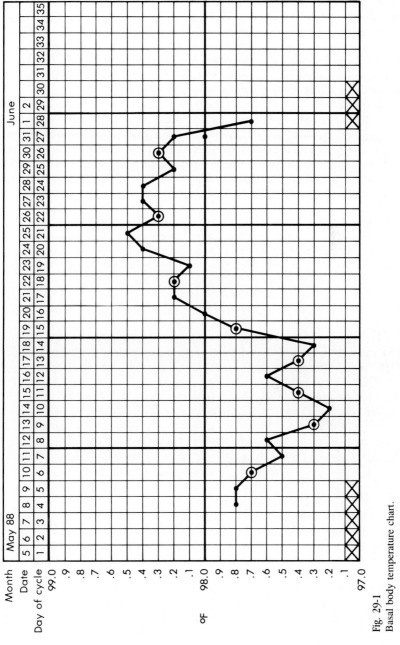

Fig. 29-1
Basal body temperature chart.

phase after the entire cycle is completed. It is not possible to predict when ovulation may occur based on BBT recordings.

The rise in BBT usually lasts for 13 to 15 days in an ovulatory cycle. A shorter luteal phase (rise in BBT lasting less than 12 days) suggests luteal phase deficiency (LPD), in which ovulation occurs but there is deficient function or shortened life of the corpus luteum, usually resulting in a deficiency of progesterone secretion and/or of the development of secretory endometrium. As both progesterone and a normal endometrial environment are important in maintaining early conception, LPD may cause poor implantation even if fertilization occurs. LPD must be confirmed by endometrial biopsy and/or a progesterone level determination.

2. Determination of serum progesterone levels. Progesterone is a major secretory product of the corpus luteum, and its level peaks at the midluteal phase of the ovulatory cycle. A serum progesterone level greater than 3 ng/ml is presumptive evidence of luteal function, and a level greater than 15 ng/ml at the midluteal phase suggests normal secretory function of the corpus luteum. However, because of considerable variation in progesterone secretion and levels on any given day, a single determination is not adequate for evaluation of the luteal phase, and it cannot represent the effect on endometrium. Thus both endometrial biopsy and the serum level of progesterone should be used in the evaluation of luteal function.

3. Endometrial biopsy. The endometrium is a target tissue for ovarian hormones; before ovulation it shows a proliferative phase under estrogen stimulation, but it develops a secretory pattern when progesterone stimulation occurs. The histologic evaluation of endometrium correlates well with the days of the ovulatory cycle. Therefore a successful endometrial biopsy gives information regarding ovulation, the functional aspect of the corpus luteum, and the normalcy of the endometrium (Table 29-6).

An endometrial biopsy can be performed at the physician's office without any anesthesia in most cases, although the patient may experience some mild discomfort. This discomfort can be relieved by an explanation of the procedure and the use of analgesics such as antiprostaglandin agents. The traditional rigid curettes have been replaced by malleable, smaller ones.

The best time to perform the endometrial biopsy has been a subject of some controversy. Because the objective of the biopsy is to evaluate the condition of endometrium in relation to luteal function and implantation of the conceptus, it is best performed during the late luteal phase (i.e., days 25 to 27 of a 28-day menstrual

Table 29-6   Evaluation of ovulatory factor

	BBT	Serum Progesterone	Endometrial Biopsy
Time for the test	Daily throughout the cycle	Midluteal phase (days 20 to 22)	Late luteal phase (days 25 to 27)
Presumptive evidence of ovulation	Biphasic pattern	>5 ng/ml (any time)	Secretory pattern
Normal luteal phase	BBT rise for >12 days	>15 ng/ml (days 20 to 22)	In-phase endometrium (within ± 2 days)
Evidence suggestive of LPD	BBT rise for <12 days	<10 ng/ml (days 20 to 22)	Out-of-phase endometrium (>3 days)

cycle). The risk of disturbing a pregnancy is apparently minimal, but the patient may be advised to avoid conception in the study cycle.

Other Infertility Tests

Numerous other tests have been described that identify the etiologic factor(s) of infertility. However, some of them have not correlated well with clinical aspects and remain more as investigational tools. All the tests discussed in this chapter are standard. The physician may perform additional diagnostic procedures—sperm immunologic tests, bacteriologic culture of the reproductive system, in vitro/in vivo sperm-mucus penetration tests, a hamster zone-free egg penetration test, and human in vitro fertilization. Unfortunately, detailed discussions of these tests are beyond the scope of this chapter.

REVIEW
QUESTIONS

1. A favorable or normal postcoital test result suggests the following except:
   a. Good quality of cervical mucus.
   b. Appropriate timing of the test.
   c. No need to get semen analysis.
   d. Absence of hostile factors in mucus.
   e. Normal coital exposure.
2. The following findings are characteristic of LPD except:
   a. Rise in BBT lasting longer than 12 days.
   b. Less than 10 ng/ml of serum progesterone at midluteal phase.
   c. Secretory endometrium out of phase by 3 or more days.
   d. Abnormal follicular development.
   e. Inadequate luteinizing hormone stimulation.
3. The following statements are correct except:
   a. The conception rates declines sharply after age of 35 years.
   b. Hysterosalpingography is best done during the midfollicular phase (menstrual day 7 to 10).
   c. Normal laparoscopic findings eliminate the need for hysterosalpingogram.
   d. Serum levels of progesterone >5 ng/ml is presumptive evidence of ovulation.
   e. Diagnostic laparoscopy is indicated in evaluating women with unexplained infertility.

ANSWERS

1. c
2. a
3. c

BIBLIOGRAPHY

Davajan V, and Mishell DR, Jr: Evaluation of the infertile couple. In Davajan V, and Mishell DR, Jr, editors: Infertility, contraception and reproductive endocrinology, Oradell, NJ, 1986, Medical Economics Books.

Hirsch MB, and Mosher WD: Characteristics of infertile women in the United States and their use of infertility services, Fertil Steril 47:618, 1987.

Kliger BE: Evaluation, therapy and outcome in 493 infertile couples, Fertil Steril 41:40, 1982.

Musich J, and Behrman JR: Infertility laparoscopy in perspective: review of five hundred cases, Am J Obstet Gynecol 143:293, 1982.

Rousseau S, et al: The expectancy of pregnancy for "normal" infertile couples, Fertil Steril 40:768, 1983.

Anatomic Defects
of the Pelvis

30

David Bell

Vaginal relaxation is a problem commonly seen by gynecologists, and it may account for 20% to 60% of gynecologic surgery. Pelvic prolapse is most often associated with multiparity and vaginal birth, especially when associated with vaginal lacerations. In addition, contributing factors include the aging process and the onset of menopause, which are associated with declining estrogen levels and atrophy of the vaginal tissues. Chronic coughing, whether related to obstructive pulmonary disease or cigarette smoking, and heavy lifting are additional sources that contribute to increased intraabdominal pressure, which is transmitted to the pelvic floor.

Patients with vaginal prolapse may often present with complaints of a vaginal mass or vaginal pressure and need to be reassured that a tumor or malignancy is not present. More common, however, is the association of urologic complaints with prolapse. Urinary stress incontinence is perhaps the most frequent urologic complaint associated with vaginal prolapse, but the gynecologist must rule out the presence of other causes of urinary incontinence before initiating therapy.

This chapter addresses the diagnosis and management of pelvic relaxation and the various anatomic abnormalities involving the vaginal canal and the surrounding structures associated with pelvic support. The management of urinary stress incontinence is particularly emphasized.

PELVIC SUPPORT (Fig. 30-1)
Muscular Support

1. The pelvic diaphragm is composed of the levator ani muscle (anteriorly), which is a blend of the pubococcygeal muscle, the iliococcygeal muscle, and the puborectal muscle; and the coccygeal muscle (posteriorly), which extends from the ischial spine to the surface of the sacrum and coccyx.
2. Internal obturator muscle.
3. Urogenital diaphragm includes the superficial and deep transverse perineal muscles.

Pelvic Ligaments

1. Pubocervical (endopelvic fascia)
2. Cardinal (Mackenrodt's)
3. Uterosacral
4. Pubourethral

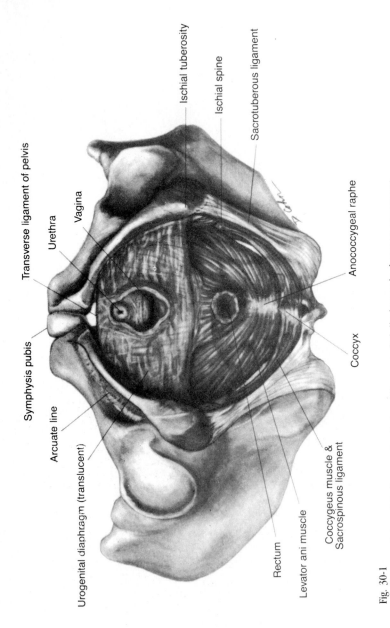

Fig. 30-1
Musculature of the pelvic floor, perineal view. The urogenital diaphragm is shown as transparent. From Jones HW III, Wentz AC, and Burnett LS, editors: Novak's textbook of gynecology, ed 11, Baltimore, 1988, Williams & Wilkins.

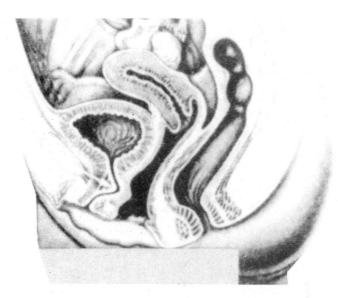

Fig. 30-2
Sagittal section of pelvis. Arrow indicates site of urethrocele.
From Howkins J: Shaw's textbook of gynaecology, ed 9, Edinburgh, 1971, Churchill-Livingstone.

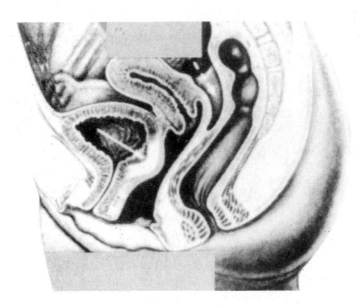

Fig. 30-3
Sagittal section of pelvis indicating site of cystocele.
From Howkins J: Shaw's textbook of gynaecology, ed 9, Edinburgh, 1971, Churchill-Livingstone.

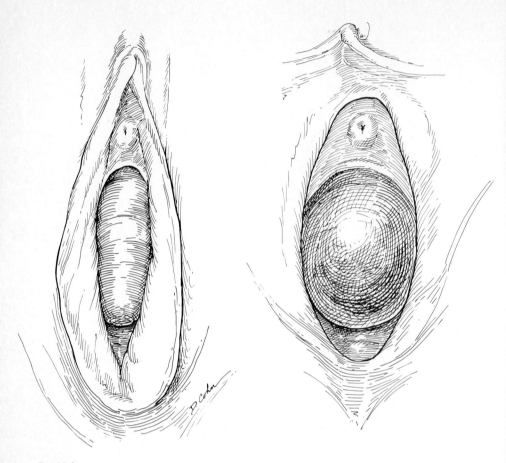

Fig. 30-4
Patient with second-degree cystocele. *Left,* without straining; *right,* with straining.
From Jones HW III, Wentz AC, and Burnett LS, editors: Novak's textbook of gynecology, ed 11, Baltimore, 1988, Williams & Wilkins.

TYPES OF VAGINAL RELAXATION
Urethrocele

1. Anatomic displacement of the urethra into the vaginal lumen (Fig. 30-2)
2. Loss of support from:
   a. Urogenital diaphragm
   b. Pubocervical ligaments
   c. Pubourethral ligaments

Cystocele

1. Anatomic displacement of the bladder into the vaginal canal (Figs. 30-3 and 30-4)
2. Represents herniation through the pubocervical fascia

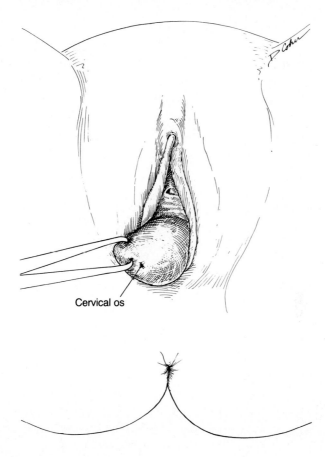

Fig. 30-5
Patient with third-degree uterovaginal prolapse.
From Jones HW III, Wentz AC, and Burnett LS, editors: Novak's textbook of gynecology, ed 11, Baltimore, 1988, Williams & Wilkins.

Uterine Prolapse

1. Descent of the cervix and uterus along the axis of the vaginal canal (Figs. 30-5 and 30-6)
2. Anatomic defect in lateral cervical ligaments
3. Associated with other forms of pelvic relaxation: descent of cervix influenced by cervical elongation
4. Degree of prolapse
   a. First degree—short of hymenal ring
   b. Second degree—the cervix reaches the level of hymenal ring
   c. Third degree—the cervix extends beyond the introitus (complete procidentia)

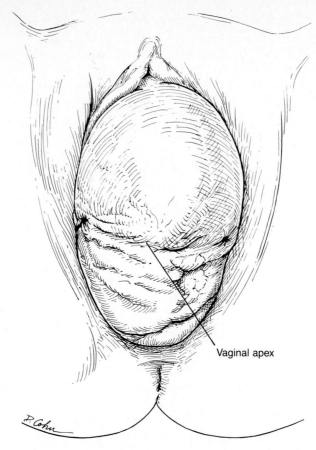

Vaginal apex

P. Cohn

Fig. 30-6
Patient with large, third-degree vaginal vault prolapse following hysterectomy. The apex of the vaginal vault is identified by a transverse scar with a "dimple" at either end. Anteriorly, there is a large
cystocele covered by smooth, shiny vaginal mucosa. Posteriorly, the rugal pattern is preserved.
From Jones HW III, Wentz AC, and Burnett LS, editors: Novak's textbook of gynecology, ed 11, Baltimore, 1988, Williams & Wilkins.

Enterocele

Enterocele represents the herniation of the cul-de-sac peritoneum through the posterior
vaginal wall (Fig. 30-7)—contains small bowel or omentum in hernia sac.

Rectocele

1. Represents the protrusion or herniation of the rectum into the vaginal lumen; associated with a defect of fascia of the posterior vaginal wall and rectovaginal septum
   (Fig. 30-8).
2. May be associated with incomplete evacuation of the rectum and require manual
   replacement.

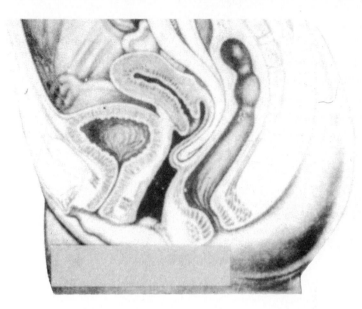

Fig. 30-7
Sagittal section of pelvis indicating enterocele.
From Howkins J: Shaw's textbook of gynaecology, ed 9, Edinburgh, 1971, Churchill-Livingstone.

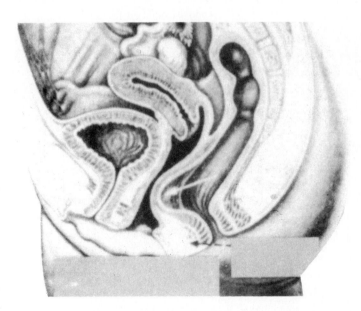

Fig. 30-8
Sagittal section of pelvis. Arrows indicate rectocele.
From Howkins J: Shaw's textbook of gynaecology, ed 9, Edinburgh, 1971, Churchill-Livingstone.

3. Must distinguish between rectocele and enterocele.
   a. Enterocele protrudes immediately posterior to the cervix
   b. Rectovaginal examination reveals enterocele contents to lie between the anterior rectal wall and posterior vagina
   c. Speculum examination reveals transverse furrow between enterocele and rectocele

DIAGNOSIS OF VAGINAL RELAXATION

See Table 30-1.

Differential Diagnosis

1. Congenital anterior vaginal wall cyst: Gartner's duct cyst
2. Pelvic mass
3. Urethral diverticulum
4. Inclusion dermoid cyst
5. Cervical fibroid
6. Cervical polyp

TREATMENT OF VAGINAL RELAXATIONS
Medical

1. Vaginal pessary may be useful:
   a. During pregnancy
   b. For poor surgical candidate
   c. As therapeutic test to confirm surgical benefit
   d. For patient who prefers conservative management
   e. For symptomatic relief while awaiting surgery
   f. As an aid in the diagnosis of urinary stress incontinence

Surgical Therapy

1. Cystourethrocele
   a. Anterior colporrhaphy
   b. Add Kelly plication if stress incontinence
   c. Complications include postoperative urinary retention and stress incontinence

Table 30-1 Symptoms of Vaginal Relaxation

	Cystourethrocele	Uterine and Vaginal Prolapse	Rectocele and Enterocele
Vaginal pressure	X	X	X
Sensation of mass in vagina	X	X	X
Low backache		X	X
Bloody discharge		X	
Incomplete evaluation of stool			X
Urinary symptoms			
Hesitancy, frequency, and urgency	X		
Retention	X	X	
Stress incontinence	X		
Chronic UTI	X		

2. Rectocele and enterocele
   a. Posterior colporrhaphy
   b. Complications include dyspareunia
3. Uterovaginal prolapse
   a. Vaginal hysterectomy
   b. McCall culdoplasty—corrects coexisting enterocele and obliterates posterior cul-de-sac
   c. Anterior and posterior colporrhaphy
   d. Sacrospinous ligament fixation
   e. Abdominal approach for vagina apex sacropexy and Moschcowitz procedure
   f. Complications include shortening of the vagina, bowel and bladder injury, ureteral injury, infection, and subsequent vault prolapse
4. Enterocele
   a. Vaginal approach involving excision of hernia sac and McCall culdoplasty plicating the uterosacral ligaments
   b. Abdominal approach using Moschcowitz procedure with pursestring sutures placed in the posterior cul-de-sac

URINARY INCONTINENCE (Fig. 30-9)

Involuntary loss of urine is a troubling and potentially disabling condition that is often, but not always, caused by pelvic relaxation. Great care in diagnosis is required to dis-

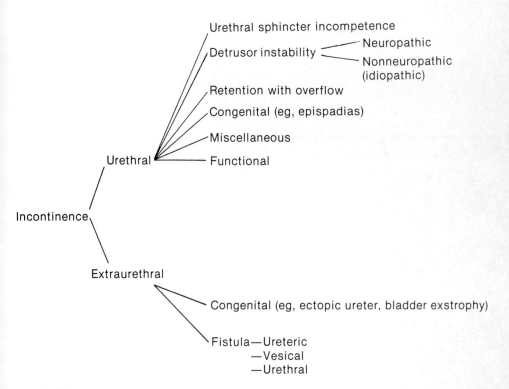

Fig. 30-9
Classification of incontinence.
From Stanton SL, editor: Clinical gynecologic urology, St. Louis, 1984, The CV Mosby Co.

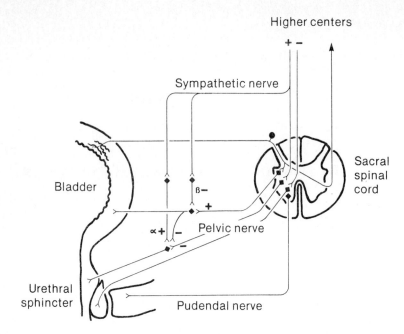

Fig. 30-10
Summary of possible organization for peripheral nervous supply to lower urinary tract. Preganglionic parasympathetic fibers and postganglionic sympathetic fibers both synapse with ganglion cells close to, and within, bladder wall. Arrangement in relation to urethra may be morphologically similar but functionally different. Somatic nerve supply to intramural urethral striated muscle runs with pelvic nerve (and is vulnerable during pelvic surgery).
From Stanton SL, editor: Clinical gynecologic urology, St. Louis, 1984, The CV Mosby Co.

tinguish the various causes, only some of which will improve with surgical therapy. Others require medical treatment and may actually worsen after surgery for presumed pelvic relaxation.

Innervation of the Bladder and Urethra (Fig. 30-10)

1. Parasympathetic
   a. Sacral nerves (S2 to S4)
   b. Contraction of the detrusor muscle
2. Sympathetic
   a. Sacral sympathetic trunk
   b. α-adrenergic: urethral contraction
   c. β-adrenergic: detrusor relaxation

Control of Micturition

1. Cerebral cortex–brain stem loop
   a. Permits voluntary control of micturition
   b. Damage results in loss of voluntary control of micturition, CNS tumors, cerebrovascular accidents
   c. Loss of control leads to uninhibited detrusor contractions

2. Brain stem—sacral pathway
   a. Results in detrusor contraction with full bladder
   b. Inhibited by cerebral cortex–brain stem loop
   c. Damaged loop results in uninhibited detrusor contractions—vesicosphincter dyssynergia, spinal-cord transection with initial detrusor paralysis or areflexia and/or delayed uninhibited detrusor reflex contractions
3. Vesical-sacral-sphincter pathway
   a. Afferent impulses—travel from bladder to sacral center
   b. Efferent impulses—directed to the smooth muscle of the bladder and urethra and the striated muscle of the pelvic floor and urethral sphincter
   c. Provides coordination between bladder and urethra for normal micturition
   d. Damaged loop leads to dyssynergia—multiple sclerosis, cord injury, diabetic neuropathy
4. Cerebral cortex–sacral pathway
   a. Coordinates cortical, spinal, and perineal function

Urinary Urge Incontinence

1. Involuntary loss of urine with strong desire to urinate
2. May be associated with involuntary detrusor contraction
3. History of urgency warrants complex urodynamic studies
4. Symptoms
   a. Urgency
   b. Frequency
   c. Nocturia
   d. Enuresis
5. Urodynamic studies reveal reduced bladder capacity
6. Causes
   a. Central nervous system diseases
   b. Multiple sclerosis
   c. Urinary infections
   d. Bladder tumors
   e. Interstitial cystitis
   f. Detrusor instability
7. Management
   a. *No* call for surgical management
   b. Anticholinergic therapy—oxybutynin hydrochloride (Ditropan) 5 mg tid; imipramine (Tofranil) 25 mg tid

Urinary Stress Incontinence

1. Involuntary loss of urine from the urethra when the intravesical pressure exceeds the maximal urethral pressure in the absence of detrusor activity
2. Symptoms
   a. Loss of urine when coughing, sneezing, or laughing
   b. Loss of urine is small—rarely emptying bladder
   c. Rarely occurs in supine position
3. Physical findings include pelvic relaxation involving cystocele and urethrocele, positive Q-tip sign (posterior rotation of the urethrovesical junction during Valsalva's maneuver)
4. Urodynamics
   a. Separate pure stress incontinence from detrusor instability

b. Uroflowmetry—usually normal flow rates (exceed 15 ml/sec); large cystocele may decrease flow rates

c. Cystometry—normal bladder compliance; absence of detrusor contraction

d. Urethral-pressure profile—decreased urethral length with bladder filling; decreased transmission of intraabdominal pressure yielding negative closure pressures

e. Residual urine—normal bladder emptying unless large cystocele is present

5. Treatment of urinary stress incontinence
   a. Conservative treatment will often suffice and should be tried first in most cases: Kegel's exercises, estrogen replacement
   b. Surgical: anterior colporrhaphy; Burch retropubic urethropexy—elevation of urethrovesical junction to Cooper's ligament; Marshall-Marchetti-Krantz operation—uses posterior surface of symphysis pubis; Stamey procedure; modified Pereyra procedure—combined vaginal-retropubic procedure

REVIEW
QUESTIONS

More than one correct answer is possible.

1. A patient with the diagnosis of urinary stress incontinence may report which of the following symptoms?
   a. Loss of urine while jogging
   b. Loss of urine at night while sleeping
   c. Inability to initiate voiding and empty bladder completely
   d. Loss of large volumes of urine at a time

2. Detrusor instability is diagnosed by which of the following?
   a. Positive Q-tip sign
   b. History of nocturnal enuresis
   c. Loss of urine while coughing
   d. Complex urodynamics

3. Urinary stress incontinence is best defined as:
   a. The involuntary loss of urine through the urethra in association with detrusor contraction.
   b. The voluntary loss of urine through the urethra in association with detrusor contraction.
   c. The involuntary loss of urine through the urethra in the absence of detrusor contraction and when intravesical pressure exceeds the maximal urethra pressure.
   d. Any loss of urine during physical exertion.

4. The major roles of complex urodynamics are:
   a. To distinguish pure stress incontinence from other forms of urinary incontinence, such as detrusor instability
   b. To predict bladder hypotonia after surgical correction
   c. To predict which patients may be better candidates for medical therapy, as compared to surgical therapy, for urinary incontinence
   d. There is no role for complex urodynamics

5. All of the following may be helpful to correct urinary stress incontinence except:
   a. Kegel's exercises
   b. Estrogen replacement
   c. Tofranil
   d. Burch retropubic urethropexy
   e. Kelly plication

6. Causes of detrusor instability could include which of the following?
   a. Parkinson's disease
   b. Urinary infections
   c. Idiopathic
   d. Radiation cystitis
   e. All of the above
7. Correction of an enterocele may include which of the following?
   a. Vaginal hysterectomy
   b. McCall culdoplasty
   c. Moschcowitz procedure
   d. Sacrospinous ligament fixation
   e. All of the above
8. Complications of an anterior colporrhaphy may include all of the following except:
   a. Urinary stress incontinence
   b. Vesicovaginal fistula
   c. Dyspareunia
   d. Rectovaginal fistula
   e. Urethrovaginal fistula

ANSWERS

1. a, c
2. b, d
3. c
4. a, b, c
5. c
6. e
7. e
8. d

BIBLIOGRAPHY

Burnett LS: Relaxations, malpositions, fistulas, and incontinence. In Jones HW, Wentz AC, and Burnett LS, editors: Novak's textbook of gynecology, ed 11, Baltimore, 1988, Williams & Wilkins.
Peters WA, and Thornton N: Surgical anatomy of the perirectal fascia: a gynecologic perspective, Obstet Gynecol Surv 42(10):605, 1987.
Stanton SL: Vaginal prolapse. In Stanton SL, editor: Clinical gynecologic urology, St. Louis, 1984, The CV Mosby Co.

Sexual Dysfunction

31

Stephen F. Pariser

Sexual issues are central to the professional concerns of the obstetrician-gynecologist. From puberty to menopause, the female patient and her sexual health are the principal concerns of good reproductive health care. Sexual development, masturbation, fertility, sexually transmitted infections, pregnancy, infertility, and maturation leading to menopause are all the province of the obstetrician-gynecologist. Because of the sensitive nature of sexual and reproductive issues, solid rapport with the patient is the cornerstone of women's good health care. Accurate information, essential for correct diagnosis and treatment, demands a comfortable physician-patient relationship. The sexual history gathering techniques given below are useful, not only in dealing with sexual problems, but also in approaching any patient.

SEXUAL HISTORY GATHERING

When establishing a new patient relationship it is helpful to inform the patient that if sexual problems develop, the physician will listen in a nonjudgmental fashion.

1. Patient comfort can be encouraged by:
   a. Attending to privacy.
   b. Avoiding "why" questions, which lead to defensive responses.
   c. Asking open-ended questions that are not threatening and give the patient the opportunity to tell her story freely.
   d. Progressing from general to specific points.
   e. Using anatomic and professional terminology, which is respectful and nonthreatening.
   f. Acknowledging verbal and body language behavioral cues suggesting anxiety, which gives the patient support and reduces anxiety.
2. Problem definition.
   a. Sexual history gathering begins with patient's description of her or her partner's problem.
   b. Clinicians need to clarify imprecise terms. For example, frigidity may be used to describe various concerns ranging from loss of desire, difficulty with arousal, orgasmic dysfunction, or a hostile relationship where a partner is averse to intimacy because of hurt and anger.
   c. Sexual difficulties are frequently situation-related. Difficulty with orgasm may be limited to coitus and not experienced during masturbation.
   d. Problem duration provides a context for exploring relationship issues, family dynamics, or associated illnesses. Sexual disinterest following childbirth may

signal libidinal changes related to breast-feeding, the stress of having a difficult newborn, or postpartum depression. Medication changes can lead to dysfunction (e.g., antihypertensives may result in anorgasmia or loss of libido). Relationships may change during family illnesses, leading to resentment and sexual disinterest.

3. Patient understanding of problem. Self-blame is rampant in dealing with sexual difficulties. A patient may develop obsessive concern about the nature of her vaginal secretion after her partner blamed his impotence on the gritty nature he felt. She may also be experiencing a major depression, which would make it difficult for her to feel well. Such patients may initially complain of chronic candidiasis, vaginitis, or dyspareunia.

4. Previous treatment approaches. Inquiry about previous interventions and their success can provide the clinician with new approaches.

5. Psychosexual history.
   a. A history of sexual assault is a common finding among women with unexplained pelvic pain.
   b. Repressive, judgmental parenting may discourage sexual maturation and comfort, which limits sexual response and interferes with arousal and orgasm.

6. Medical/surgical history. Good sexual relationships benefit from good health. Mood disorders, diabetes, multiple sclerosis, heart disease, and endocrine disorders such as hypothyroidism are among the many medical ailments that can impair healthy sexual response.

Sensitivity, patience, and concern enable the physician to inspire rapport and thus hear about sexual concerns from patients. The breadth of obstetrics and gynecology is so sexually centered that the value of rapport and the ability to direct patients with sexual concerns are invaluable and essential.

CATEGORIES OF SEXUAL DISORDERS

Sexual disorders are separated into psychophysiologic categories by the American Psychiatric Association (see Bibliography).

1. Sexual desire disorders.
   a. Hypoactive sexual desire disorder. Diminished sexual desire or fantasy not secondary to a major depression that may lead to lowered libido. Drugs and medical illnesses such as arthritis and heart disease can inhibit desire. Relationships troubled with conflict often suffer from low levels of desire; however, loss of desire is often not global but rather is partner-specific.
   b. Sexual aversion disorder. Extreme aversion to genital contact with a sexual partner. This disorder suggests traumatic sexual experience or other severe psychiatric syndromes.

2. Sexual arousal disorders.
   a. Female sexual arousal disorder. This often manifests as difficulty in attaining or maintaining the physiologic vasocongestive response to arousal, which leads to natural vaginal lubrication. Many women experience difficulty with this arousal disorder because they permit themselves to undergo coitus without the necessary comfortable mind-set with regard to their partner or adequate precoital nurturing.
   b. Male erectile disorder. Difficulty in attaining and maintaining an erection to permit coital completion. This disorder is common among diabetic men. Some estimates suggest that up to 60% of adult male diabetics will experience impotence. Physical examination and sleep laboratory studies are useful in determin-

ing the presence of organic impotence by examining nocturnal penile tumescence. Performance anxiety is often a major contributing factor in psychogenic impotence. Drugs such as antihypertensive agents and psychotropic agents are among the many sources of drug-induced impotence. A careful drug history is essential in evaluating impotence.
3. Orgasm disorders.
   a. Inhibited female orgasm. Delay or absence of orgasm following an adequate phase of excitement. In some women it will be a problem limited to coitus; in others it will also involve masturbatory (self or partner) activity. It may sometimes be a symptom of a depressive illness, an adverse drug reaction, or inhibition.
   b. Inhibited male orgasm.
   c. Premature ejaculation.
4. Sexual pain disorders.
   a. Dyspareunia. Genital pain related to precoital, coital, or postcoital activity that is not caused by inadequate vasocongestive arousal response or vaginismus. Careful gynecologic and, in some instances, lower genital colposcopic examination may be indicated to exclude organic factors. Psychiatric syndromes such as a major depression or an obsessive-compulsive disorder may be factors in this disorder. Antidepressant medication and supportive psychotherapy using behavioral techniques are often helpful.
   b. Vaginismus. Involuntary spasm of the muscles of the outer third of the vagina that impairs coitus. Often begins after a painful coital experience, such as forced penetration or coitus during an infection. May be associated with inhibition and fear. When physical examination excludes an organic source of pain, behavioral techniques, including the progressive use of dilators, may be helpful. Often the patient's own fingers will be the least-threatening desensitizing device.

PREGNANCY

Evidence suggests that sexual activity declines during pregnancy, requiring some time to return to prepregnancy levels.
1. Decreased sexual desire.
2. Decreased coital and noncoital contact.
3. Diminished orgasmic response.
Breast-feeding mothers may show a reduction of sexual interest as compared with nonlactating mothers. Elevated prolactin levels in lactating mothers may lead to vaginal dryness by lowering estrogen levels. Coital activity merits discussion during prenatal visits and, in certain instances, will be restricted (e.g., preterm labor).

MENOPAUSE

Sexual comfort can be enhanced with estrogen replacement therapy, reducing atrophic lower genital changes. Sexual intimacy, coital or noncoital, can continue with maturity as long as health and interest permit.

INFERTILITY

Infertility evaluations are incomplete without a sexual history. Sexual causes of infertility include the following:
1. Lack of coital frequency.
2. Improper coital technique.
3. Inappropriate timing of coitus.

4. Sexual dysfunction.
   a. Hypoactive sexual desire disorder.
   b. Sexual aversion disorder.
   c. Male erectile disorder.
   d. Inhibited male orgasm.
   e. Premature ejaculation.
   f. Dyspareunia.
   g. Vaginismus.
Sexual complications of infertility include the following:
1. Loss of spontaneity and relaxation.
2. Performance anxiety can lead to impotence.
3. Anger, resentment, and blame can interfere with relationship.

GYNECOLOGIC ONCOLOGY

Preinvasive and invasive disease can cause significant anxiety, impairing both the libido and sexual relationships. Viral changes associated with lower genital cervical, vulvar, and vaginal intraepithelial neoplasias can disrupt sexual relationships.
1. Treatment can be disruptive, restricting sexual intercourse.
2. Concern about recurrence of invasive and or preinvasive disease provokes anxiety.
Radical surgery or radiation can interfere with sexual function in some cases.
1. Radical Wertheim hysterectomy for cervical cancer results in vaginal shortening.
2. Vulvectomy may require clitorectomy, which does not necessarily cause anorgasmia.
3. Body-image changes need to be addressed.
4. Preoperative and preradiation therapy sexual assessment is important to offer assistance with recovery and resumption of sexual and other intimate relationships.

SUMMARY

1. Sexual concerns are intertwined with obstetric and gynecologic care.
2. Open-ended interviewing with appropriate use of anatomic terms facilitates patient comfort during discussions.
3. Preoperative and prenatal interviews will benefit by appropriate education and referral for sexual dysfunctions and marital problems.

REVIEW QUESTIONS

1. A 32-year-old woman has been married for 9 years and presents with a complaint of pain with intercourse for the last several months. What is the first step in her evaluation?
   a. Pelvic examination for vulvar and vaginal infection
   b. Laparoscopy to look for endometriosis
   c. Referral to a marriage counselor
   d. An open-ended history of the problem
2. Common causes of pain with intercourse in the female include which of the following:
   a. Inadequate lubrication
   b. Vaginal or vulvar infection
   c. Previous history of sexual trauma
   d. Depressive mood disorders
   e. All of the above

3. Which of the following are associated with inadequate sexual lubrication in the female?
   a. Menopause
   b. Lactation
   c. Danazol therapy for endometriosis
   d. a, b, and c
   e. a and c
4. Libido can be inhibited by
   a. Lactation
   b. Cervical intraepithelial neoplasia
   c. Both
   d. Neither

ANSWERS

1. d
2. e
3. d
4. c

BIBLIOGRAPHY

Alder EM, et al: Hormones, mood and sexuality in lactating women, Br J Psychiatr 148:74, 1986.
American Psychiatric Association: Diagnostic and statistical manual, III-R, Washington, DC, 1986, American Psychiatric Association.
Anderson BL, et al: Sexual dysfunction and signs of gynecologic cancer, Cancer 57:1880, 1986.
Pariser SF, Levine SB, and Gardner ML, editors: Clinical sexuality, New York, 1983, Marcel Dekker, Inc.

Menopause and Osteoporosis

Frederick P. Zuspan

The human female is the only mammal that lives beyond her reproductive-age span. There is no good animal model for studying menopause, which should be considered as an endocrinopathy. Menopause is a disease of the twentieth century because, at the turn of the century, the white female lived for an average of 47 years and the black female for an average of 38 years. There are currently 120 million women living in the United States; 35 million have no ovarian function, and approximately 24 million are on some form of hormone replacement therapy.

Osteoporosis will afflict at least 20 million of the women living today. There will be 1.5 million fractures per year at a cost of $6 billion, and 35% of the women who have major fractures will die within 6 months of the fracture. Osteoporosis, a preventable disease, is a major health hazard (Table 32-1) in this country because the lifespan of women is now 82 years.

PHYSIOLOGY OF MENOPAUSE

The average age at which menopause occurs is 51 years. The 5 to 8 years preceding menopause are known as the *climacteric,* which is associated with the following:
1. Fluctuating changes in ovarian function.
2. Occasional prolonged or absent menstrual cycles.
3. The presence of occasional anovulation.
4. Occasional premenstrual hot flushes.

Once menses have ceased, the condition is known as *menopause* and the endocrinopathy that began in the previous years now becomes gradually more apparent, as evidenced both by clinical symptoms (Table 32-2) and by laboratory findings as follows:
1. FSH level greater than 40 mU/ml—an accepted indicator of the onset of menopause.
2. An increase in gonadotropin-releasing hormone.
3. Decrease in estradiol levels from an average of 120 pg/ml to 18 pg/ml—after cessation of ovarian function.
4. Decrease in androstenedione—produced in equal quantities by ovaries and adrenal glands before menopause, but after menopause, 80% is produced by adrenal glands. Postmenopausal level is 900 pg/ml, down from 1500 pg/ml.
5. Decrease in sex hormone binding globulin (SHBG).

DIAGNOSIS OF MENOPAUSE

See Table 32-2.
1. Absence of menses for 1 year.
2. FSH greater than 40 mU/ml.

Table 32-1   Estimated female deaths per year

Disease	New Cases	Number of Deaths	Mortality (per 100,000)
Carcinoma of endometrium	35,000	2,900	2.6
Fracture—osteoporosis	700,000	30,000	27.2
Carcinoma of breasts*	130,000	41,000	36.8
Carcinoma of lungs†	51,000	44,000	39.4

*One in ten women in the U.S. will have breast cancer during her lifetime, but ERT does not increase this risk.
†Carcinoma of the lungs is now statistically the number one killer of women; the change in incidence is allegedly because of cigarette smoking.

Table 32-2   Symptoms of menopause

Target Organ	Symptoms
Bladder and urethra	Urethritis, frequency or urgency, emergence of stress incontinence, development of cystoure-throcele
Breasts	Decrease in size and are less firm, loss of elasticity with drooping
Brain	Psychologic changes, forgetfulness, inability to concentrate, behavioral changes (60% of women), development of depression
Cardiovascular system	Enhancement of atherosclerosis, increased incidence of coronary heart disease
Neuroendocrine	Hot flushes (75% of women), psychologic changes
Skeleton	All osteoporosis related: loss of height, backache, fractures
Skin and mucous membranes	Dryness, decreased resiliency and loss of elastic tissue, atrophy, minor hirsutism of face
Uterus and pelvic structures	Decrease in size of fibroids, loss of elasticity and onset of prolapse, development of cystocele/rectocele/urethrocele
Vagina	Increase in pH, atrophic vaginitis, dyspareunia (75% of women)
Vulva	Atrophic dystrophy, pruritus vulvae

NOTE: Obese women have greater availability of estrogen because (1) lower SHBG concentrations result in higher levels of free estradiol and (2) they have more adipose tissue with greater peripheral aromatization of both estradiol and estrone.

TREATMENT OF MENOPAUSE

Treatment of menopause is discussed in the Estrogen Replacement Therapy section.

OSTEOPOROSIS

Not all women develop osteoporosis, even in the absence of estrogen. A risk-profile evaluation is essential for the individual patient when estrogen replacement therapy (ERT) is under consideration. The risk profile follows:

1. Genetic: Positive family history; small, slender physique; Caucasian or Oriental race.

2. Sex hormonal evaluation: Early menopause or ovariectomy, nulliparity, history of amenorrhea or frequent anovulation.
3. Diet: Low calcium intake; excessive intake of animal protein, alcohol, and caffeine.
4. Life-style: Lack of exercise, cigarette smoking.
5. Associated disorders: Long-term heparin therapy, glucocorticosteroid therapy, diabetes mellitus, thyrotoxicosis, hyperthyroidism, Cushing's syndrome, hypopituitarism.

Physiology

Bone loss begins 5 to 7 years before menopause (i.e., at age 45 to 52) at a rate of 3% a year. After menopause the rate of loss is 1% per year, with slightly increased serum calcium and decreased parathormone (PTH).

Diagnosis

Most often, osteoporosis has no symptoms, so suspicion of osteoporosis is frequently based on risk factors. Factors to look for include:
1. Decrease in height
2. Periodontal disease
3. Dowager's hump
4. Compression fractures of spine

No single laboratory method is good for diagnosis, but methods include CT scan of weight-bearing bones (i.e., spine and hip) and single- or double-beam densitometry. Spine and radius fractures are frequently seen before age 60, and hip fractures are most commonly seen after age 70.

Prevention

The major indication for ERT is prevention of osteoporosis. Other preventive factors include the following:
1. Eliminate risk components
2. Exercise
3. Increase calcium to 1000 to 1500 mg per day along with ERT.

Estrogen stops bone loss but does not replace calcium in the bone. Estrogen's mechanism is most likely indirect, and recent evidence suggests it works by increasing PTH.

ESTROGEN REPLACEMENT THERAPY

Not all women need ERT. Assume they do and work backwards. Close monitoring is needed for migraine headaches, uterine leiomyoma, and gall bladder disease. ERT is not associated with increased risk of thromboembolic disease, stroke, hypertension, or benign breast disease.

Contraindications for ERT

1. Pregnancy
2. Breast cancer
3. Active liver disease
4. Active or recent deep-vein thrombophlebitis

Indications for ERT

1. Vasomotor
2. Osteogenic

3. Cardiovascular
4. Genitourinary
5. Psychologic

Complications of ERT

1. Hyperplasia of endometrium
2. Endometrial cancer: risk with no ERT—1 per 1000 women per year; risk with ERT in the absence of progesterone—5 per 1000 women per year. The use of progesterone for 10 to 13 days either monthly, bimonthly, or concurrently with estrogen decreases risk to 1 per 1000 women per year.

Beneficial Effects of ERT

1. Prevents or stops progression of osteoporosis
2. Decreases risk of myocardial infarction by 50%
3. Antiatherogenic—increases HDL cholesterol
4. Relieves vasomotor symptoms
5. Prevents genitourinary system atrophy
6. Enables estrogen target organ to reestablish normality

Workup Needed Before ERT

1. Evaluate each patient on her own merit.
2. Develop risk-profile evaluation for osteoporosis.
3. Detailed history and physical examinations with identification for contraindications to ERT.
4. Cervical Pap smear.
5. Blood-lipid profile.
6. Height recorded and compared to previous height.
7. Mammogram.
8. Consent and understanding for ERT. If patient has a history of abnormal or unusual bleeding, a sample of the endometrium is necessary.
   Once all data are evaluated, consider ERT unless an absolute contraindication is present.

Types of Estrogen Therapy Available

1. Oral medications
2. Vaginal creams
3. Subcutaneous pellets
4. Injections
5. Dermal patch
   Oral medication is the least expensive type of ERT, and many forms are available. The dermal patch and subcutaneous implants are both ethinyl estradiol.

Therapy Regimens for ERT

Unopposed ERT may result in endometrial hyperplasia or abnormal bleeding, necessitating uterine sampling for as many as 25% of patients. But if used in conjunction with progesterone (i.e., gestagen therapy), the results are only slightly higher than those for the control group.
1. Estrogen Monday through Friday, stop on Saturday and Sunday. Then administer a gestagen every 2 months for at least 10 days. Expect a menstrual period 3 to 5 days after the gestagen is stopped.

2. Estrogen and gestagen to be taken concurrently on a daily basis Monday through Friday. Example: conjugated estrogen 0.625 mg and medroxyprogesterone acetate 2.5 mg or norethindrone 0.3 mg. (More than 90% of women whose endometrium was sampled after being on this regimen for at least 4 months had uterine atrophy and no menstrual spotting. This results in a high compliance rate.)
3. Estrogen to be taken on day 1 through 25, and gestagen on days 16 through 25. This will usually result in a menstrual period following the cessation of hormonal therapy, and hot flushes will often recur before the beginning of the next cycle. Compliance may be less.
4. Vaginal creams may be used for temporary relief of atrophic vaginitis or vaginal atrophy. Usual dose application results in 50% absorbed systemically. Medication is not sufficient to prevent osteoporosis.
5. Dermal patch contains either .05 or .1 mg of ethinyl estradiol. Applied twice a week. Gestagen required in some form in conjunction with patch if the uterus is present.
6. Subcutaneous pellets of 25 mg ethinyl estradiol—two used for a total of 50 mg— have a duration of action of 7 to 12 months. Inserted as an outpatient procedure under local anesthesia with trocar stab wound in abdomen. May be used in conjunction with 75 mg testosterone pellet.
7. Injection—episodic use gives high peak level and lasts less than 4 weeks.

It is not known whether or not gestagen should be used in conjunction with estrogen if uterus is absent, but it should be used if uterus is present to prevent estrogen end-organ stimulation of the uterus.

Ancillary Considerations for Therapy

1. Exercise—walk, swim, aerobics—to maintain normal body weight.
2. Supplemental calcium—up to 1000 mg per day.
3. Positive outlook on life: Love yourself so you can love others.
4. Baby aspirin daily to prevent increase in thromboxane—decreases platelet adhesiveness—may be recommended in future.
5. The above measures are *not* a substitute for ERT.

REVIEW
QUESTIONS

1. The risk of endometrial cancer for postmenopausal women who take estrogen may be reduced by:
   a. Decreasing the dose of estrogen.
   b. Including 4 or more estrogen-free days each month.
   c. Decreasing the duration of estrogen therapy.
   d. Adding a gestagen with the estrogen therapy.
   e. All of the above.
2. During the postmenopausal years without therapy:
   a. Bone formation is increased.
   b. Bone formation is decreased.
   c. Bone resorption is increased.
   d. Bone resorption is decreased.
   e. Bone formation and resorption are unchanged.

3. The use of gestagens in postmenopausal women:
   a. Opposes the action of estrogen on relief of vasomotor symptoms.
   b. Opposes the action of estrogen on bone metabolism.
   c. Opposes the action of estrogen on the endometrium.
   d. All of the above.
   e. None of the above.
4. During the postmenopausal years, estrogen therapy will:
   a. Delay vaginal atrophy but not urethral atrophy.
   b. Delay urethral atrophy but not vaginal atrophy.
   c. Delay both vaginal and urethral atrophy.
5. Estrogen therapy for postmenopausal women results in:
   a. Increased bone formation.
   b. Decreased bone formation.
   c. Increased bone resorption.
   d. Decreased bone resorption.
   e. All of the above.
   f. None of the above.
6. The etiology of hot flushes is:
   a. Declining estrogen levels.
   b. Rising gonadotropin levels.
   c. Histamines.
   d. Unknown.
7. Hot flashes:
   a. Generally have no effect on the pulse rate.
   b. Generally begin in the face.
   c. Are experienced by nearly 100% of postmenopausal women.
   d. May occur before actual cessation of menses.
   e. Seldom occur more than once or twice a day.
8. Genital changes associated with menopause:
   a. May include dyspareunia and blood-tinged leukorrhea.
   b. Are unresponsive to topical estrogens.
   c. Include a shift toward cornified cells in the vaginal smears.
   d. Are seldom detected grossly.
9. Postmenopausal osteoporosis may be:
   a. Significant in 50% of postmenopausal women after age 60.
   b. Caused by reduced estrogen levels.
   c. Caused by high FSH levels.
   d. Treated with estrogens, which increase bone responsiveness to PTH.
   e. Treated with calcium, which increases circulating PTH.
10. The risk factors for coronary heart disease and atherosclerosis in postmenopausal women are probably:
    a. Increased by reduced estrogen levels.
    b. Not altered by reduced estrogen levels.
    c. Decreased because of reduced estrogen levels.
    d. Altered by exogenous therapy.
    e. Not reduced after long-standing premenopausal use of oral contraceptives.

ANSWERS

1. e
2. c

3. c
4. c
5. d
6. d
7. d
8. a
9. a
10. a

BIBLIOGRAPHY

Albright F, Smith PH, and Richardson AM: Postmenopausal osteoporosis: its clinical features, JAMA 116:2465, 1941.

Barlow DH et al: Long-term hormone implant therapy: hormonal and clinical effects, Obstet Gynecol 67:321, 1986.

Davis ME: Long-term estrogen substitution after the menopause, Clin Obstet Gynecol 7:558, 1964.

Davis MR: Screening for postmenopausal osteoporosis, Am J Obstet Gynecol 156:1, 1987.

Gambrell RD et al: Reduced incidence of endometrial cancer among postmenopausal women treated with progestogens, J Am Geriatr Soc 27:389, 1979.

Hammond CB, and Maxson WS: Estrogen replacement therapy, Clin Obstet Gynecol 29(2):407, 1986.

Judd H, and Utin WH, editors: Current Perspectives in the Management of the Menopausal and Postmenopausal Patient Symposium, Am J Obstet Gynecol 156:1279, 1987.

Riis B, Thomsen K, and Christiansen C: Does calcium supplementation prevent postmenopausal bone loss? N Engl J Med 316:173, 1987.

Breast Disease

33

Nicholas J. Teteris

One fourth of all American women who consult a physician do so because of some breast problem. Many of these women visit the physician with an underlying fear of malignancy.

The importance of early diagnosis and treatment of breast cancer is well publicized. Carcinoma of the breast develops in 10% of American women during their lifetime. Breast cancer represents 28% of all malignancies seen in women and accounts for 18% of all cancer deaths. Every 13 minutes in the United States, a woman dies of breast cancer and 3 new cases are discovered. Annually, approximately 130,000 new cases are diagnosed and 41,000 deaths occur from this disease.

ANATOMY AND PHYSIOLOGY
Anatomy

See Fig. 33-1.
1. Paired modified sebaceous glands (ectoderm) enveloped within superficial pectoral fascia.
2. Ten to twenty triangularly shaped lobes, further subdivided into lobules and acini.
3. Ducts dilate into ampullae, converge, and open onto the nipple.
4. Glandular ducts are surrounded by fat and fibrous septa (Cooper's ligaments) that attach to the skin and superficial fascia.
5. The three major pathways of lymphatic drainage are axillary (75% of drainage), transpectoral, and internal mammary.

Hormonal Influences

1. Breast development is dependent primarily on the presence of estrogen and progesterone and is dependent to a lesser degree on the presence of normal levels of insulin, cortisol, thyroxine, growth hormone, and prolactin.
2. Mature breast epithelium responds to changing levels of estrogen and progesterone in a manner similar to that of the endometrium, accompanied by tenderness and fullness during the luteal phase of the menstrual cycle.

Anomalies

Asymmetric development is the most common anomaly involving the mammary glands. Accessory breasts (polymastia) and supernumerary nipples (polythelia) are common anomalies along the embryologic mammary ridge and can be functional or rudimentary.

SAGITTAL SECTION

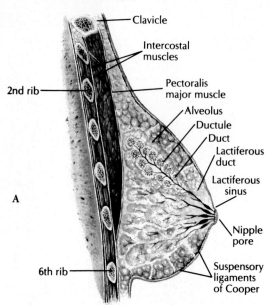

- Clavicle
- Intercostal muscles
- Pectoralis major muscle
- Alveolus
- Ductule
- Duct
- Lactiferous duct
- Lactiferous sinus
- Nipple pore
- Suspensory ligaments of Cooper

2nd rib

6th rib

A

ANTERIOR DISSECTION

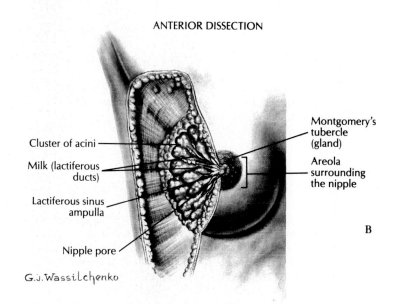

Cluster of acini

Milk (lactiferous ducts)

Lactiferous sinus ampulla

Nipple pore

Montgomery's tubercle (gland)

Areola surrounding the nipple

B

G.J.Wassilchenko

Fig. 33-1
Anatomy of the breast. A from Seidel et al: Mosby's guide to physical assessment, St Louis, 1987, The CV Mosby Co. B from Bobak et al: Maternity and gynecologic care, ed 4, St Louis, 1989, The CV Mosby Co.

DISEASES OF THE BREASTS
Symptoms

The common symptoms of breast disease are pain and tenderness, and the usual pathologic physical findings are the presence of a mass and/or discharge from the nipple. These symptoms and physical findings are the *same* for both benign and malignant disease. Only 10% of patients with early breast carcinoma present with a complaint of pain.

Presenting symptoms are shown in Table 33-1.

Physical Examination

1. Ability to detect breast masses is a function of mass size, experience of examiner, thoroughness (examination should take 3 to 5 minutes), and amount of breast tissue present.
2. Examination should consist of:
   a. Inspection and palpation of the breasts with patient in supine position, in sitting position with and without pectoral muscles contracted (hands on iliac crests, exerting pressure), and with breasts dependent (bending forward with arms raised).
   b. Palpation should be performed with flat of the hand and should include complete examination of the breast, nipple, axilla, and supraclavicular area.
   c. Look for asymmetry, skin dimpling, edema, deformity, nipple retraction, inflammation, discharge, and masses. Records should reflect location and characteristics of pathologic condition.

Breast Self-Examination

1. Ideally, physician should teach breast self-examination (BSE) while performing the physical examination.
2. Majority of breast masses are first discovered by the patient. Early diagnosis may contribute to improved prognosis and survival.
3. BSE should be done on day 6 of the menstrual cycle or on the same calendar day of each month for nonmenstrual women.

DIAGNOSTIC METHODS IN BREAST DISEASE
Mammography

1. Radiographic method of accurately detecting breast carcinoma at an early and potentially curable stage.
2. Physical examination is capable of detecting carcinomas that are 1 cm in diameter or larger. Mammography may pick up microcalcification in breast cancer months, or even years, before it becomes clinically palpable (less than 1 cm). Aggressive tumors double in volume in 60 days; average doubling time is 100 days. It takes 30 doubling times to reach 1-cm size, and a carcinoma that size probably has been present for 6 to 8 years.
3. Mammography should be part of the diagnostic workup of women with breast complaints and/or abnormal findings.
4. Mammography should be performed on most women before biopsy.
5. Mammography does not replace carefully performed breast examination; the converse is also true.
6. Mammography is indispensable in localizing and removing for biopsy nonpalpable (occult) lesions.
7. Two-view mammographic examination should deliver .1 to .8 rad to the breast and,

Table 33-1   Synopsis of common diseases and conditions of the breast

Disease/Frequency (%)	Age Range (Median Age)	Symptoms and Findings
Fibroadenoma (19%)	15-40 (20)	Firm, painless, mobile, rubbery mass; may be large, multiple (14% of cases), and bilateral (25% of cases); predominantly in young women; benign
Fibrocystic changes (34%)	20-50 (30)	Lesions are commonly bilateral and multiple, of variable sizes that are described as granular to nodular, and in more advanced form present as cystic or diffuse masses; usually larger before menstrual period—rapid change and fluctuation of size is characteristic; symptoms of dull, heavy pain and a sense of fullness and tenderness to touch—usually worse before menstrual period
Intraductal papilloma (6%)	35-55 (40)	Serous or serosanguineous watery nipple discharge—usually spontaneous and unilateral from a single duct
Duct ectasia (4%)	35-55 (40)	Multicolored, sticky, bilateral nipple discharge from multiple ducts; burning, itching, or dull drawing pain around nipple and areola with palpable tortuous tubular swellings under the areola
Carcinoma (27%)	30-90 (54)	Solitary, unilateral, solid, hard, nonmobile, irregular, poorly delineated, painless mass—usually in upper outer quadrant of breast; advanced disease associated with nipple retraction, discharge, skin dimpling, and irregular axillary nodes

theoretically, could produce one excess breast carcinoma per year per 1 million women examined (after 10-year latency period).

8. American Cancer Society and American College of Radiology guidelines on mammographic screening of asymptomatic women:
   a. Baseline mammogram at age 35.
   b. Mammogram every year or every other year for women aged 40 to 50.
   c. Annual mammogram for women age 50 or older.

Ultrasonography

1. Lacks the sensitivity and specificity to be used as a screening tool.
2. Main application is to distinguish cystic from solid lesions when mass cannot be aspirated.

Table 33-1—cont'd

Treatment

Aspiration to rule out cyst—then surgically remove, especially if large

Aspiration of palpable cysts; excisional biopsy if mass persists or recurs; mastalgia treatment; good support bra; reduce consumption of methylxanthines and tobacco; diuretic during premenstrual phase (Diuril .5 g/day); danazol 100-400 mg daily for 4-6 months; 600 IU of vitamin E daily; bromocriptine 2.5 mg/day first week of cycle, 5 mg/day for next 3 weeks of cycle; tamoxifen 10 mg/day fifth through twenty-fifth days of cycle for 4 months; simple mastectomy reserved for cases of intractable pain or if biopsy shows evidence of premalignant lesion

Location of involved duct and excision

Location and excision of involved ducts

Therapy is individualized and depends on histology of lesion, involvement of nodes, receptor status of tumor, and wishes of patient after clear enunciation of options, risks, and benefits; therapeutic options include radical, modified radical, and simple mastectomy with axillary node dissection, tumor excision (wedge resection) with radiation, hormonal manipulation, and adjuvant chemotherapy; consideration of reconstructive surgery may provide considerable psychologic benefit to patient

Thermography

1. May have a role as a prognostic indicator in that aggressive tumors tend to be more thermogenic.
2. Breast cancer with a negative thermogram has a better prognosis than if thermogram is positive.

Needle Aspiration

See Fig. 33-2.
1. Aspiration under aseptic conditions can be safely performed in an office setting.
2. Local skin anesthesia can be used but is seldom necessary.
3. Cytologic evaluation of cystic fluid is rarely of any diagnostic benefit (Fig. 33-3).

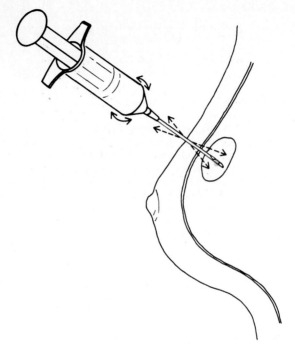

Fig. 33-2
Needle biopsy and aspiration with negative pressure. The needle is rotated, and moved back and
forth and slightly in and out to aspirate a representative specimen.
From Vorherr H: Am J Obstet Gynecol 148:128, 1984.

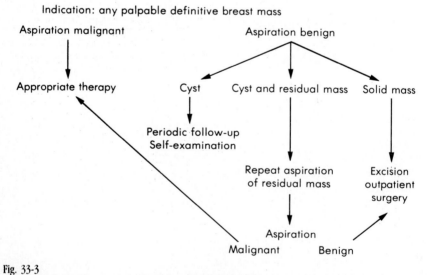

Fig. 33-3
Algorithm for fine-needle aspiration biopsy of the breast.
From Frable WJ: Fine needle biopsy of breast lesions. Paper presented at The American Board of Obstetrics
and Gynecology Conference on Breast Disease, Chicago, May 13, 1986.

Biopsy

1. Indications for biopsy:
   a. Persistent dominant mass, with or without nipple discharge.
   b. Mammographic changes suggestive of malignancy.
   c. Persistent erythema or edema of skin.
2. Most can be done as outpatient procedure under local anesthesia.
3. Minimize disfiguring scar formation by using circumareolar incision and by following Langer's lines.
4. Determine estrogen receptor (ER) and progesterone receptor (PR) status of tumor.
5. A 12-day delay from time of biopsy until definitive therapy does not adversely affect prognosis and gives patient time to consider therapeutic options.
6. Fine-needle aspiration (cytology) or biopsy (core specimen) yields 85% accuracy of diagnosis, with false-negative rate of 15%.
7. Negative mammogram and negative fine-needle aspiration gives 95% assurance that mass is not malignant (5% false-negative rate).
8. Biopsy must be performed on all solid dominant lesions.
9. Open biopsy is the only way to prove that a mass is *not* malignant.

BREAST CARCINOMA
Pathology and Pathogenesis (Table 33-2)

Epithelial tumors account for 96% of breast malignancies, and 4% are sarcomas. Causal hypotheses include viral, genetic, and endocrine factors.

Risk factors identify only one fourth of the women who will develop breast cancer. These risk factors are:

1. Family history of breast cancer (highest genetic risk is first-degree relatives of premenopausal women with bilateral breast cancer).
2. Frequency increases with age; breast carcinomas are uncommon before age 30, and 85% of breast carcinomas occur after age 40 (Fig. 33-4).
3. Exposure to unopposed, endogenous estrogen.
4. Obesity in postmenopausal years. (It is postulated that increased peripheral conversion of androstenedione to estrone is a causative factor.)
5. American and European women have a higher incidence of breast cancer than African, Asian, or Middle Eastern women. Why this is so is not clear.
6. Exposure to ionizing radiation.

Table 33-2   Simplified classification of breast carcinoma

Type of Carcinoma	Percentage of All Cases Diagnosed
Ductal carcinoma	
In situ	5%
Infiltrating	80%
Lobular carcinoma	
In situ	3%
Infiltrating	9%
Paget's disease	1%
Inflammatory carcinoma	2%

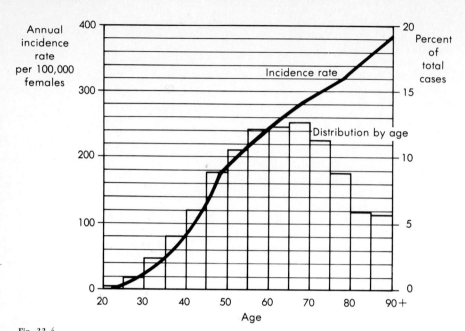

Fig. 33-4

Incidence in the United States, by age, of female breast cancer.

From Seidman H, and Mushinski MH: Breast cancer incidence, mortality, survival, and prognosis. In Feig SA, and McLelland R, editors: Breast carcinoma: current diagnosis and treatment, New York, 1983, Masson Publishing. Copyright by American College of Radiology.

7. Carcinoma of one breast (risk of developing cancer in other breast is 1% per year).
8. Delivery of first child after age 35.

Putative risk factors that are no longer thought to play a role in the genesis of breast cancer include cigarette smoking, drugs that raise prolactin levels (e.g., reserpine), and exogenous estrogen, as in oral contraceptives or estrogen replacement.

Diagnosis of Breast Cancer

1. Symptoms: Pain, discharge, palpable mass. The frequency of cancer as a cause of discharge increases with age (Table 33-3).The distribution of the location of breast cancers is: 50% are located in upper outer quadrant, 10% in each of the other 3 quadrants, and 20% are located centrally, in the area of the areola.
2. Mammography—see under Diagnostic Methods in Breast Disease
3. Biopsy—see under Diagnostic Methods in Breast Disease

Treatment of Breast Cancer

1. Objectives of therapy are:
   a. Control local disease.
   b. Treat metastases.
   c. Improve quality of life for the afflicted to achieve the best prognosis with the least anatomic disfigurement and to allow for the possibility of reconstructive surgery.
2. Metastases: Breast carcinoma metastasizes most frequently to the lungs, liver, and bones. Micrometastases occur early by hematogenous and lymphatic routes. Two

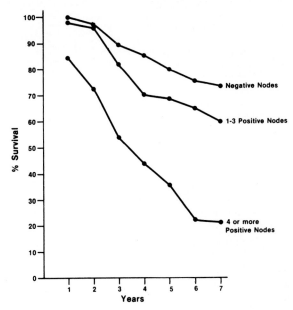

Fig. 33-5
Survival with breast carcinoma in relation to positive nodes.
From Gambrell RD: AM J Obstet Gynecol 150:122, 1984.

Table 33-3   Nipple discharge

Age (years)	Incidence of Cancer (%)
Less than 50	7
50 - 60	13
Greater than 60	32

thirds of all women with breast carcinoma will eventually develop distant metastasis regardless of the type of initial therapy. Many women with breast carcinoma
have systemic disease at the time that the diagnosis is made.
3. Treatment options: Until recently, the only form of therapy for this disease was radical mastectomy. Today therapy is individualized, and women are offered alterna-
tives such as lumpectomy, simple mastectomy, or radical surgery with and without
chemotherapy and/or radiation. These decisions are based on:
   a. Histologic grading and size of primary lesion.
   b. Presence or absence of axillary node metastases.
   c. Hormone receptor status of the tumor (Fig. 33-5).
      (1) ER positive tumors are usually well differentiated and behave clinically in
          a less aggressive manner than ER negative neoplasms. A 60% response to
          hormonal therapy is expected if a tumor is ER positive and 80% response
          is expected if the tumor is also PR positive.
      (2) If tumor is ER negative, less than 10% response to hormonal manipula-
          tion can be anticipated, and chemotherapy becomes the treatment of
          choice.
      (3) Hormonal therapy can consist of either ablative surgery, such as bilateral

Table 33-4 Stages and survival of women with breast cancer

Clinical Staging*	5-Year Survival (%)	Range of Survival (%)
Stage I		
Tumor less than 2 cm in diameter; nodes, if present, not thought to contain metastases; without distant metastases	85	82-94
Stage II		
Tumor less than 5 cm in diameter; nodes, if palpable, not fixed; without distant metastases	66	47-74
Stage III		
Tumor greater than 5 cm or of any size with invasion of skin or attached to chest wall; nodes in supraclavicular area; without distant metastases	41	7-80
Stage IV		
With distant metastases	10	—

*American Joint Committee

oophorectomy, or the use of drugs to prevent hormonal synthesis or to block receptor sites. Tamoxifen, aminoglutethimide, danazol, depomedroxyprogesterone, estrogens, and androgens are examples of such drugs.

(4) Combinations of cytotoxic drugs are superior to single-agent therapy. Drugs known to be effective in the treatment of breast carcinoma are cyclophosphamide, Adriamycin, methotrexate, 5-fluorouracil and vinblastine.

(5) Of those women treated with combined chemotherapy, 55% will respond to therapy and 15% will experience complete remission for about a year and a half (Table 33-4).

4. Breast cancer and pregnancy: A small percentage—2.8%—of women with breast cancer are pregnant, and the survival figures, stage for stage, for gravid and nongravid women who are adequately treated are about the same.

5. Mortality: Sadly, the mortality from breast carcinoma has not changed significantly in the last 40 years. Women are living longer after the diagnosis is made. Some investigators argue that although improved diagnostic methodology permits earlier diagnosis, current therapy is not appreciably altering the course of the disease, lending support to the thesis of early micrometastasis. A more optimistic point of view is held by other investigators; they suggest that improved diagnostic and therapeutic technology has not had sufficient time to affect mortality statistics. Time will soon tell which of these divergent opinions is correct.

REVIEW
QUESTIONS

1. Mastalgia of fibrocystic change can be treated by:
   a. Diuretics
   b. Vitamin E
   c. Tamoxifen
   d. Danazol
   e. All of the above
2. The majority of breast masses are first detected by:
   a. Thermography
   b. Physician examination
   c. Mammography
   d. The patient

Match the following:

3. _____ Intraductal papilloma
4. _____ Duct ectasia
5. _____ Fibroadenoma
6. _____ Carcinoma
7. _____ Fibrocystic change

a. Disease of young women
b. Serosanguineous unilateral nipple discharge
c. Bilateral, sticky, multicolored nipple discharge
d. Mean age of 30 years
e. Mean age of 54 years

True or False

8. Breasts are modified sebaceous glands of endodermal origin.
9. Pain is a frequent symptom associated with cancer of the breast.

Match the following:

10. _____ Mammogram
11. _____ Thermogram
12. _____ Ultrasonography
13. _____ Fine needle

a. Distinguish solid from cystic
b. Used to localize occult malignancies
c. Prognostic tool
d. 85% specificity

ANSWERS

1. e
2. d
3. b
4. c
5. a
6. e
7. d
8. F
9. F
10. b
11. c
12. a
13. d

BIBLIOGRAPHY

American Board of Obstetrics and Gynecology: Conference on breast disease, Seattle, 1987, The Board.

Berg JW: Clinical implications of risk factors for breast cancer, Cancer 53:589, 1984.

Carlile T: Breast cancer detection, Cancer 47:1164, 1981.

DeWard F: Epidemiology of breast cancer: a review, Eur J Cancer Clin Oncol 19:1671, 1983.

Holleb AI, editor: Cancer statistics 1988, CA 38(1):1, 1988.

Korenman SG: Estrogen window hypothesis of the etiology of breast cancer, Lancet 1:700, 1980.

Minton JP: Methylxanthines in breast disease. In Swartz GF, and Marchant D, editors: Breast disease, diagnosis and treatment, New York, 1980, Symposia Specialists.

Townsend CM, Jr: Management of breast cancer: surgery and adjuvant therapy, Clin Symp 39(4), 1987.

Veronesi V et al: Comparing radical mastectomy with quadrantectomy, axillary dissection, and radiotherapy in patients with small cancers of the breast, N Engl J Med 305:6, 1981.

Vorherr H: Breast aspiration biopsy, Am J Obstet Gynecol 148:127, 1984.

Vulvar Diseases

Larry J. Copeland

Most vulvar diseases can be categorized as congenital, inflammatory, dystrophic, or neoplastic. Congenital and inflammatory problems (Table 34-1) occur predominantly in young women, and dystrophic (Table 34-2) and neoplastic (Table 34-3) abnormalities are most commonly found in women during the postmenopausal years. Benign tumors of the vulva (Table 34-4) are uncommon.

Unfortunately, delays in the diagnosis of vulvar neoplasms are common. The primary reason for delay is the reluctance of older women to seek medical care for vulvar complaints, usually because they deny that a significant problem exists or are too embarrassed to draw attention to it. Physicians may also contribute to delays in diagnosis by delaying histologic evaluations of atypical areas. Dystrophic abnormalities are usually generalized and respond well to hormonal therapy. Localized lesions or lesions unresponsive to conservative therapy require one or more biopsies. Colposcopic evaluation or the use of a 1% toluidine blue stain may help identify occult vulvar abnormalities.

Table 34-1   Vulvar diseases of young women

Condition	Signs and Symptoms	Treatments/Comments
Developmental Abnormalities		
Cyst of the canal of Nuck (hydrocele)	A fluctuant cystic mass present in the labium majus pudendi or inguinal area	A peritoneal cyst (diverticulum) adjacent to the round ligament; simple excision; will recur if only drained
Mesonephric duct remnant	Cyst extending up lateral vagina	Excise if symptomatic
Accessory breast tissue	Small nonspecific subcutaneous nodule, usually not noticed until pregnancy when the tissue is stimulated	Excision is recommended to avoid discomfort during pregnancy and also to prevent breast tumors of the vulva
Inflammatory Infections/Problems		
Bartholin's cyst or abscess	Painful swelling adjacent to introitus, usually at the 4 to 5 o'clock or 7 to 8 o'clock positions; may spontaneously drain	The abscess develops within the duct, probably as a result of distal obstruction of the duct; best managed by marsupialization; antibiotics—broad spectrum; usually a mixed bacterial flora with gram-negative and anaerobic organisms; may be related to previous or current gonococcal infection; unless infected or symptomatic, no treatment necessary
Epidermal (sebaceous, inclusion) cysts	Usually multiple, less than 1 cm in diameter; when palpated, they feel solid; they contain white-yellow sebaceous material; unless infected, they are usually nontender; may develop in episiotomy scars from "buried" epithelium	Unless infected or tender, no treatment needed
Sexually transmitted diseases (syphilis, lymphogranuloma venereum, chancroid, condyloma)	See Chapter 22	—

Table 34-1   Vulvar diseases of young women—cont'd

Condition	Signs and Symptoms	Treatments/Comments
Behçet's syndrome	Painful superficial serpiginous-like ulcers; lesions tend to be deeply ulcerated and tender; concurrent oral ulcerations and, occasionally, ocular inflammation; arthritis, ulcerative colitis, thrombophlebitis, acne, and neurologic abnormalities may be associated	Bacteriologic, viral, and serologic studies are negative; biopsy shows nonspecific inflammation and vasculitis; may respond to a short course of corticosteroids; considered an autoimmune disease and may overlap clinically with Crohn's disease; remissions after treatment with estrogen-dominant oral contraceptives have been reported

Table 34-2   Vulvar dystrophy

Type	Signs and Symptoms	Evaluation	Treatment/Comments
Hypertrophic dystrophy (with and without atypia)	Pruritis, commonly of extended duration; vulvar skin appears thickened, irregular, and may or may not be erythematous or white	Punch biopsy	Topical steroidal therapy for inflammation; topical estrogen therapy to reverse hyperplasia; if unresponsive, excision or laser diathermy may be necessary (be aware of not missing a diagnosis of invasive tumor)
Atrophic dystrophy (lichen sclerosus)	Pruritis; thin white shiny epithelium; intraepithelial hemorrhage and ecchymosis may be present	Unless clinically certain of nature of lesion, punch biopsy; biopsy absolutely necessary if not promptly responsive to topical therapy	Topical-steroid therapy initially to reduce inflammatory reaction; topical testosterone (2% testosterone dipropionate in white petrolatum bid to promote thickening of the epithelium
Mixed dystrophy (with and without atypia)	Pruritis; white or pigmented epithelium	Punch biopsy	Same as atrophic dystrophy

Table 34-3 Premalignant and malignant vulvar neoplasms

Condition	Signs and Symptoms	Evaluation	Treatment/Comments
Intraepithelial Neoplasia			
Squamous carcinoma in situ (Bowen's disease, bowenoid papulosis)	Pruritis; white or pigmented epithelium; isolated or multifocal	Biopsy	Wide local excision; laser diathermy is acceptable if invasive disease has been ruled out (multiple biopsies); 5-fluorouracil (Efudex) topical therapy may reverse some lesions
Paget's disease	Pruritis; velvety red epithelium with interspersed white patches	Biopsy; evaluate for occult carcinoma of colon or breast	Simple vulvectomy to treat the intraepithelial lesion and evaluate for a breast-underlying apocrine-gland carcinoma (20% of patients)
Squamous Carcinoma	Pruritis, pain, burning, bloody discharge; nodule or ulceration	Biopsy; also evaluate for lesions of other areas of genital tract, especially cervix and vagina; assess regional lymphadenopathy (inguinal nodes); staging evaluation to include a chest x-ray examination and CT scan of pelvis to evaluate for pelvic lymphadenopathy	Depends on diameter and the depth of the primary tumor; small superficial lesions (less than 1 mm) are considered microinvasive, and a wide local excision is the treatment; if the lesion is more deeply invasive but still small, a wide excision and node sampling are appropriate; a radical vulvectomy and bilateral inguinal lymphadenectomy has been considered standard therapy

for most frankly invasive vulvar lesions—however, the trend is toward more conservative surgery combined with irradiation therapy

Malignant Melanoma	Usually pigmented; raised, may ulcerate	Biopsy	Wide local excision and regional (inguinal) lymphadenopathy; prognosis significantly decreases if lesions invade beyond a depth of 0.75 mm
Bartholin's Gland Carcinoma	Soft fluctuant mass may ulcerate and bleed	Biopsy (numerous histologic types—squamous, adenocarcinoma, adenoid cystic carcinoma, transitional cell carcinoma)	Wide local excision often requiring a hemivulvectomy; ipsilateral inguinal lymphadenectomy; postoperative irradiation therapy
Basal Cell Carcinoma	Ulcerated lesion with firm rolled edges	Biopsy; carefully evaluate for a squamous element	Wide local excision; rarely metastasizes
Verrucous Carcinoma	Exophytic tumor; may resemble a vulvar condyloma	Biopsy; lacks malignant histologic features and therefore may require repeat biopsies or generous biopsies	Wide local excision to obtain tumor-free margins; this tumor is considered relatively resistant to radiation
Vulvar Sarcomas	Mass	Biopsy	Depends on histologic type; except for alveolar rhabdomyosarcoma, most vulvar sarcomas metastasize late

Table 34-4   Benign vulvar tumors

Condition	Signs and Symptoms	Evaluation	Treatment/Comments
Hidradenoma	Usually single lesions on the labia; may ulcerate; usually between 0.5 and 1.5 cm	Wide local excision	Wide local excision; these benign tumors are sometimes misdiagnosed as adenocarcinomas, occasionally resulting in unnecessary treatment
Endometriosis	Firm nodules; if superficial, the nodules appear bluish; usually occur at posterior fourchette or in episiotomy scars; a history of cyclic enlargement may be given	Wide local excision	Wide local excision
Fibroma/lipoma	Variable size; usually painless, mobile, and slow-growing.	Excision	Rapid growth causes concern for the possibility of a sarcoma

REVIEW
QUESTIONS

More than one correct answer is possible.
1. Firm nodular lesions prone to develop in episiotomy scars include:
   a. A mesonephric duct remnant
   b. An epidermal cyst
   c. A basal cell carcinoma
   d. A hidradenoma
   e. An endometriotic cyst
2. Atrophic vulvar dystrophy lesions are best treated with:
   a. 5-fluorouracil (5%)
   b. Podophyllin (25% solution in compound tincture of benzoin)
   c. Topical estrogen therapy (conjugated estrogen cream)
   d. 2% testosterone dipropionate in white petrolatum
   e. Betamethasone cream 0.05%
3. A 74-year-old patient presented with a complaint of vulvar pruritis. Physical examination revealed a 1-cm thickened area of reddened skin on the right labium minus pudendi. No lymphadenopathy was noted. A punch biopsy was taken, and an invasive squamous carcinoma, invading to a depth of 2.5 mm, was identified. Appropriate primary therapy for this lesion is:
   a. Radical vulvectomy and bilateral inguinal lymphadenectomy.
   b. Wide local excision.
   c. Wide local excision and a right superficial inguinal lymphadenectomy.
   d. Laser diathermy to a depth and lateral margin of 5 mm.
   e. Radical vulvectomy and irradiation therapy to the vulva and inguinal lymph nodes.

ANSWERS

1. b, e
2. d
3. c

BIBLIOGRAPHY

Boronow RC: Combined therapy as an alternative to exenteration for locally advanced vulvovaginal cancer: rationale and results, Cancer 49:1085, 1982.

Boyce J et al: Prognostic factors in carcinoma of the vulva, Gynecol Oncol 20:364, 1985.

Copeland LJ: Neoplasms of the vulva. In Rakel RE, editor: 1989 Conn's current therapy, Philadelphia, 1989, WB Saunders Co.

Copeland LJ et al: Bartholin gland carcinoma, Obstet Gynecol 67:794, 1986.

Figge DC, Tamimi HK, and Greer BE: Lymphatic spread in carcinoma of the vulva, Am J Obstet Gynecol 152:387, 1985.

Friedrich EG, Jr: Vulvar disease, vol 9, Major problems in obstetrics and gynecology, Philadelphia, 1983, WB Saunders Co.

Hacker NF et al: Individualization of treatment for stage I squamous cell vulvar carcinoma, Obstet Gynecol 63:155, 1984.

Hoffman JS, Kumar NB, and Morley GW: Prognostic significance of groin lymph node metastases of squamous carcinoma of the vulva, Obstet Gynecol 66:402, 1985.

Homesley HD et al: A randomized study of radiation therapy versus pelvic node resection for patients with invasive squamous cell carcinoma of the vulva having positive groin nodes. A Gynecologic Oncology Group study, Obstet Gynecol 68:733, 1986.

International Society for the Study of Vulvar Disease: New nomenclature for vulvar disease, Obstet Gynecol 47:122, 1976.

Podratz KC et al: Melanoma of the vulva: an update, Gynecol Oncol 16:153, 1983.

Woodruff JD: Diseases of the vulva. In Jones HW, Jr, and Jones GS, editors: Novak's textbook of gynecology, ed 10, Baltimore, 1981, Williams & Wilkins.

Diagnosis of Common Gynecologic Cancers

Larry J. Copeland

Lower genital tract tumors (vulva, cervix, and endometrium), while possibly asymptomatic in the early developmental stages, usually become symptomatic and clinically evident during the early invasive stages (Table 35-1). Unfortunately, the same cannot be said for malignant neoplasms of the ovary. Ovarian carcinomas characteristically present with vague symptoms, and at the time of diagnosis, most patients have an advanced stage of disease (Table 35-2). Unlike cervical or endometrial carcinoma, both of which can usually be diagnosed with relatively simple outpatient procedures, ovarian neoplasms require surgical intervention to establish the diagnosis.

Table 35-1 Clinical characteristics of the common lower genital tract tumors

Site and Histologic Type	Most Common Age Group	Risk Factors	Presenting Complaints	Diagnosis
Cervix				
Squamous cell carcinoma (80%–95% of cervical cancers)	Wide range—20s to 80s; most are between 30 and 60 years of age	"Epidemiologically" considered a venereal disease; rare in women who have never been sexually active; once thought to be related to herpes, now more strongly associated with human papilloma virus (HPV) infections	Vaginal bleeding; vaginal discharge; pelvic pain is usually a late symptom	Cervical cytology screening (Pap smear); if a lesion is clinically obvious, perform a biopsy; a conization may be required for occult or microinvasive lesions; it is inappropriate and potentially harmful to perform conization on clinically obvious lesions when a biopsy would establish the diagnosis
Adenocarcinoma (arising from the endocervical glands; 5%–20% of cervical cancers)	Similar to squamous	Seems less related to sexual activity	Tends to be less symptomatic than squamous lesions	Biopsy; endocervical curettage; may require conization
Small cell neuroendocrine	Variable age groups	Unknown	Vaginal bleeding Tends to grow rapidly and metastasize early	Biopsy
Endometrium				
Adenocarcinoma (grade 1, 2, or 3*), adenosquamous,* clear cell carcinoma,* papillary serous*	Most patients are over age 40, usually postmenopausal; when diagnosed in younger patients, there is usually a history of anovulation	Anovulation (nulligravida), obesity, continuous unopposed estrogen	Irregular vaginal bleeding	Endometrial biopsy and endocervical curettage; fractional D & C if unable to do outpatient biopsies

*These histologic types are poor prognostic types.

Table 35-2 Clinical characteristics of the ovarian tumors

Histologic Type	Most Common Age Group	Signs and Symptoms	Diagnosis
Epithelial Tumors (Analogous Epithelium) Serous (fallopian tube), mucinous (endocervix), mesonephric (glomerular), Brenner (transitional), mixed, undifferentiated	40-70; patients under age 40 usually have low-grade tumors	Symptoms characteristically vague—abdominal swelling, weight gain, weight loss, gastrointestinal (upper and lower) symptoms; pelvic mass; nodulous cul de sac; ascites	Exploratory laparotomy; CA-125 may be elevated; over two thirds of patients have metastatic disease at diagnosis
Germ cell tumors *Malignant (tumor marker)* Dysgerminoma (LDH), endodermal sinus tumor (AFP), immature teratoma, embryonal cell carcinoma (AFP, hCG), choriocarcinoma (hCG), polyembryoma (hCG, AFP), mixed (hCG, AFP), malignant transformation of mature teratoma	Young—most patients are 12-30	Acute lower abdominal distention or pain; pelvic mass	Tumor markers AFP, hCG, LDH; exploratory laparotomy

Benign

Gonadoblastoma	—	Bilateral adnexal masses—primary amenorrhea; dysgenetic gonads (45 XO or 46 XY)	Pelvic x-ray—microcalcification; exploratory laparotomy
Mature teratoma (including dermoids, carcinoids, and stroma ovarii; rarely transform to malignant	—	Pelvic mass, persistent while patient is on oral contraceptives; hyperthyroidism may occur with struma ovarii; carcinoid syndrome may occur with carcinoids	Pelvic x-ray—calcification (teeth in dermoids); exploratory laparotomy
Stromal tumors			
Granulosa	All ages	Pelvic mass; abdominal distention; signs of estrogen production may be evident; in the prepubertal patient, pseudoprecocious puberty may develop; in the postmenopausal patient, vaginal bleeding is common	Exploratory laparotomy; also evaluate endometrium and breasts, both of which are at increased risk for neoplasia
Theca	Usually over 35	Same as granulosa	Same as granulosa
Sertoli-Leydig cell tumor (arrhenoblastoma)	Usually 18-50	Pelvic mass; defeminization (amenorrhea, loss of feminine fat distribution, poor breast development) followed by masculinization (hirsutism, clitoromegaly, temporal balding, hoarseness)	Serum testosterone; exploratory laparotomy

LDH, Lactic dehydrogenase; *AFP*, alpha-fetoprotein; *hCG*, human chorionic gonadotropin.

REVIEW QUESTIONS

1. The primary role of the Pap smear is:
   a. To screen an asymptomatic patient for preinvasive or early invasive cervical neoplasms
   b. To confirm the diagnosis of a suspicious cervical lesion
   c. To assist in the evaluation of postmenopausal bleeding
   d. To evaluate vaginal infections
   e. To screen for upper genital tract cancer cells from tubal or ovarian cancers
2. Which of the following histologic types of endometrial carcinoma is not associated with a poor prognosis?
   a. Poorly differentiated adenocarcinoma (grade 3)
   b. Secretory carcinoma
   c. Adenosquamous carcinoma
   d. Clear cell carcinoma
   e. Papillary serous carcinoma
3. The tumor markers associated with these germ cell tumors—dysgerminoma/endodermal sinus tumor/choriocarcinoma—are, respectively:
   a. AFP/hCG/None
   b. hCG/None/hCG
   c. None/None/hCG
   d. LDH/AFP/hCG
   e. LDH/None/hCG

ANSWERS

1. a
2. b
3. d

BIBLIOGRAPHY

Anderson DG et al: The cytologic diagnosis of endometrial adenocarcinoma, Am J Obstet Gynecol 125:376, 1976.
Berg JW, and Lampe JG: High-risk factors in gynecologic cancer, Cancer 48:429, 1981.
Frenczy A, and Winkler B: Cervical intraepithelial neoplasia and condyloma. In Kurman RJ, editor: Blaustein's pathology of the female genital tract, ed 3, New York, 1987, Springer-Verlag New York Inc.
Hawwa ZM, Nahhas WA, and Copenhaver EH: Postmenopausal bleeding, Lahey Clin Found Bull 19:61, 1970.
Henson D, and Tarone R: An epidemiologic study of cancer of the cervix, vagina, and vulva based on the Third National Cancer Survey in the United States, Am J Obstet Gynecol 129:525, 1987.
Kawada CY, and An-Foraker SH: Screening for endometrial carcinoma, Clin Obstet Gynecol 22:713, 1979.
Kurman RJ, and Norris HJ: Endometrial carcinoma. In Kurman RJ, editor: Blaustein's pathology of the female genital tract, ed 3, New York, 1987, Springer-Verlag New York Inc.
Kurman RJ, and Norris HJ: Endometrial hyperplasia and metaplasia. In Kurman RJ, editor: Blaustein's pathology of the female genital tract, ed 3, New York, 1987, Springer-Verlag New York Inc.
MacMahon B: Risk factor for endometrial cancer, Gynecol Oncol 2:122, 1974.
Mahboubi E, Eyler N, and Wynder EL: Epidemiology of cancer of the endometrium, Clin Obstet Gynecol 25:5, 1982.
Weiss RS, and Lucas WE: Adenocarcinoma of the cervix, Cancer 57:1996, 1986.
Welander C et al: Staging and treatment of endometrial carcinoma, J Reprod Med 8:41, 1972.
Winkler B et al: Pitfalls in the diagnosis of endometrial neoplasia, Obstet Gynecol 64:185, 1984.

Cancer Staging

36

John G. Boutselis

Staging is a means of communicating and comparing treatment and outcomes between institutions. Staging also allows an evaluation of the treatment plans that are used within one institution. For these reasons, a patient's stage at the time of diagnosis remains constant throughout her life and does not change even if the disease progresses. Staging does not limit the treatment plan, and therapy can be tailored to the characteristics of the malignancy in each patient. Unfortunately, clinical staging provides only a rough estimate of prognosis.

Methods of staging must be available to all institutions and include physical examination, routine radiographs, colposcopy, cystoscopy, sigmoidoscopy, IVP, and barium enema.

Carcinoma of the vulva, cervix, and vagina, and gestational trophoblastic neoplasia are staged on clinical criteria alone. Cancer of the endometrium, tube, and ovary are staged using a combination of clinical and pathologic findings.

This chapter outlines the International Federation of Gynecology and Obstetrics (FIGO) staging criteria for common gynecologic cancers.

FIGO CLINICAL STAGING OF CARCINOMA OF THE VULVA

See Table 36-1.
1. Stage I
   a. All tumors 2 cm or less (T1) with clinically negative nodes (N0 or N1)
   b. T1 N0 M0, T1 N1 M0
2. Stage II
   a. All tumors more than 2 cm without involvement of urethra, vagina, or anus (T2), with clinically negative nodes (N0 or N1)
   b. T2 N0 M0, T2 N1 M0

Table 36-1 Survival rates with carcinoma of the vulva

FIGO Stage	Number	Cases in Stage (%)	Corrected 5 Years (%)
I	306	35.1	91.1
II	352	28.9	80.9
III	213	24.4	48.4
IV	101	11.6	15.3
TOTAL	972	100	58.9

407

3. Stage III
   a. Tumors involving the urethra, anus, or vagina (T3) and all T1-3 tumors with suspicious nodes (N2)
   b. T3 N0 M0, T3 N1 M0, T3 N2 M0, T1 N2 M0, T2 N2 M0
4. Stage IV
   a. *All* tumors extending to bladder or rectal mucosa (T4), *all* tumors with fixed or ulcerated nodes (N3), and *all* tumors with distant metastases (M1)
   b. T4 N0 M0, T4 N1 M0, T4 N1 M0, all others containing N3 of M1a or M1b

FIGO CLINICAL STAGING OF CARCINOMA OF THE VAGINA

1. Stage I
   a. Limited to vaginal mucosa
2. Stage II
   a. Extends into the submucosa
   b. May involve paravaginal, but not lateral, pelvic wall
3. Stage III
   a. Extends to lateral pelvic wall
4. Stage IV
   a. Bladder or rectal mucosa
   b. Extrapelvic metastases

Five-Year Survival Rates (estimated)

1. Stage I: 80% to 85%
2. Stage II: 60% to 65%
3. Stage III: 30% to 40%
4. Stage IV: 0% to 5%

FIGO STAGING OF CERVICAL CANCER*

See Table 36-2.
1. Stage 0: Intraepithelial carcinoma (carcinoma in situ) (preinvasive).

Table 36-2 Five-year survival rate based on 2000 cases of cervical cancer at the M. D. Anderson Hospital and Tumor Institute

Stage	Survival Rate (%)
Stage I	91.5
Stage IIa	83.5
Stage IIb	66.5
Stage IIIa	45
Stage IIIb	36
Stage IV	14

From DiSaia PJ, and Creasman WT: Clinical gynecologic oncology, ed 3, St. Louis, 1989, The CV Mosby Co.

*Data from FIGO (see bibliography).

2. Stage I: Confined to the cervix.
   a. Ia: Preclinical carcinoma of cervix (microinvasion).
   b. Ia1: Minimal microscopically evident stromal invasion.
   c. Ia2: Stromal invasion of 5 mm or less from basement membrane; lateral spread of 7 mm or less.
   d. Ib: Lesions greater than Ia that are confined to cervix.
3. Stage II: Cancer extends into parametrial, but not to lateral, pelvic wall. Involves vaginal mucosa, excluding the lower third.
   a. IIa: No obvious parametrial invasion.
   b. IIb: Obvious parametrial invasion that does not extend to lateral pelvic wall.
4. Stage III: Tumor extends to lateral pelvic wall or lower third of vaginal mucosa. All cases with hydronephrosis or nonfunctioning kidney caused by cancer are included.
   a. IIIa: No extension to lateral pelvic wall or lower third of vagina.
   b. IIIb: Extension to pelvic wall, hydronephrosis, or nonfunctioning kidney.
5. Stage IV: Extends beyond the pelvis or clinical rectal or bladder mucosa invasion. Bullous edema excluded.
   a. IVa: Cancer spread to adjacent organs.
   b. IVb: Distant-organ spread.

FIGO CLINICAL STAGING OF ENDOMETRIAL CARCINOMA

See Table 36-3.
1. Stage 0
   a. Atypical hyperplasia or carcinoma in situ
   b. Histologic findings suspicious of malignancy
2. Stage I: Cancer involving corpus uteri
   a. Ia: Length of uterine cavity is 8 cm or less
   b. Ib: Length of uterine cavity is more than 8 cm
   c. Cases subgrouped into histologic grades
      (1) Grade 1: Well-differentiated adenocarcinoma
      (2) Grade 2: Moderately well-differentiated with partially solid areas
      (3) Grade 3: Predominantly solid or entirely undifferentiated carcinoma
3. Stage II: Carcinoma involving corpus and cervix but confined to uterus
4. Stage III: Extrauterine extension but confined to pelvis
5. Stage IV: Extrapelvic metastasis or invading mucosa of the bladder or rectum; bullous edema excluded
   a. IVa: Spread of growth to adjacent organs
      IVb: Spread of growth to distant organs

Table 36-3   Five-year survival rate in endometrial cancer

Stage	Number of Patients	5 Years (%)
I	6340/8550	74.2
II	970/1690	57.4
III	240/822	29.2
IV	30/314	9.6

From Kottmeier H, editor: Annual report on the results of treatment in gynecologic cancer, vol 18, Stockholm, 1982, FIGO.

FIGO CLINICAL STAGING OF FALLOPIAN TUBE CARCINOMA

There is no official FIGO staging of fallopian tube carcinoma. Most physicians use the FIGO system of staging of the ovary.

Five-Year Survival

1. Stage I: 60%
2. Stage II: 30%
3. Stage III: 10%
4. Stage IV: 5% to 10%
5. Overall: 20% to 25%

FIGO STAGING OF PRIMARY CARCINOMA OF THE OVARY*

See Table 36-4.
1. Stage I: Growth limited to ovaries.
   a. Ia: One ovary, no ascites, capsule intact; no surface tumor.
   b. Ib: Both ovaries, no ascites, capsule intact; no surface growth.
   c. Ic: One or both ovaries with tumor on surface, capsule is ruptured, or ascites contain malignant cells or have positive peritoneal washings.
2. Stage II: Growth on one or both ovaries with pelvic extension.
   a. IIa: Metastases to tubes and/or uterus.
   b. IIb: Metastases to other pelvic tissues.
   c. IIc: Tumor is either stage IIa or IIb with the addition of tumor on the surface of one or both ovaries, a ruptured capsule, or ascites with malignant cells or positive peritoneal washings.
3. Stage III: Growth on one or both ovaries with extrapelvic metastasis, positive retroperitoneal nodes, or inguinal nodes or with metastases to liver surface, omentum, or small bowel.
   a. IIIa: Tumor in true pelvis, negative nodes, and microscopic seedling on peritoneal su faces.
   b. IIIb: Tumor of one or both ovaries with implants less than 2 cm on abdominal peritoneal surfaces; nodes are negative.
   c. IIIc: Abdominal implants greater than 2 cm in diameter and/or positive peritoneal or inguinal nodes.
4. Stage IV: Growth involving one or both ovaries with distant metastases. If pleural effusion is present, cytology must be positive. Liver parenchymal metastasis equals Stage IV.

Table 36-4   Survival rates in ovarian epithelial carcinoma

Stage	2-Year (%)	5-Year (%)
I	80	70
II	40	25
III	18	12
IV	5	0

From DiSaia PJ, and Creasman WT: Clinical gynecologic oncology, ed 3, St. Louis, 1989, The CV Mosby Co.

*From FIGO (see bibliography).

STAGING OF GESTATIONAL TROPHOBLASTIC NEOPLASIA

The staging system for gestational trophoblastic neoplasia is defined by the International Society for the Study of Trophoblastic Neoplasms (see box below).

The FIGO definitions of the clinical stages of gestational trophoblastic tumors (see box below) are currently used by most physicians.

Staging System for Gestational Trophoblastic Neoplasia (International Society for the Study of Trophoblastic Neoplasms)

Stage 0: Molar pregnancy: low or high risk
Stage I: Confined to corpus uteri
Stage II: Metastases to pelvis and vagina
Stage III: Metastases to lung
Stage IV: Distant metastases to liver, brain, and intestine

From Goldstein and Berkowitz: Gestational trophoblastic neoplasia: clinical principles of diagnosis and management, Philadelphia, 1982, WB Saunders Co.

FIGO Definitions of the Clinical Staging of Gestational Trophoblastic Tumors

Stage I: Gestational trophoblastic tumor strictly contained to the uterine corpus
Stage II: Gestational trophoblastic tumor extends to the adnexa outside the uterus but is limited to the genital structures
Stage III: Gestational trophoblastic tumor extends to the lung with or without genital tract involvement
Stage IV: All other metastatic sites

From DiSaia PJ, and Creasman WT: Clinical gynecologic oncology, ed 3, St. Louis, 1989, The CV Mosby Co.

CLASSIFICATION AND REMISSION OF GESTATIONAL TROPHOBLASTIC NEOPLASIA

See Table 36-5 and box on pp. 36-6.

Table 36-5 Classification and remission of gestational trophoblastic neoplasia

Class	Remission
I	
Nonmetastatic	139/139 (100%)
II	
Metastatic (good prognosis)	55/55 (100%)
Metastatic (poor prognosis)	42/63 (66%)
TOTAL	236/257 (92%)

Modified from Hammond C, Weed J, and Currie J: Am J Obstet Gynecol 136:844, 1980.

Poor-Prognosis Metastatic Disease

Long duration (last pregnancy more than 4 months)

High pretreatment titre (greater than 100,000 IU/24 hr or greater than 40,000 mIU/ml); hCG (40,000+ mIU/cc)

Brain or liver metastases

Significant prior chemotherapy

Choriocarcinoma following term pregnancy

From DiSaia PJ, and Creasman WT: Clinical gynecologic oncology, ed 3, St. Louis, 1989, The CV Mosby Co.

REVIEW
QUESTIONS

Indicate which of the following are appropriate methods for clinical staging of cervical carcinoma (True or False).

1. Physical examination and IVP
2. Colposcopy and cystoscopy
3. Laparoscopy
4. Barium enema and sigmoidoscopy
5. Lymphangiography or venography

Using True or False, note which of the following descriptions of each clinical stage of cervical cancer are correct.

6. Stage I: Cancer confined to the cervix
7. Stage Ib: Cancer of the cervix with parametrial invasion
8. Stage II: Parametrial invasion but no extension to lateral pelvic wall; cancer involving the lower third of the vaginal mucosa
9. Stage IIb: Obvious parametrial invasion that does not extend to the pelvic wall; bilateral hydronephrosis is present
10. Stage IIIb: Tumor extends to pelvic wall or parametrial invasion with hydronephrosis or nonfunctioning kidney

Indicate (True/False) which of the following descriptions for each clinical pathologic stage of endometrial carcinoma are correct.

11. Stage 0: Atypical hyperplasia or carcinoma in situ. Histologic findings suspicious of malignancy.
12. Stage Ia: Cancer confined to the corpus uteri. The length of the uterine cavity is greater than 8 cm.
13. Stage II: Cancer involving the corpus uteri and cervix and confined to the uterus.
14. Stage III: Endometrial carcinoma with extrapelvic metastasis.
15. Stage IV: Extrapelvic metastasis or involves the mucosa of the bladder or rectum. Bullous edema is not included.

Indicate (True or False) which of the following descriptions for each clinical pathologic stage of ovarian carcinoma are correct.

16. Stage I: Growth limited to the ovaries.
17. Stage Ia: Growth involving one ovary, no ascites, capsule of ovary intact, and no ovarian capsule surface growth.

18. Stage Ib: Both ovaries involved with cancer, no ascites, capsule of ovarian tumor intact, and no ovarian surface growth.
19. Stage IIa: Cancer involves one or both ovaries with extension or metastasis to the uterus or tubes.
20. Stage IV: Growth involving one or both ovaries with distant metastasis. If pleural effusion is present, cytology must be positive. Metastasis to the liver parenchyma is included in stage IV.

Select the correct (True or False) 5-year survival rates for cervical carcinoma on a stage-specific basis.

21. Stage I: 91%
22. Stage IIb: 85%
23. Stage IIIa: 65%
24. Stage IIIb: 36%
25. Stage IV: 14%

Indicate which patients (True or False) are considered to have a poor prognosis with gestational trophoblastic neoplasia.

26. Long duration (last pregnancy more than 4 months)
27. Low hCG pretreatment titre
28. Brain or liver metastasis
29. Lung metastasis only
30. Failure to respond to significant prior chemotherapy

ANSWERS

1. T	16. T
2. T	17. T
3. F	18. T
4. T	19. T
5. F	20. T
6. T	21. T
7. F	22. F
8. F	23. F
9. F	24. T
10. T	25. T
11. T	26. T
12. F	27. F
13. T	28. T
14. F	29. F
15. T	30. T

BIBLIOGRAPHY

Averette H et al: Surgical staging of gynecologic malignancies, Cancer 60:2010, 1987.

Beahrs OH, and Myers MH, editors: American Joint Committee on Cancer: manual for staging of cancer, ed 2, Philadelphia, 1983, JB Lippincott Co.

DiSaia PJ, and Creasman WT: Clinical gynecologic oncology, ed 3, St. Louis, 1989, The CV Mosby Co.

Kottmeier H, editor: Annual report on gynecologic cancer, vol 19, Stockholm, 1985, FIGO.

Morrow CP, and Townsend DE: Synopsis of gynecologic oncology, ed 3, New York, 1987, John Wiley & Sons Inc.

Trophoblastic Disease

Larry J. Copeland

Although choriocarcinoma is the most malignant aspect of the spectrum of trophoblastic disease, it is one of the few metastatic malignant tumors that is curable by chemotherapy. Even patients with multiple organ involvement, including the liver and brain, are potentially curable when managed optimally. Unfortunately, delays in the diagnosis of early disease remain a problem. Delays occur because of the rarity of the disease and the diverse symptomatology.

Because of the multiple nuances of this disease, a physician who is thoroughly familiar with the disease, usually a gynecologic oncologist, should be directing the care of these patients.

CLASSIFICATION
Clinical

1. Germ cell tumor of ovary (choriocarcinoma—pure or mixed)
2. Gestational
    a. Benign—hydatidiform mole, partial mole
    b. Malignant
        (1) Nonmetastatic
            (a) Persistent hydatidiform mole
            (b) Invasive mole (chorioadenoma destruens)
            (c) Placental-site trophoblastic disease
            (d) Choriocarcinoma
        (2) Metastatic
            (a) Low risk
            (b) High risk
                • Traditional criteria
                • WHO scoring

Pathologic

1. Hydatidiform mole (classic, complete)
    a. Avascular hydropic villi
    b. Proliferation of trophoblastic tissue (syncytiotrophoblasts/cytotrophoblasts)
    c. Empty-egg theory: chromosomal make-up all paternal (usually 46, XX)

2. Partial mole
   a. Normal villi intermingled
   b. Villi contain vessels, red blood cells
   c. Minimal hyperplasia
   d. Fetus, cord, or amniotic membranes often identified
   e. Triploid/trisomy
3. Chorioadenoma destruens (invasive mole)
   a. Proliferation of trophoblasts
   b. Usually limited to uterus but may be metastatic
   c. Invasion into adjacent tissue (myometrium)
   d. Persistence of villi
4. Placental-site trophoblastic tumor
   a. Arises from the placental-bed trophoblast (choriocarcinoma arises from villous trophoblast)
   b. Can follow any type of gestation
   c. Predominantly cytotrophoblasts with few syncytial elements
   d. Few cells stain for hCG; most cells stain for human placental lactogen (hPL)
   e. Minimal hemorrhage and necrosis
5. Choriocarcinoma
   a. Sheets of proliferative trophoblasts
   b. Hemorrhage and necrosis common
   c. No villi

HYDATIDIFORM MOLE

1. Incidence
   a. Orient, Mexico: 1 in 150 pregnancies
   b. United States: 1 in 1500 to 2000 pregnancies
   c. Highest risk: young women (teens) and older women (in their 30s and 40s)
2. Clinical presentation
   a. Bleeding, uterine size (half are large for dates, a quarter are small for dates, and a quarter are appropriate for dates)
   b. Hyperemesis, toxemia
   c. Absent fetal heart tones
   d. Adnexal mass, theca-lutein cysts (clinically recognized in 15% to 20% of patients with hydatidiform mole)
3. Diagnosis
   a. Ultrasonography (beware tangential cuts of placenta, fibroids, missed abortion, and multiple gestation)
   b. hCG: 40,000 mIU/ml (beware multiple gestations)
   c. Serial hCG, normally expect a decline after 10 weeks
   d. Tissue
   e. Amniogram (historic interest)
4. Management
   a. Evacuation—suction curettage; if no suction apparatus is available, then:
      (1) D & C if less than or equal to 12-week size uterus
      (2) Hysterotomy if greater than 12-week size uterus
   b. Avoid contractions because of the risk of tissue deportation
   c. Conservative management of theca-lutein cysts
   d. Hysterectomy acceptable treatment in older patient

e. Surveillance after evacuation
  (1) Contraception (birth control pill recommended)
  (2) Weekly β-hCG until three normal—then monthly for 6 to 12 months
f. Chemotherapy: initiate if β-hCG plateaus or rises

PARTIAL MOLE

1. Incidence
   a. Difficult to assess, relatively uncommon
2. Clinical presentation
   a. Epidemiology of complete moles not applicable
   b. Average gestational age is 20 weeks gestation (mole average is 16 weeks)
   c. Uterus less likely to be large for dates
3. Diagnosis
   a. Usually after tissue passed, abortion, premature labor
   b. Ultrasonography
4. Management after evacuation of uterus
   a. Follow with β-hCG titres
   b. Effective contraception
   c. About 2% may require treatment

CHORIOADENOMA DESTRUENS

1. Incidence
   a. Difficult to assess, probably 10% to 15% of moles
2. Clinical presentation
   a. Bleeding—vaginal, intraperitoneal, other sites
3. Diagnosis
   a. Usually not made until after hysterectomy
   b. Villi must be present
4. Management
   a. Although the disease may be self-limiting, all should receive chemotherapy

PLACENTAL-SITE TROPHOBLASTIC TUMOR

1. Incidence
   a. Rare, diagnosis is being made more frequently in recent years
2. Clinical presentation
   a. Persistent postpartum bleeding
   b. Produces small amounts of hCG
   c. Can be associated with toxemia or a nephrotic syndrome
   d. Tends to metastasize later than choriocarcinoma
3. Management
   a. Response to chemotherapy may be poor
   b. Give early consideration to hysterectomy

CHORIOCARCINOMA

1. Incidence
   a. After 1 in 20,000 to 40,000 term pregnancies
   b. Of all hydatidiform moles, 3% to 4% develop into choriocarcinoma

2. Clinical presentation
   a. Precursor gestation (half with hydatidiform mole, a quarter with term pregnancy, and a quarter with abortion)
   b. Variable—may masquerade as other diseases (neurologic, gastrointestinal, urologic, pulmonary)
   c. Delays in diagnosis common
   d. Bleeding—vaginal, postpartum—cannot rely on D & C producing a histologic diagnosis (hemorrhage and necrosis)
3. Diagnosis
   a. Clinical suspicion—β-hCG
   b. Metastatic survey—chest x-ray examination; CT of brain, abdomen, and pelvis
   c. Avoid biopsy of vaginal metastases
4. Management
   a. Chemotherapy—regimen varies with "risk" level
   b. Radiotherapy—for prevention of hemorrhage (brain metastases)
   c. Surgery—to manage hemorrhagic complications and to resect resistant foci (uterus, lung)

STAGING (FIGO, 1982)

1. I: confined to uterine corpus
2. II: metastases to pelvis or vagina
3. III: metastases to lung
4. IV: other distant metastases

PROGNOSTIC SCORING

See Table 37-1.

Table 37-1   Scoring system for prognosis of gestational trophoblastic disease

Factor	Score* 0	1	2	4
Age	39 or younger	Older than 39	—	—
Antecedent pregnancy	Mole	Abortion, ectopic pregnancy	Term pregnancy	—
Time interval (months)	Less than 4	4-6	7-12	More than 12
Initial hCG	Less than 10^3	10^3-10^4	10^4-10^5	Greater than 10^5
Blood group	—	OxA	B or AB	—
Largest tumor (cm)	Less than 3	3-5	Greater than 5	—
Sites of metastases	—	Spleen, kidney	GI, liver	Brain
Number of metastases	—	1-4	4-8	More than 8
Previous chemotherapy	—	—	Single drug	2 or more

*Low risk: 4; medium risk: 5-7; high risk: 8

TRADITIONAL "HIGH-RISK" CRITERIA (FOR PATIENTS WITH METASTATIC DISEASE)

1. Very elevated β-hCG
   a. Urinary hCG: 100,000 IU/L (24-hour collection)
   b. Serum hCG: 40,000 mIU/ml
2. Duration of disease: 4 months
3. Liver or brain metastases
4. Previous chemotherapy resistance
5. Following a term pregnancy

CHEMOTHERAPY
Nonmetastatic or "Low-Risk" Metastatic

1. Single agents
   a. Methotrexate 0.3 mg/kg/day × 5 or actinomycin D 10 to 12 mcgm/kg/day × 5 (maximum of 0.5 mg/day)
   b. Repeat with recovery of blood counts and stomatitis (usually 7- to 9-day window)
2. Treat one cycle past a normal titre
3. Monitor blood counts and liver function tests (if elevated, avoid methotrexate)
4. Change to combination therapy if there is a plateau or rise of titre

"High-Risk" Metastatic

1. Referral center (gynecologic oncologist)
2. Combination chemotherapy:
   a. Methotrexate, actinomycin D, and cyclophosphamide (MAC)
   b. Vinblastine, bleomycin, and cisplatin (VBP)
   c. Etoposide, methotrexate, actinomycin D, cyclophosphamide, and vincristine (EMA-CO)
3. Monitor toxicities closely
4. Depending on clinical profile, most patients receive three courses past a normal titre

RADIOTHERAPY

1. Role
   a. May reduce risk of bleeding from metastases
   b. Traditional treatment for liver and brain metastases
   c. Less commonly used now for liver metastases because percutaneous embolization is available for bleeding from liver metastases
   d. Usual dose is 2000 to 3000 rad over 2 to 3 weeks

SPECIAL SITUATIONS
CNS Metastases

1. Lung metastases occurs also in 94% of patients
2. MRI better than CT
3. Steroidal therapy and anticonvulsant therapy
4. If intracranial pressure is normal, intrathecal chemotherapy may be advisable
5. Radiotherapy

Extensive Pulmonary Metastases

1. Aggressive therapy can accelerate respiratory failure (possible mechanism is bleeding or edema)

2. Recommend starting with "light" therapy (e.g., 2 days of MAC or 1 day of EMA-CO)
3. Improvement in arterial oxygenation should guide therapy

REVIEW
QUESTIONS

More than one correct answer is possible.

1. What variant of gestational trophoblastic disease is characterized by the following: low β-hCG titres, tends to remain within the uterus, metastasizes late, and has a poor response to chemotherapy. Histologically, cytotrophoblastic or intermediate cells predominate (syncytial trophoblastic cells are absent or rare), and hemorrhage and necrosis are usually absent.
   a. Hydatidiform mole
   b. Partial mole
   c. Chorioadenoma destruens
   d. Placental-site trophoblastic tumor
   e. Choriocarcinoma

2. Approximately what percentage of hydatidiform moles develop into choriocarcinoma?
   a. 0.5%
   b. 3% to 4%
   c. 10%
   d. 18%
   e. 30%

3. A 24-year-old patient develops a choriocarcinoma after a term pregnancy. The diagnosis was not made until 5 months after delivery, at which time she had persistent vaginal bleeding. Large metastatic nodules were present in the right lower lung lobe, and smaller metastases were present throughout the left lung. The patient has received five cycles of MAC chemotherapy, and the only focus of clinical disease is two 4-cm nodules in the right lower lung. Although the titre before her fifth cycle was within normal (for the first time since starting chemotherapy), she presents now with a β-hCG titre of 250 mIU/ml (confirmed on repeating). A repeat staging evaluation reveals no new metastatic lesions. The most appropriate approach to treatment is:
   a. Radiation therapy to a right lower lung field
   b. Continue with MAC chemotherapy
   c. Perform a hysterectomy
   d. Change to another chemotherapy combination
   e. Resect the right lower lung lobe and follow this with a different combination of chemotherapy

ANSWERS

1. d
2. b
3. d or e (author's choice would be e rather than d)

BIBLIOGRAPHY

Bagshawe KD: Treatment of high-risk choriocarcinoma, J Reprod Med 29:813, 1984.

DiSaia PJ, and Creasman WT: Clinical gynecologic oncology, ed 2, St. Louis, 1984, The CV Mosby Co.

Goldstein DP, and Berkowitz RS: Gestational trophoblastic neoplasms, vol 14, Major problems in obstetrics and gynecology, Philadelphia, 1982, WB Saunders Co.

Gordon AN et al: High-risk metastatic gestational trophoblastic disease, Obstet Gynecol 65:550, 1985.

Hammond CB, and Soper JT: Poor-prognosis metastatic gestational trophoblastic neoplasia, Clin Obstet Gynecol 27:228, 1984.

Morrow CP: Postmolar trophoblastic disease: diagnosis, management, and prognosis, Clin Obstet Gynecol 27:211, 1984.

Surwit EA et al: Poor prognosis gestational trophoblastic disease: an update, Obstet Gynecol 64:21, 1984.

Twiggs LB: Nonneoplastic complications of molar pregnancy, Clin Obstet Gynecol 27:199, 1984.

Young RH, and Scully RE: Placental-site trophoblastic tumor: current status, Clin Obstet Gynecol 27:248, 1984.

Index

Genetic defects, 46t
Genetic disorders, 45-47
  prenatal diagnosis of, with amniocentesis, 79
Genetics of Rh antigen, 149-150
Genital organs
  external, anatomy of, 1-3
  internal, anatomy of, 5-13
Genital tract, lower
  clinical characteristics of tumors of, 403t
  infections in; see Vulvovaginitis
  presence or absence of symptoms in, 291
Genitalia, fetal, ultrasound image of, 70
Gestagen therapy, 378-379
Gestation(s)
  abnormal, levels of hCG in, 25-26
  anesthetics given during, 217
  dating, ultrasonography used for, 24
  ectopic, 27-28
    location of, 24
  multiple, incompetent cervix and, 137
Gestational age
  assessment of, 39-40
    ultrasonography used for, 58, 62
  estimated, 39
  neonatal assessment of, 40
Glands, Bartholin's, 3
Glomeruloendotheliosis, 174
Glomerulonephritis, acute, 104
Glucocorticoids
  with betamethasone or dexamethasone, 185
  immune thrombocytopenic purpura treated with, 112
  preterm labor managed with, 132
Glycopyrrolate, 227
Glycosuria, physiologic, 33
GnRH analogs; see Gonadotropin-releasing hormone analogs
Gonadoblastoma, 405t
Gonadotropin-releasing hormone analogs, 305
  amenorrhea treated with, 343
Grandmother theory, 151
Granulosa, 405t
Graves' disease, 108
  hyperthyroidism in offspring of women with, 107
Greater vestibular glands, 3
Growth
  fetal, antepartum factors associated with, 168
  intrauterine retardation of; see Intrauterine growth retardation
Growth retardation, intrauterine, cordocentesis used to evaluate, 82

H

Haemophilus vaginalis, 294-295
Hair, 32
Halban's syndrome, abnormal bleeding in reproductive years due to, 333t

Hardy-Weinberg equation, gene frequency estimated with, 46-47
hCG; see Human chorionic gonadotropin
hCG doubling times, 26
HDL; see High-density lipoprotein
Headaches, spinal, 226
Heart, four-chamber, ultrasound image of, 68
Heart disease, 97-101
  congenital, 54, 97
  diagnosis of, during pregnancy, 97-98
  findings of normal pregnancy that mimic, 33-34
  rheumatic, 97
Heart murmurs, systolic outflow, 97-98
Heart rate, fetal
  acceleration of, 210
  baseline, 210
  decelerations of, 210-212
  irregularities in, 212-213
  monitored during labor, 210
  variability in, 212
Heartbeat, fetal, auscultation of, 40
Hematologic disease, 110-112
Hematologic system, changes in, during pregnancy, 37
Hematomas, 209
Hemihematocolpos, bicolus, abnormal bleeding in adolescents due to, 331t
Hemodialysis, 105
Hemoglobin S, 111
Hemoglobin SC, 111
Hemoglobinopathies, 111-112
Hemolytic disease, 149-153
  caused by irregular antibodies, 154-155
  cordocentesis used to evaluate, 82
Hemolytic uremic syndrome, 105
Hemorrhage
  fetal-maternal, measurement of, 152-153
  postpartum, management of, 249-250
  subarachnoid, 120
  uterovaginal, management of, 334
Heparin, breast-feeding and, 261
Hepatitis
  maternal, breast-feeding and, 262
  viral, 117-118
Hepatobiliary diseases, 116-118
Herpes, maternal, 52
Herpes, vulvovaginal infections and, 293t
Herpes simplex virus, vulvovaginitis caused by, 276-277
Herpes virus Type II, 296-297
Herpes viruses, maternal, breast-feeding and, 262
Hidradenoma, 400t
HIV; see Human immunodeficiency virus
hMGs; see Human menopausal gonadotropins
Hobbit nipple shell, inverted nipples treated with, 254
Hodgkin's disease, 121-122
Hoffman technique, inverted nipples treated with, 254